Homemade Hand Sanitizer Recipes to Kill Off Germs in Style

Table of Contents

Table of Contents 2

Introduction 7

Note While Making Sanitizers 9

Homemade Hand Sanitizer Recipes 12

Basic Homemade Hand Sanitizer # 1 12

Basic Homemade Hand Sanitizer # 2 14

Basic Hand Sanitizer # 3 16

Alcohol Hand Sanitizer 18

Hand Sanitizer using Vinegar 19

Alcohol-free Sanitizer with Lemon and Tea Tree Oil 20

Essential Oils Sanitizer 21

Sanitizer with Thieves Oil 23

OnGuard Sanitizer 24

Eucalyptus and Rosemary Hand Sanitizer 25

Tea Tree Oil Sanitizer 27

Citrus and Cinnamon Sanitizer Spray 28

Strong Hand Sanitizer 30

Citronella and Rose Oil Sanitizer 31

Customized Hand Sanitizer with Gel Base 33

Witch Hazel and Tea Tree Oil Sanitizer 34

Isopropyl Alcohol Hand Sanitizer 36

Moisturizing Hand Sanitizer Spray 37

Lemon and Peppermint Sanitizer Spray 39

"Thieves Oil" Natural Hand Germ Busters 41

Sanitizer with Aloe Vera Juice 42

Neem and Tea tree Hand Sanitizer with Hydrogen Peroxide 44

Aloe Vera Hand Sanitizer 46

Naturally Emulsified Sanitizer 47

Instant Hand Sanitizer Using Dettol 49

Clove and Tea Tree Sanitizer 50

Natural Citrus Sanitizing Spray 52

Herbal "Thieves" Vinegar Hand Sanitizer Spray 54

Natural Hand Sanitizer using Flax Gel 56

All Herbal Hand Sanitizer 58

Gel Hand Cleanser 60

Herbal Hand Sanitizer 62

Lemony -Orangy Hand Sanitizer 64

Hand Sanitizer using Astringent 66

Foaming Hand Sanitizer 67

Homemade Sanitizer for Kids 68

Lemony Tea Tree Sanitizer with Aloe Vera Juice 68

Gentle Hand Sanitizer 70

Aloe Vera Gel Sanitizer 72

Little Tykes Hand Sanitizer 74

"Thieves" Hand Sanitizer for Kids 76

Disinfecting Citrus Mint Hand Sanitizer 78

Homemade Hand Sanitizer Spray for Kiddos 80

Sanitizer Wipes (Hand and Surface) 81

Herbal Antibacterial Wipes 81

Disinfectant Wipes 82

Reusable Disinfecting Baby Wipes 84

Apple Cider Vinegar Wipes 86

Antibacterial Kitchen Wipes using Vinegar 88

Re-usable Hydrogen Peroxide Cleaning Wipes 90

"Clorox" Wipes 92

Disinfecting Cleaning Wipes 94

Disinfecting Bathroom Wipes 96

Homemade Baby Wipes 97

Surface Sanitizer Recipes 99

Homemade Multi-Purpose Disinfectant Spray 99

Disinfectant Spray 101

Vinegar Disinfectant Spray 103

Toilet Bowl Cleaner 105

Sanitizing Solution for Floors 106

Natural Granite Cleaner 108

Toilet Seat Cleaner 110

Sanitizing Glass Cleaner 111

Natural Antibacterial Surface Spray with Witch Hazel 113

Antibacterial Surface Cleaner 115

Miscellaneous Sanitizer Recipes 117

Mattress Sanitizer with Vodka 117

Mattress Sanitizer with Vinegar 119

Sanitizer Spray for Toys 121

All-purpose Sanitizer for Babies, their Surroundings and their Toys 123

Disinfectant Spray for Fabrics #1 125

Disinfectant Spray for Fabrics #2 126

Room Sanitizer # 1 128

Room Sanitizer # 2 129

Conclusion 130

Introduction

Modern epidemics, like the one going on right now, have shown that we are more vulnerable now than ever despite the progress in technology and medicine. A microorganism, as small as a virus can bring the economy to its knees. It can also affect your health. So, how do you protect yourself? The best way to do this is to keep your hands clean and free of germs.

Your hands are susceptible to bacteria and viruses because you touch random objects. You use the same hands to eat food and can easily transfer these bacteria and viruses into your body. It is difficult to wash your hands at every point. You also cannot expect to avoid touching surfaces, either. You are probably always on the go, so you need to have a convenient way to keep your hands clean and healthy. It is during these times that you need to use hand sanitizers. These products are gel-like and have some alcohol in them. This alcohol will kill the bacteria and virus on your skin.

People often choose to avoid store-bought hand sanitizers. They complain that these products make their skin dry. The alcohol in the sanitizers makes their skin dry. Some companies choose to give their customers complimentary moisturizers on the purchase of their sanitizer, but this does not help either. Some sanitizers also have a pungent or bad odor since they are mass-produced. It is for this reason people believe they should avoid purchasing sanitizers. How will they protect themselves otherwise? They can make them at home.

If you also do not like purchasing hand sanitizers at the store, you can make them at home. This book has different sanitizer recipes. The recipes are extremely simple to follow, and the ingredients are available in every supermarket. Since a child's skin is more sensitive, you need to use different proportions of alcohol and gel to avoid hurting their skin. This book also has some kid-friendly sanitizer recipes that you can use. You must understand that you cannot protect yourself if the surfaces at home are piled with dust and germs. There are some recipes in this book that you can use to disinfect your house.

You can also add essential oils to the recipes, so you can decide how you want the sanitizer to smell. You can also tweak the recipes and the proportions of the ingredients to suit your skin. When you use sanitizers, you can decrease the chances of falling ill. Remember to sanitize whenever you touch surfaces in any public place or even at home.

Thank you for purchasing the book. I hope you get all the information you are looking for.

Note While Making Sanitizers

- Use isopropyl alcohol and sanitize all the things that you are using to make sanitizer like, countertop, container, bowls, measuring cup, spatula etc.
- Wash your hands with soap and water whenever possible. Use sanitizers only when you do not have access to soap and water.
- If you have **just** washed with an alcohol-based sanitizer, be careful if you have to work with flame.
- Keep sanitizers that are made with alcohol, out of reach of children. This is important.
- Using sanitizer after washing hands will kill more germs. If you have dry skin, it is a great idea to use some moisturizer after using sanitizer.
- If you are making sanitizer with alcohol, concentration of alcohol should be more than 60%. Lesser concentration will not help in killing germs. Higher the concentration, better the results. The American Food and Drug Administration recommends a concentration between 60-95%.

- Use the right quantity of ingredients as mentioned in the recipe. Measure the ingredients properly before making the sanitizer.
- Alcohol-free sanitizers may not kill as many germs as an alcohol-based sanitizer would.
- Adding natural preservatives like Vitamin E and alcohol will increase the shelf life of the sanitizers. Without the natural preservatives, the effect of sanitizer will not last more than a month. So do not make a large batch if you are not using natural preservatives.
- Store sanitizers in a suitable container.
- For dirty or greasy hands, wash your hands with water and soap initially and then use the sanitizer to kill germs if any.
- It is better to use store bought aloe Vera gel than using fresh aloe Vera because using fresh aloe Vera will reduce the shelf life drastically. It will not last longer than a couple of days at room temperature. If you place it in the refrigerator, it will not last for more than 4 – 5 days.
- If you are wearing rings on your fingers, remove the rings before using sanitizers.
- Make sure not to use hydrogen peroxide along with vinegar.
- Do not use vinegar-based surface sanitizer over natural stones or expensive stones like marble or granite.

- Once you spray on surfaces, allow it air dry.

Homemade Hand Sanitizer Recipes

Basic Homemade Hand Sanitizer # 1

Makes: 2 ounces

What you need:

- 8 teaspoons 95% alcohol
- 2 teaspoons unscented castile soap
- 2 teaspoons organic aloe Vera gel
- 2-ounce spray bottle
- Bowl
- Hand whisk
- Small funnel
- Label

Directions:

1. Pour alcohol into the bowl along with castile soap and aloe Vera gel.
2. Whisk until smooth using the hand whisk.
3. Place the funnel in the bottle. Pour the mixture into the bottle. Tighten the cap and label the bottle with date and name.

How to use:

Spray on your hands, fingers, in between the fingers, palms, nails, back of the hands and fingertips. Rub your hands together. Let it air dry.

Basic Homemade Hand Sanitizer # 2

Makes: 8 ounces

What you need:

- 6 tablespoons isopropyl alcohol or rubbing alcohol (99%)
- 5 drops lavender essential oil or lemon juice
- 2 tablespoons aloe Vera gel
- Glass bowl
- Measuring cup
- 8 ounce flip top bottle
- Label
- Small funnel
- Hand whisk

Directions:

1. Firstly, measure isopropyl alcohol and add into the glass bowl. Next measure aloe Vera gel and add into the bowl. Add essential oil as well.
2. Whisk the mixture with a hand whisk until smooth and free flowing.
3. Pour the mixture into the bottle using the funnel.
4. Label the bottle with name and date.

How to use: Squeeze 2 – 3 drops of the sanitizer on one of your palms and rub it all over your hands, fingers, in between your fingers, back of the hands and nails. Then rub your palms together until dry. If the sanitizer evaporates within 15 seconds, you have used insufficient sanitizer. If it evaporates after 15 seconds, you have used the right amount.

Basic Hand Sanitizer # 3

Makes: 4 ounces

What you need:

- 4 teaspoons aloe Vera gel
- 91 % rubbing alcohol or 160+ proof grain alcohol, as required
- 1 teaspoon carrier oil of your choice like fractionated coconut oil or jojoba oil or sweet almond oil
- 20 – 25 drops essential oil
- 1 teaspoon glycerin
- 5 – 6 drops vitamin E oil
- 4 ounces spray bottle
- Glass bowl
- Small funnel
- Hand whisk

Directions:

1. Add carrier oil and aloe Vera gel into the glass bowl.
2. Whisk until smooth using the hand whisk.
3. Add essential oil, vitamin E oil and glycerin and whisk until smooth and well combined.

4. Place the funnel in the bottle. Pour the mixture into the bottle.

5. Pour enough alcohol to fill the bottle, up to the neck of the bottle. Tighten the spray cap and label the bottle with date and name.

How to use:

Spray on your hands, fingers, in between the fingers, palms, back of the hands, nails and fingertips. Rub your hands together for a few seconds. Let it air dry.

Alcohol Hand Sanitizer

Makes: 2 ounces

What you need:

- 2 ounces 190 proof grain alcohol
- 10 drops bergamot essential oil
- 10 drops eucalyptus essential oil
- Small funnel
- 2 ounces flip top bottle

Directions:

1. Add alcohol and essential oils into the bottle.
2. Tighten the cap and shake the bottle until well combined.

How to use: Squeeze a few drops of the sanitizer on one of your palms and rub it all over your hands, fingers, in between your fingers, back of your hands and nails. Then rub your palms and back of your hands until dry.

Hand Sanitizer using Vinegar

Makes: 8 ounces

What you need:

- 1 cup white vinegar
- Small funnel
- Spray bottle

Directions:

1. Pour vinegar into a spray bottle. Tighten the spray cap.

How to use:

Spray on your hands, fingers, in between the fingers, palms, back of your hands, nails and fingertips. Rub your hands together for a few seconds. Let it air dry.

Alcohol-free Sanitizer with Lemon and Tea Tree Oil

Makes: 2 ounces

What you need:

- 4 tablespoons alcohol-free witch hazel
- 10 drops tea tree essential oil
- 10 drops lemon essential oil
- 5 – 6 drops vitamin E oil
- 2 ounces glass spray bottle
- Small funnel

Directions:

1. Pour witch hazel into the spray bottle. Add essential oils and vitamin E oil.
2. Tighten the spray cap and shake the bottle until well combined.

How to use:

Shake the bottle each time before using. Spray on your hands, fingers, in between the fingers, palms, nails and fingertips. Rub your hands together for a few seconds. Let it air dry.

Essential Oils Sanitizer

Makes: 12 ounces

What you need:

- 11.5 ounces water
- 10 drops lemon essential oil
- 4 drops cinnamon essential oil
- 4 drops rosemary essential oil
- 4 drops clove essential oil
- 4 drops eucalyptus essential oil
- 2 teaspoons aloe Vera gel
- 12 ounces spray bottle
- Measuring cup

Directions:

1. Measure water and pour into the spray bottle. Add all the essential oils and aloe Vera gel.
2. Fasten the spray cap. Shake the bottle until well combined.
3. Use when required.

How to use:

Spray on your hands, fingers, in between the fingers, palms, back of your hands, nails and fingertips. Rub your hands together for a few seconds. Let it air dry.

Sanitizer with Thieves Oil

Makes: 2 ounces

What you need:

- 3 ½ tablespoons alcohol-free witch hazel
- 10 drops thieves essential oil
- 10 drops bergamot essential oil
- 2 drops eucalyptus essential oil
- 2 ounces glass spray bottle

Directions:

1. Add essential oils into the spray bottle.
2. Pour witch hazel. Tighten the spray cap and shake the bottle until well combined.

How to use:

Shake the bottle each time before using. Spray on your hands, fingers, in between the fingers, palms, nails and fingertips. Rub your hands together for a few seconds. Let it air dry.

OnGuard Sanitizer

Makes: 3.5 ounces

What you need:

- 2.7 ounces aloe Vera gel liquid
- 20 drops OnGuard blend
- 20 drops tea tree oil
- 0.7 ounce witch hazel
- Small funnel
- 4 ounces amber colored glass gel pump bottle

Directions:

1. First add essential oils into the bottle.
2. Pour aloe Vera gel liquid and witch hazel.
3. Tighten the cap and shake the bottle until well incorporated

How to use: Pump a few drops of the sanitizer on one of your palms and rub it all over your hands, fingers, in between your fingers, back of your hands and nails. Then rub your palms together until dry.

Eucalyptus and Rosemary Hand Sanitizer

Makes: 4 ounces

What you need:

- 4 teaspoons aloe Vera gel
- 91 % rubbing alcohol or 160+ proof grain alcohol, as required
- 1 teaspoon carrier oil of your choice like fractionated coconut oil or jojoba oil or sweet almond oil
- 8 drops eucalyptus essential oil
- 6 drops rosemary essential oil
- 8 drops lavender essential oil
- 1 teaspoon glycerin
- 5 – 6 drops vitamin E oil
- 4 ounces spray bottle
- Glass bowl
- Funnel
- Hand whisk

Directions:

1. Add carrier oil and aloe Vera gel into the glass bowl.
2. Whisk until smooth using the hand whisk.

3. Add all the essential oils, vitamin E oil and glycerin and whisk until smooth and well combined.

4. Place the funnel in the bottle. Pour the mixture into the bottle.

5. Pour enough alcohol to fill the bottle, up to the neck of the bottle. Tighten the spray cap and label the bottle with date and name.

How to use:

Spray on your hands, fingers, back of the hands, in between the fingers, palms, nails and fingertips. Rub your hands together for a few seconds. Let it air dry.

Tea Tree Oil Sanitizer

Makes: 13 ounces

Ingredients:

- 12 ounces water
- 2 teaspoons liquid castile soap
- 20 drops tea tree essential oil
- 2 teaspoons vitamin E oil
- Spray bottle
- Small funnel

Directions:

1. Add water into the spray bottle.
2. Add liquid castile soap, vitamin E oil and essential oil.
3. Tighten the spray cap and shake the bottle until well incorporated.
4. Use as required. Using this much tea tree oil may not suit all skin types. So add lesser if it irritates your skin.

How to use:

Spray on your hands, back of the hands, fingers, in between the fingers, palms, nails and fingertips. Rub your hands together for a few seconds. Let it air dry.

Citrus and Cinnamon Sanitizer Spray

Makes: 4 ounces

What you need:

- 4 teaspoons aloe Vera gel
- 91 % rubbing alcohol or 160+ proof grain alcohol, as required
- 1 teaspoon carrier oil of your choice like fractionated coconut oil or jojoba oil or sweet almond oil
- 4 drops eucalyptus essential oil
- 4 drops rosemary essential oil
- 4 drops cinnamon essential oil
- 4 drops lemon essential oil
- 4 drops orange essential oil
- 4 drops clove essential oil
- 1 teaspoon glycerin
- 5 – 6 drops vitamin E oil
- 4 ounces spray bottle
- Glass bowl
- Funnel

- Hand whisk

Directions:

1. Add carrier oil and aloe Vera gel into the glass bowl.
2. Whisk until smooth using the hand whisk.
3. Add all the essential oils, vitamin E oil and glycerin and whisk until smooth and well combined.
4. Place the funnel in the bottle. Pour the mixture into the bottle.
5. Pour enough alcohol to fill the bottle, up to the neck of the bottle. Tighten the spray cap and label the bottle with date and name.

How to use:

Spray on your hands, fingers, in between the fingers, palms, back of the hands, nails and fingertips. Rub your hands together for a few seconds. Let it air dry.

Strong Hand Sanitizer

Makes: 12 – 15 ounces

What you need:

- 40 drops germ destroyer essential oil
- 4 tablespoons aloe Vera gel
- 1 teaspoon vegetable glycerin (optional)
- Distilled water, as required
- 2 tablespoons rubbing alcohol
- Essential oil of your choice for fragrance
- Glass bowl
- Squeeze bottle
- Label
- Small funnel
- Hand whisk

Directions:

1. Add aloe Vera gel into a glass bowl. Whisk it with a hand whisk until smooth and free flowing.
2. Add germ destroyer oil, glycerin, rubbing alcohol and essential oil. Whisk until smooth.

3. Add distilled water, a little at a time and whisk well each time, until the consistency you desire is achieved.
4. Pour into a squeeze bottle. Label the bottle with name and date.

How to use:

Squeeze a few drops of the sanitizer on one of your palms and rub it all over your hands, fingers, in between your fingers, back of the hands and nails. Then rub your palms together until dry.

Citronella and Rose Oil Sanitizer

Makes: 10 – 11 ounces

What you need:

- 1 cup aloe Vera gel
- 2 tablespoons rubbing alcohol
- 20 drops citronella essential oil
- 20 drops clove essential oil
- 6 drops rose essential oil
- 4 teaspoons olive oil
- Glass bowl
- 12 ounces pump bottle

- Measuring cup
- Label
- Funnel
- Whisk

Directions:

1. Measure aloe Vera gel and add into the glass bowl.
2. Add rubbing alcohol and olive oil. Whisk well with the hand whisk.
3. Add the essential oils and whisk until smooth.
4. Pour into the bottle. Label the bottle with name and date.

How to use:

Pump a few drops of the sanitizer on one of your palms and rub it all over your hands, fingers, in between your fingers, back of the hands and nails. Then rub your palms together until dry.

Customized Hand Sanitizer with Gel Base

Makes: 8 ounces

What you need:

- 8 ounces hand sanitizer gel base
- 2 – 3 drops water soluble color of your choice
- 5 – 6 drops essential oil of your choice like tea tree oil, lavender oil, eucalyptus oil etc.
- Flip top bottle or pump bottle
- Small funnel

Directions:

1. Measure out the gel base and add into the bottle.
2. Add essential oils and color.
3. Tighten the cap and shake the bottle until well incorporated.

How to use:

Squeeze or pump a few drops of the sanitizer on one of your palms and rub it all over your hands, fingers, in between your fingers, back of the hands and nails. Then rub your palms together until dry.

Witch Hazel and Tea Tree Oil Sanitizer

Makes: 32 ounces

What you need:

- 1 ¼ cups aloe Vera gel
- 10 tablespoons witch hazel
- 4 teaspoons tea tree essential oil
- 1 teaspoon vitamin E oil
- 40 drops lavender essential oil
- Glass bowl
- Measuring cup
- Pump bottle
- Label
- Small funnel
- Hand whisk

Directions:

1. Add aloe Vera gel and witch hazel into the glass bowl. Whisk well using the hand whisk.
2. Add ass the essential oils and whisk until smooth.
3. Pour into a bottle. Label the bottle and use whenever required.

How to use:

Pump a few drops of the sanitizer on one of your palms and rub it all over your hands, fingers, in between your fingers, back of the hands and nails. Then rub your palms together until dry.

Isopropyl Alcohol Hand Sanitizer

Makes: 4 ounces

What you need:

- 3 – 4 drops tea tree essential oil
- ½ cup isopropyl alcohol
- 4 ounces spray bottle
- Small funnel

Directions:

1. Pour isopropyl alcohol into the spray bottle. Add tea tree essential oil.
2. Tighten the cap and shake the bottle until well combined.

How to use:

Shake the bottle before using the spray. Spray on your hands, fingers, in between the fingers, palms, back of the hands, nails and fingertips. Rub your hands together for a few seconds. Let it air dry.

Moisturizing Hand Sanitizer Spray

Makes: 4 ounces

Ingredients:

- 1 teaspoon vegetable glycerin
- ½ teaspoon vitamin E oil
- 1 teaspoon almond oil
- 2 tablespoons witch hazel
- 6 drops tea tree essential oil
- 10 drops thieves essential oil
- Distilled water, as required
- Amber or cobalt glass spray bottle
- Small funnel
- Label

Directions:

1. Pour vegetable glycerin, almond oil, vitamin E oil, witch hazel and essential oils into the glass spray bottle with the help of the funnel.
2. Pour enough distilled water to fill up the bottle. Tighten the spray cap and shake the bottle until well combined.
3. Label the bottle with name and date.

4. Place the bottle in your purse or in the cupboard.

How to use:

Spray on your hands, fingers, in between the fingers, palms, back of the hands, nails and fingertips. Rub your hands together for a few seconds. Let it air dry.

Lemon and Peppermint Sanitizer Spray

Makes: 7 ounces

What you need:

- 2 tablespoons white vinegar
- 10 tablespoons water
- 3 – 4 drops peppermint essential oil
- 3- 4 drops lemon essential oil
- 2 tablespoons vodka
- Glass measuring cup
- Glass spray bottle
- Label

Directions:

1. Measure water, vinegar, vodka and essential oils and pour into the glass measuring cup.
2. Pour into the glass spray bottle. Tighten the spray cap and shake the bottle vigorously until well combined.
3. Label the bottle with name and date.

How to use:

Shake the bottle before using the spray. Spray on your hands, fingers, in between the fingers, palms, back of the hands, nails and fingertips. Rub your hands together for a few seconds. Let it air dry.

"Thieves Oil" Natural Hand Germ Busters

Makes: 7 – 8 ounces

What you need:

- 6 tablespoons distilled water or boiled and cooled water
- 0.2 ounce lemon essential oil
- 0.1 ounce cinnamon bark or leaf essential oil
- 0.2 ounce eucalyptus essential oil
- 8 ounces spray bottle
- Small funnel

Directions:

1. Pour water into the spray bottle.
2. Drop the essential oils into the bottle. Tighten the spray cap and shake the bottle vigorously until well combined.
3. Label the bottle with name and date.

How to use:

Shake the bottle before using the spray. Spray on your hands, fingers, in between the fingers, palms, back of the hands, nails and fingertips. Rub your hands together for a few seconds. Let it air dry.

Sanitizer with Aloe Vera Juice

Makes: 8 – 9 ounces

What you need:

- 6 tablespoons aloe Vera juice
- 0.2 ounce tea tree essential oil
- 0.14 ounce cinnamon essential oil
- 0.2 ounce lemon or lemongrass essential oil
- 2 tablespoons rubbing alcohol
- Spray bottle
- Small funnel

Directions:

1. Pour aloe Vera juice and alcohol into the spray bottle.
2. Add essential oils. Tighten the spray cap. Shake the bottle well.
3. Label the bottle with name and date.

How to use:

Shake the bottle before using the spray. Spray on your hands, fingers, in between the fingers, palms, back of the hands, nails and fingertips. Rub your hands together for a few seconds. Let it air dry.

Neem and Tea tree Hand Sanitizer with Hydrogen Peroxide

Makes: 6 ounces

What you need:

- 2/3 cup rubbing or isopropyl alcohol
- ½ tablespoon hydrogen peroxide
- 1 teaspoon glycerol
- 10 drops tea tree essential oil
- 10 drops neem essential oil
- 2 tablespoons distilled water
- Glass measuring cup
- Glass spray bottle
- Label

Directions:

1. Measure water, alcohol, glycerol, hydrogen peroxide and essential oil and add into the glass measuring container with spout.
2. Pour into the glass spray bottle. Fasten the cap and shake the bottle vigorously until well combined.
3. Label the bottle with name and date.

How to use:

Spray on your hands, back of the hands, fingers, in between the fingers, palms, nails and fingertips. Rub your hands together for a few seconds. Let it air dry.

Aloe Vera Hand Sanitizer

Makes: 4 ounces

What you need:

- 4 ounces aloe Vera gel
- 6 drops tea tree essential oil
- 8 drops lavender essential oil
- 4 ounces spray bottle
- Hand whisk
- Glass bowl

Directions:

1. Add aloe Vera gel into a bowl. Also add tea tree essential oil and lavender essential oil.
2. Whisk well with a hand whisk. Pour into the spray bottle. Tighten the spray cap. Label the bottle with name and date.

How to use:

Spray on your hands, back of the hands, fingers, in between the fingers, palms, nails and fingertips. Rub your hands together for a few seconds. Let it air dry.

Naturally Emulsified Sanitizer

Makes: 8 ounces

What you need:

- 1 cup aloe Vera gel
- 40 drops white thyme essential oil
- 80 drops orange essential oil
- 40 drops litsea essential oil
- 1 teaspoon lecithin
- 8 ounces pump bottle
- Glass bowl
- Small bowl
- Immersion blender
- Pump bottle
- Label
- Small funnel
- Spoon

Directions:

1. Add essential oils and lecithin into a small bowl. Stir with a spoon until well combined.

2. Add aloe Vera gel into the glass bowl. Whisk with the immersion blender until smooth.

3. With the immersion blender running, pour essential oils mixture into the glass bowl. Keep blending until emulsified. It will be like a thick lotion.

4. Pour into the pump bottle. Tighten the cap. Label the bottle with name and date.

How to use:

Pump a few drops of the sanitizer on one of your palms and rub it all over your hands, fingers, in between your fingers, back of the hands and nails. Then rub your palms together until dry.

Instant Hand Sanitizer Using Dettol

Makes: 4 ounces

What you need:

- ½ cup water (preferably distilled)
- ½ tablespoon Dettol or any other antiseptic liquid
- Spray bottle
- Small funnel

Directions:

1. Pour water and Dettol into the spray bottle with the help of the funnel. Fasten the spray cap and shake the bottle until well combined.
2. Spray on your hands, palms, fingers, fingertips, in between fingers
3. Use it within 2 – 3 days after preparing it.

How to use:

Spray on your hands, back of the hands, fingers, in between the fingers, palms, nails and fingertips. Rub your hands together for a few seconds. Let it air dry.

Clove and Tea Tree Sanitizer

Makes: 18 ounces

What you need:

- 16 ounces aloe Vera gel
- 50 – 60 drops tea tree essential oil
- 18 drops clove essential oil
- 18 drops lavender essential oil
- 2 tablespoons witch hazel
- Glass bowl
- Measuring cup
- Pump bottle
- Label
- Small funnel
- Hand whisk

Directions:

1. Add aloe Vera gel and witch hazel into the glass bowl. Whisk well using the hand whisk.
2. Add ass the essential oils and whisk until smooth.
3. Pour into the pump bottle. Tighten the bottle cap. Label the bottle with name and date.

How to use:

Pump a few drops of the sanitizer on one of your palms and rub it all over your hands, fingers, in between your fingers, back of the hands and nails. Then rub your palms together until dry.

Natural Citrus Sanitizing Spray

Makes: 16 ounces

What you need:

- 1 1/3 cups 99% isopropyl alcohol
- 10 drops pink grapefruit essential oil
- 10 drops mandarin orange essential oil
- 2/3 cup aloe Vera gel
- 16 ounces spray bottle
- Hand whisk
- Glass bowl
- 16 ounces spray bottle
- Measuring cup
- Small funnel

Directions:

1. Measure isopropyl alcohol and aloe Vera gel and add into the glass bowl.
2. Whisk with a hand whisk until smooth.
3. Add essential oils and whisk until well combined.
4. Pour into the spray bottle. Tighten the spray cap.
5. Tighten the spray cap. Label the bottle with name and date.

How to use:

Spray on your hands, back of the hands, fingers, in between the fingers, palms, nails and fingertips. Rub your hands together for a few seconds. Let it air dry.

Herbal "Thieves" Vinegar Hand Sanitizer Spray

Makes: About 12 ounces

What you need:

- 1 tablespoon chopped, fresh lavender flowers
- 1 tablespoon chopped, fresh mint
- 1 tablespoon chopped, fresh marjoram
- 1 tablespoon chopped, fresh rosemary
- 1 tablespoon chopped, fresh sage
- 1 tablespoon chopped, fresh anise hyssop
- 2 cups white vinegar
- 2 cloves garlic, peeled, crushed
- Mason's jar
- Strainer
- Bowl
- Small funnel
- Spray bottle

Directions:

1. Place all the herbs and garlic in the Mason's jar. Pour vinegar over it.

2. Tighten the lid. Place the bottle on your window sill where you have sun falling on the bottle. Let it steep for 7 – 10 days.

3. Place a strainer over a bowl. Strain the vinegar into the bowl. Discard the herb mixture.

4. Pour into the spray bottle using the funnel. Label the bottle with name and date.

How to use:

Spray on your hands, back of the hands, fingers, in between the fingers, palms, nails and fingertips. Rub your hands together for a few seconds. Let it air dry.

Natural Hand Sanitizer using Flax Gel

Makes: 18 – 19 ounces

What you need:

- ¼ cup whole flaxseeds
- 1 ½ cups water
- ½ cup vodka or 99% rubbing alcohol
- 1 tablespoon vegetable glycerin
- 3 drops tea tree essential oil
- 2 drops lavender essential
- 2 drops rose geranium essential oil
- Mixing bowl of the stand mixer
- Pump bottles or squeeze
- Label
- Saucepan
- Strainer
- Stand mixer

Directions:

1. Pour water into a saucepan. Add flaxseeds and place the saucepan over medium-low heat. Stir frequently and cook

for about 12 – 15 minutes. Now the mixture will resemble gel and will be jiggly.

2. Place a strainer over the bowl and strain the mixture into the bowl. Throw off the solids. You should be left with around 1 cup of flax gel.
3. Beat with the stand mixer until smooth.
4. Pour vodka and beat until well combined.
5. Add glycerin and all the essential oils. Beat until well incorporated.
5. Pour into the pump bottle. Label the bottle with name and date.

How to use:

Spray on your hands, back of the hands, fingers, in between the fingers, palms, nails and fingertips. Rub your hands together for a few seconds. Let it air dry.

All Herbal Hand Sanitizer

Makes: 10 – 12 ounces

What you need:

- 3 cups water
- 3 handfuls neem leaves (margosa leaves)
- Few sprigs holy basil with the dried flowers and seeds
- 1 ½ tablespoons powdered alum
- 1 ½ tablespoons powdered camphor
- Spray bottle
- Saucepan with lid
- Strainer
- Bowl
- Small spray bottle

Directions:

1. Pour water into a saucepan. Place the saucepan over medium heat and let it heat.
2. Once it begins to boil, add neem leaves and holy basil and let it sink down into the water. Push the leaves if required.
3. Cover and simmer on low heat for about 10 minutes.
4. Place a strainer over a bowl. Strain the herbal mixture into the bowl and discard the leaves.

5. Add alum and camphor into the hot steeped water and stir until it dissolves completely.
6. Let it cool completely.
7. Transfer into the spray bottle. Tighten the spray cap.
8. Label the bottle with name and date. Refrigerator until use.

How to use:

For your daily use, pour some into a small spray bottle. Spray on your hands, back of the hands, fingers, in between the fingers, palms, nails and fingertips. Rub your hands together for a few seconds. Let it air dry.

Gel Hand Cleanser

Makes: 16 – 17 ounces

Ingredients:

- 10 ounces 190 proof vodka
- 6 ounces aloe Vera gel
- 34 drops lemon essential oil
- 16 drops eucalyptus essential oil
- 40 drops clove bud essential oil
- 20 drops cinnamon leaf essential oil
- 10 drops rosemary essential oil
- Bowl
- Flip top bottle or squeeze bottle
- Hand whisk
- Large Mason's jar
- Pump bottle

Directions:

1. Add all the essential oils and vodka into the Mason's jar. Tighten the lid and shake the jar until well combined.
2. Add aloe Vera gel and whisk with a hand whisk until well combined.

3. Pour into a pump bottle.

4. Label the bottle with name and date.

How to use:

Spray on your hands, back of the hands, fingers, in between the fingers, palms, nails and fingertips. Rub your hands together for a few seconds. Let it air dry.

Herbal Hand Sanitizer

Makes: 8 ounces

What you need:

- 4 teaspoons aloe Vera gel
- 7 ounces isopropyl alcohol
- 3 teaspoons Gaia Herbs lemon balm certified organic liquid extract
- 3 teaspoons Gaia Herbs Usnea Uva Ursi Supreme liquid extract
- 20 drops holy basil essential oil
- 4 drops eucalyptus essential oil
- 16 drops lavender essential oil
- 8 drops rosemary essential oil
- Spray bottle

Directions:

1. Add isopropyl alcohol, aloe Vera gel, Gaia herbs lemon balm and Usnea Uva Ursi liquid extract into the spray bottle.
2. Tighten the cap and shake the bottle until well incorporated.

3. Add essential oils and tighten the cap. Shake the bottle well.
4. Label the bottle with name and date.

How to use:

Spray on your hands, back of the hands, fingers, in between the fingers, palms, nails and fingertips. Rub your hands together for a few seconds. Let it air dry.

Lemony -Orangy Hand Sanitizer

Makes: 4 ounces

What you need:

- 6 tablespoons witch hazel with aloe Vera or vodka or 190 proof grain alcohol
- Distilled water or boiled and cooled water, as required
- 10 drops vitamin E oil
- 10 drops lemon essential oil
- 10 drops tea tree essential oil
- 10 drops orange essential oil
- Label
- 4 ounce spray bottle
- Small funnel

Directions:

1. Pour witch hazel into the spray bottle with the help of the funnel. Add vitamin E oil and all the essential oils.
2. Tighten the spray cap and shake the bottle until well mixed.
3. Pour enough water to fill the bottle up to the neck.
4. Tighten the spray cap and shake until well combined.
5. Label the bottle with name and date.

How to use:

Spray on your hands, back of the hands, fingers, in between the fingers, palms, nails and fingertips. Rub your hands together for a few seconds. Let it air dry.

Hand Sanitizer using Astringent

Makes: 11 – 12 ounces

What you need:

- 1 cup isopropyl alcohol
- 2.1 ounces neem – aloe Vera astringent
- 2.1 ounces glycerin
- Bowl
- Small funnel
- Spoon
- 12 ounces spray bottle

Directions:

1. Pour alcohol, astringent and glycerin into a bowl and stir with a spoon.
2. Pour into the spray bottle using the funnel. Tighten the spray cap and shake until well combined.
3. Label the bottle with name and date.

How to use:

Spray on your hands, back of the hands, fingers, in between the fingers, palms, nails and fingertips. Rub your hands together for a few seconds. Let it air dry.

Foaming Hand Sanitizer

Makes: 8 ounces

What you need:

- 1 teaspoon liquid castile soap
- 10 drops thieves essential oil
- 10 drops peppermint essential oil
- Water, as required
- 8 ounces pump bottle

Directions:

1. Add castile soap into the pump bottle.
2. Add essential oils. Fill with water, to slightly below the neck of the bottle.
3. Tighten the cap. Shake the bottle until well combined.

How to use:

Pump a few drops of the sanitizer on one of your palms and rub it all over your hands, fingers, in between your fingers, back of the hands and nails. Then rub your palms together until dry.

Homemade Sanitizer for Kids

Lemony Tea Tree Sanitizer with Aloe Vera Juice

Makes: 3 – 4 ounces

What you need:

- 6 tablespoons aloe Vera juice
- 0.27 ounce tea tree essential oil
- 0.18 ounce white thyme essential oil
- 0.33 ounce lemon or lemongrass essential oil
- Spray bottle
- Small funnel

Directions:

1. Pour aloe Vera juice into the spray bottle using the funnel.
2. Add essential oils. Tighten the spray cap. Shake the bottle well.
3. Label the bottle with name and date.

How to use:

Shake the bottle before using the spray. Spray on your hands, fingers, in between the fingers, palms, back of the hands, nails and fingertips. Rub your hands together for a few seconds. Let it air dry. This sanitizer can be used on furniture as well.

Gentle Hand Sanitizer

Makes: 4 ounces

What you need:

- 40 drops germ destroyer essential oil
- ½ cup aloe Vera gel
- Glass bowl
- Flip top bottle
- Label
- Hand whisk
- Small funnel

Directions:

1. Measure out aloe Vera gel and add into the glass bowl.
2. Add germ destroyer essential oil. Whisk the mixture with a hand whisk until it resembles gel.
3. Pour into the bottle with the help of the funnel. Label the bottle with name and date.

How to use:

Squeeze or pump a few drops of the sanitizer on one of your palms and rub it all over your hands, fingers, in between your fingers, back of the hands and nails. Then rub your palms together until dry.

Aloe Vera Gel Sanitizer

Makes: 16 ounces

What you need:

- 2 cups aloe Vera gel
- 48 drops lavender essential oil
- 48 drops tea tree essential oil
- 16 ounces glass pump bottle or squeeze bottle
- Label
- Hand whisk
- Small funnel

Directions:

1. Measure out aloe Vera gel and add into the glass bowl.
2. Add germ destroyer essential oil. Whisk the mixture with a hand whisk until it resembles gel.
3. Pour into the bottle with the help of the funnel. Label the bottle with name and date.

How to use:

Squeeze or pump a few drops of the sanitizer on one of your palms and rub it all over your hands, fingers, in between your fingers, back of the hands and nails. Then rub your palms together until dry.

Little Tykes Hand Sanitizer

Makes: 2 ounces

What you need:

- 8 teaspoons 95% alcohol
- 2 teaspoons unscented castile soap
- 2 teaspoons organic aloe Vera gel
- 2 drops tea tree essential oil
- 4 drops lavender essential oil
- 2 ounce spray bottle
- Small funnel
- Label

Directions:

1. Pour alcohol into the spray bottle with the help of the funnel. Add essential oils. Tighten the spray cap and shake the bottle until well combined.
2. Set aside for 2 – 3 hours. Do not disturb the bottle during this time.
3. Now add castile soap and aloe Vera gel into the bottle.
4. Tighten the cap and shake the bottle until well incorporated.

5. Label the bottle with date and name.

How to use:

Spray on your kid's hands, fingers, in between the fingers, palms, nails, back of the hands and fingertips. Ask them to rub their hands together. Let it air dry.

"Thieves" Hand Sanitizer for Kids

Makes: 2 ounces

What you need:

- 8 teaspoons 95% alcohol
- 2 teaspoons unscented castile soap
- 2 teaspoons organic aloe Vera gel
- 6 drops orange essential oil
- 10 drops cinnamon leaf essential oil
- 4 drops pine essential oil
- 2 ounce spray bottle
- Small funnel
- Label

Directions:

1. Pour alcohol into the spray bottle with the help of the funnel. Add essential oils. Tighten the spray cap and shake the bottle until well combined.
2. Set aside for 2 – 3 hours. Do not disturb the bottle during this time.
3. Now add castile soap and aloe Vera gel into the bottle.
4. Tighten the cap and shake the bottle until well incorporated.

5. Label the bottle with date and name.

How to use:

Spray on your kid's hands, fingers, in between the fingers, palms, nails, back of the hands and fingertips. Ask them to rub their hands together. Let it air dry.

Disinfecting Citrus Mint Hand Sanitizer

Makes: 2 ounces

What you need:

- 8 teaspoons 95% alcohol
- 2 teaspoons unscented castile soap
- 2 teaspoons organic aloe Vera gel
- 6 drops lemon essential oil
- 10 drops rosemary essential oil
- 4 drops peppermint essential oil
- 2 ounce spray bottle
- Small funnel
- Label

Directions:

1. Pour alcohol into the spray bottle with the help of the funnel. Add essential oils. Tighten the spray cap and shake the bottle until well combined.
2. Set aside for 2 – 3 hours. Do not disturb the bottle during this time.
3. Now add castile soap and aloe Vera gel into the bottle.
4. Tighten the cap and shake the bottle until well incorporated.

5. Label the bottle with date and name.

How to use:

Spray on your kid's hands, fingers, in between the fingers, palms, nails, back of the hands and fingertips. Ask them to rub their hands together. Let it air dry.

Homemade Hand Sanitizer Spray for Kiddos

Makes: 4 ounces

- 1 teaspoon vegetable glycerin
- 6 – 8 tablespoons 190 proof vodka or rubbing alcohol
- 20 drops spruce essential oil
- 40 drops tea tree essential oil
- 12 drops lemon essential oil
- Glass spray bottle
- Label
- Small funnel

Directions:

1. Pour glycerin, followed by essential oils and finally alcohol into the glass spray bottle, with the help of funnel. Tighten the spray cap. Shake the bottle until well incorporated.
2. Label the bottle with name and date.

How to use:

Spray on your kid's hands, fingers, in between the fingers, palms, nails, back of the hands and fingertips. Ask them to rub their hands together. Let it air dry.

Sanitizer Wipes (Hand and Surface)

Herbal Antibacterial Wipes

Makes: 80

What you need:

- 20 heavy paper towels, cut into 4 pieces each, separate the papers
- 1 ¼ teaspoons tea tree essential oil
- 1 ¼ teaspoons eucalyptus essential oil
- ¾ teaspoon rosemary essential oil
- 1 ¼ teaspoons lavender essential oil
- ¾ teaspoon clove essential oil
- 5 tablespoons thieves vinegar or 99% isopropyl alcohol
- 1 large jar
- Measuring cup

Directions:

1. For "thieves" vinegar, follow the recipe of Herbal "thieves" vinegar hand sanitizer spray recipe.
2. Roll one piece of the quartered paper.
3. Now place the next paper below the edge of the end of the first roll and roll over the 2nd paper.

4. Repeat this process (step 3) until all the papers are rolled together into 1 large roll. This way, when you pull out one sheet, the end of the next sheet will be the first sheet each time.
5. Place the rolled paper roll in the jar.
6. Add "thieves" vinegar into the measuring cup. Add essential oils and stir.
7. Pour over the paper towels. Close the lid and shake the jar so that the mixture is absorbed by the towels.
8. Let it rest for 30 minutes.

How to use:

Pull out a sheet of paper. Wipe your hands, fingers, in between the fingers, palms, nails, back of the hands and fingertips.

Disinfectant Wipes

Makes: 1-roll paper towels

What you need:

- 4 cups warm water
- 2 tablespoons dish soap
- 2 cups rubbing alcohol
- 15 drops lemon essential oil

- 1 roll paper towels
- Tupperware container or any other plastic container
- Bowl

Directions:

1. Place the roll of paper towels in the container.
2. Mix together in a bowl, alcohol, dish soap, lemon essential oil and warm water. Pour over the paper towels.
3. Close the lid and store until use.
4. Pull out as many as needed and keep the lid closed.
5. If you do not want to use paper towels, you can use re-usable washcloths.

How to use:

Pull out a sheet of paper. Wipe your hands, fingers, in between the fingers, palms, nails, back of the hands and fingertips.

Reusable Disinfecting Baby Wipes

Makes: 10

What you need:

- ½ cup warm filtered water or distilled water
- ¼ cup rubbing alcohol
- ½ tablespoon liquid castile soap
- 2 – 3 drops lavender essential oil
- 2 – 3 drops tea tree essential oil
- 10 flannel baby wipes, 1 or 2 ply (8 inches each), folded in half or quarter
- Measuring cup
- Spoon
- Baby wipe container

Directions:

1. Place baby wipe in the baby wipe container.
2. Measure water in the measuring cup. Add liquid castile soap, essential oils and rubbing alcohol.
3. Stir with a spoon until well combined.
4. Drizzle over the wipes. Close the box and let it sit undisturbed for 15 minutes.

How to use:

Pull out a wipe. Wipe your baby's hands, fingers, in between the fingers, palms, nails, back of the hands, legs, feet and fingertips.

Once used, wash and dry them for future use.

Apple Cider Vinegar Wipes

Makes: 80

What you need:

- ½ cup water
- ½ cup witch hazel
- ½ cup aloe Vera gel
- 2 tablespoons apple cider vinegar
- 20 drops tea tree essential oil
- 10 drops eucalyptus essential oil
- 10 drops ylang ylang oil
- 40 paper towels, 2 ply
- Baby wipe container or any other container
- Large bowl
- Spoon

Directions:

1. Place the paper towels in a pile and cut into 2 halves.
2. Add water, witch hazel, aloe Vera and essential oils into a bowl and stir with a spoon.
3. Roll each piece of paper towel and place it in the bowl.
4. Once soaked, transfer into the re-sealable container.

How to use:

Pull out a sheet of paper. Wipe your hands, fingers, in between the fingers, palms, nails, back of the hands and fingertips.

Antibacterial Kitchen Wipes using Vinegar

Makes: 40

What you need:

- ½ cup white vinegar
- 1 ½ cups water
- 20 drops tea tree essential oil
- 1 teaspoon Dr. Bronner's Organic Sal Suds Liquid Cleaner
- 20 drops eucalyptus essential oil
- 20 drops lemon essential oil
- Airtight container or baby wipe box
- 40 paper towels, 2 or 3 ply
- Bowl
- Spoon

Directions:

1. Place the paper towels in the airtight container.
2. Add water, detergent and vinegar into a bowl and stir with a spoon until detergent dissolves.
3. Add essential oils and stir well.
4. Drizzle the mixture over the paper towels. Close the lid and let it soak for a while.

How to use:

First clean the surface with a microfiber cloth.

Pull out a sheet of paper. Wipe the cleaned surface to sanitize.

Re-usable Hydrogen Peroxide Cleaning Wipes

Makes: 60

What you need:

- 6 cups warm water
- 1/3 cup hydrogen peroxide
- 12 drops lavender essential oil
- 12 drops lemongrass essential oil
- 5 tablespoons liquid castile soap
- Hand whisk
- Large airtight glass container
- 30 reusable cloth wipes, cut into 2 halves

Directions:

1. Pour half the water into the glass container.
2. Whisk in the liquid castile soap and the essential oils.
3. Roll each half of the cloth wipe and place it standing, in the glass container.
4. Pour remaining water and hydrogen peroxide over the wipes. Cover the container and shake until the cloth halves are well soaked.

How to use:

Pull out a cloth wipe and wipe the required surface. Used cloth wipes should be washed in the washing machine. Once they are dried, you can place it back in the container. This will work as long there is liquid in the container.

When there is no more liquid, make a new batch.

"Clorox" Wipes

Makes: 40

What you need:

- 1 ½ cups rubbing alcohol
- 6 cups distilled water
- 12 teaspoons "Dawn" dishwashing soap
- 20 drops lemon essential oil
- Glass jar with lid
- 20 washcloths, cut into 2 halves
- Bowl

Directions:

1. Stack the jar with washcloths.
2. Pour alcohol into the bowl. Add essential oil and stir well.
3. Drizzle over the washcloths. Close the lid.

How to use:

Pull out a washcloth and wipe the required surface. Used cloth wipes should be washed in the washing machine. Once they are dried, you can place it back in the container. This will work as long there is liquid in the container.

When there is no more liquid, make a new batch.

Disinfecting Cleaning Wipes

Makes: 30 wipes

What you need:

- 1 ½ cups white vinegar
- 1 ½ cups filtered water
- 30 drops lemon essential oil
- 8 drops bergamot essential oil
- 16 ounces lavender essential oil
- 30 washcloths (10 x 10 inches each)
- Large Mason's jar or a glass jar with a tight fitting lid
- Spoon

Directions:

1. Add water, vinegar and all the essential oils into the jar. Stir with a spoon until well incorporated.
2. Roll the washcloths and place them in the jar. Tighten the lid of the jar. Upturn the jar for a minute so that all the cloth pieces are well soaked.
3. Place the jar in a cupboard.

How to use:

Pull a wipe and squeeze it of excess moisture, in the jar itself.

Clean the surface with it. Once you are done with cleaning, rinse the washcloth and you can use it again if required. Used cloth wipes should be washed in the washing machine. Once they are dried, you can place it back in the jar. This solution will work as long there is liquid in the jar.

Disinfecting Bathroom Wipes

Makes: 20

What you need:

- 2 cups warm water
- 5 drops thyme essential oil
- 2 – 3 drops sweet orange essential oil
- 2 – 3 drops lemon essential oil
- 1 tablespoon liquid castile soap
- 20 disposable wipes
- Bowl
- Mason's jar or glass jar with lid or airtight container

Directions:

1. Stack the disposable wipes in the container.
2. Mix together in a bowl, castile soap, essential oils and warm water. Pour over the wipes.
3. Close the lid and let the wipes soak the solution.

How to use:

Use as the way you normally do.

Homemade Baby Wipes

Makes: 40

What you need:

- 3 ½ cups boiled water, cooled until warm
- 2 tablespoons pure Witch hazel
- 20 drops grapefruit seed extract or 4 capsules vitamin E
- 12 drops orange essential oil
- 12 drops lavender essential oil
- 2 tablespoons aloe Vera gel
- 2 teaspoons liquid castile soap
- 2 teaspoons almond oil or olive oil (optional)
- Old baby wipe container
- 20 sheets heavy duty paper towels, cut into 2 halves

Directions:

1. Fold the paper towels and stack them in the container.
2. Mix together in a bowl, castile soap, almond oil, witch hazel, aloe Vera gel, grapefruit seed extract, essential oils and warm water. Pour over the wipes. Do not add these essential oils if your baby has very sensitive skin. You can use chamomile or calendula essential oils instead.

3. Close the lid and let the wipes soak the solution. Upturn the container to soak well. These wipes can last for a month.

How to use:

Use as the way you normally do.

Surface Sanitizer Recipes

Homemade Multi-Purpose Disinfectant Spray

Makes: 32 ounces

What you need:

- 2 cups white distilled vinegar or extra alcohol
- 2 cups 100 proof alcohol or higher alcohol
- 100 – 120 drops tea tree essential oil or lavender essential oil
- Spray bottle
- Label
- Measuring cup

Directions:

1. Add alcohol into the spray bottle followed by the essential oils using funnel. Tighten the spray cap and shake the bottle until well combined.
2. Next add vinegar and shake once again.
3. Label the bottle with name and date.

Disinfectant Spray

Makes: 64 ounces

What you need:

- 3 – 4 lemons
- Water, as required
- 4 cups vodka
- Large Mason's jar or any other jar
- Glass spray bottle
- Label
- Small funnel

Directions:

1. Peel the lemons. Add lemon peels into the jar. Pour vodka over the lemon peels.
2. Fasten the lid tightly and set aside on your countertop 12 – 15 days.
3. Discard the lemon peels and pour steeped vodka into the glass spray bottle. Add equal quantity of water. Suppose steeped vodka is 2 cups, add 2 cups water.
4. Fasten the nozzle tightly. This spray is good general surfaces.

5. For areas that should not remain moist for too long, reduce the water to half the water in step 3.
6. Label the bottle with name and date.

Vinegar Disinfectant Spray

Makes: 16 ounces

What you need:

- ½ cup white vinegar
- 1 ½ cups water
- 14 drops tea tree essential oil
- 14 drops lavender essential oil
- 16 ounces spray bottle
- Label
- Measuring cup
- Small funnel

Directions:

1. Add vinegar into the spray bottle followed by the essential oils and water, using funnel. Tighten the spray cap and shake the bottle until well combined.
2. Label the bottle with name and date.

How to use:

Spray generously on the surface that needs to be cleaned, after initially wiping the surface clean with a cloth. Wipe off the sprayed area with a microfiber cloth, after 2 – 3 minutes.

Toilet Bowl Cleaner

Makes: 1 use

What you need:

- 6 – 7 tablespoons baking soda
- 8 drops tea tree essential oil
- 3 tablespoons vinegar
- Toilet brush

How to use:

Add baking soda, essential oil and vinegar into the toilet bowl.

Once it fizzes, scrub the bowl with the toilet brush.

Sanitizing Solution for Floors

*** Important: Keep this solution away from children***

Makes: 32 ounces

What you need:

- ½ teaspoon unscented chlorine bleach
- 4 cups water
- 32 ounces spray bottle
- Label
- Measuring cup

Directions:

1. Measure water and pour into the spray bottle. Add chlorine bleach.
2. Tighten the spray cap.
3. Shake the bottle until well combined.
4. Label the bottle with name and date, also mentioning to keep away from children.

How to use:

Spray generously on the floor, after initially wiping the surface clean with a cloth. Wipe off the sprayed area with a microfiber mop, after 2 – 3 minutes.

Natural Granite Cleaner

Makes: 32 ounces

What you need:

- 1 cup rubbing alcohol
- 3 cups warm water
- 1 teaspoon dish soap
- 20 drops lavender or basil or cinnamon essential oil
- Piece of cloth
- Microfiber cloth or mop
- Glass spray bottle
- Label

Directions:

1. Add alcohol, dish soap, water and essential oils into the spray bottle.
2. Tighten the spray cap. Shake the bottle until well combined.
3. Label the bottle with name and date.

How to use:

Wipe the granite surfaces to be cleaned with a cloth. Spray generously on the granite surfaces. After a couple of minutes, wipe off the sprayed area with a microfiber cloth.

For floors, first clean the floor with a mop. Spray on the flour generously. After a couple of minutes wipe off with microfiber mop.

Toilet Seat Cleaner

Makes: 16 ounces

Ingredients:

- 2 cups vinegar
- 10 drops lemon essential oil
- 10 drops tea tree essential oil
- Spray bottle

Directions:

1. Pour vinegar into the spray bottle. Add essential oils and fasten the cap.
2. Shake the bottle well.

How to use:

Spray daily on the toilet seat. Wipe off after 5 – 6 minutes.

Sanitizing Glass Cleaner

Makes: 14 ounces

Ingredients:

- 1 cup water
- 2 tablespoons rubbing alcohol
- ¼ cup white vinegar or cider vinegar
- 1 drop orange essential oil
- 16 ounces spray bottle
- Label

Directions:

1. Add water, alcohol vinegar and essential oil into the spray bottle.
2. Tighten the spray cap.
3. Label the bottle with name and date.

How to use:

Spray on the glass directly. Wipe off with a cloth.

Natural Antibacterial Surface Spray with Witch Hazel

Makes: 17 ounces

What you need:

- 2 cups water, distilled or filtered
- 20 drops orange or lavender or eucalyptus essential oil
- 60 drops tea tree oil
- 2 tablespoons witch hazel
- 18 ounces spray bottle
- Measuring cup

Directions:

1. Pour witch hazel and essential oils into a spray bottle.
2. Churn the mixture by moving the bottle in a swirling manner.
3. Add water. Tighten the spray cap.
4. Shake the bottle until well combined. Label the bottle with name and date.
5. Place it in a cool and dark place until use.

How to use:

Spray generously on the surface that needs to be cleaned, after initially wiping the surface clean with a cloth. Wipe off the sprayed area with a microfiber cloth, after 2 – 3 minutes.

Antibacterial Surface Cleaner

Makes: 30 ounces

What you need:

- 4 cups vinegar
- 8 lemons
- 10 drops oregano essential oil
- 10 drops tea tree essential oil
- 10 drops lemon essential oil
- Large glass jar with a lid
- Glass bowl
- Small funnel
- 32 ounces glass spray bottle
- Metal strainer

Directions:

1. Measure out the vinegar and pour into the glass jar.
2. Slice a few of the lemons and add into the jar. Juice the remaining lemons and add the juice as well as lemon rinds into the jar.
3. Place the jar in a cupboard. For about 18 – 21 days. During this period of steeping, if you happen to use lemons, add

the lemon rinds into the bottle. The more the lemon rinds, fragrance will smell of lemon.

4. After 18 – 21 days, place a strainer over the glass measuring container. Strain the mixture into the jar. Discard the lemon rinds.
5. Add all the essential oils into the mixture and stir until well combined.
6. Pour into a glass spray bottle using funnel. Tighten the spray cap.
7. Shake the bottle until well combined. Label the bottle with name and date.
8. Place it in a cool and dark place until use.

How to use:

Spray generously on the surface that needs to be cleaned, after initially wiping the surface clean with a cloth. Wipe off the sprayed area with a microfiber cloth, after 2 – 3 minutes.

Miscellaneous Sanitizer Recipes

Mattress Sanitizer with Vodka

Makes: 9 ounces

What you need:

- 1 cup vodka or 99% rubbing alcohol
- 8 drops lemon essential oil
- 15 drops tea tree essential oil
- 8 drops eucalyptus essential oil
- 8 drops lavender essential
- Glass spray bottle
-

Directions:

1. Pour vodka into the spray bottle. Add all the essential oils.
2. Tighten the spray cap.
3. Shake the bottle until well combined. Label the bottle with name and date.

How to use:

Spray lightly all over the mattress. Turn the mattress over and spray on the other side as well. Let it air dry. This is good for pillows as well.

Mattress Sanitizer with Vinegar

Makes: 9 ounces

What you need:

- ½ cup vinegar
- ½ cup boiled and cooled water
- 4 drops eucalyptus essential oil
- 4 drops peppermint essential oil
- 4 drops lavender essential
- Glass spray bottle

Directions:

1. Pour vinegar into the spray bottle. Add all the essential oils.
2. Tighten the spray cap.
3. Shake the bottle until well combined. Label the bottle with name and date.

How to use:

Spray lightly all over the mattress. Turn the mattress over and spray on the other side as well. Let it air dry. It can take a few hours.

Sanitizer Spray for Toys

Makes: 8 – 9 ounces

What you need:

- ½ cup distilled water
- ½ cup white vinegar
- 15 drops lavender essential oil
- 5 drops germ destroyer essential oil (optional)
- Spray bottle
- Label
- Funnel

Directions:

1. Pour vinegar and water into the spray bottle using funnel. Add all the essential oils.
2. Tighten the spray cap.
3. Shake the bottle until well combined. Label the bottle with name and date.

How to use:

Spray generously all over the toys. Let it air dry for a couple of minutes.

Take a clean, moist cloth and wipe the toys with it. Let it air dry.

All-purpose Sanitizer for Babies, their Surroundings and their Toys

Makes: 9 ounces

What you need:

- ½ cup seltzer water
- ½ cup white vinegar
- 1 tablespoon hydrogen peroxide
- 4 drops tea tree oil
- Small funnel
- Spray bottle

Directions:

1. Pour vinegar, seltzer water, hydrogen peroxide and tea tree oil, just before using this solution to spray. The sanitizing effect will not last for long.
2. Tighten the spray cap.
3. Shake the bottle until well combined.

How to use:

Spray generously all over the toys, and their surroundings. Let it air dry for a couple of minutes.

Take a clean, moist cloth and wipe the toys and their surroundings like crib, room etc. with it. Let it air dry.

Disinfectant Spray for Fabrics #1

Makes: 8 ounces

What you need:

- ½ cup vodka or vinegar or witch hazel
- Boiled and cooled water, as required
- 10 drops essential oils of your choice
- Small funnel
- 8 ounces spray bottle

Directions:

1. Pour vodka, water and essential oils into the spray bottle.
2. Tighten the spray cap.
3. Shake the bottle until well combined. Label the bottle with name and date.

How to use:

Initially spray on one of the edges to see if it is going to stain your fabric. If it does not, go ahead and spray generously all over desired fabric. Let it air dry.

Disinfectant Spray for Fabrics #2

Makes: 5 ounces

What you need:

- 4 ounces distilled water
- 2 tablespoons baking soda
- 15 drops lemon essential oil
- 5 drops tea tree essential oil
- 5 drops palmarosa essential oil
- 5 drops eucalyptus essential oil
- Small funnel
- Spray bottle

Directions:

1. Place funnel in the bottle. Add baking soda and water.
2. Tighten the spray cap.
3. Shake the bottle until well combined.
4. Next drop the essential oils into the bottle.
5. Tighten the spray cap.
6. Shake the bottle until well combined.

How to use:

Initially spray on one of the edges to see if it is going to stain your fabric. If it does not, go ahead and spray generously all over desired fabric. Let it air dry. It works well on carpets and couches as well.

Room Sanitizer # 1

What you need:

- 40 drops lemongrass essential oil
- 40 drops tea tree essential oil
- 40 drops eucalyptus essential oil
- Small, dark glass dropper bottle
- Diffuser

Directions:

1. Add all the essential oils into a clean, dark bottle. Tighten the cap of the bottle.
1. Shake the bottle well until the oils are well combined.
2. Store the bottle in a dark and cool place.

How to use:

Shake the bottle well before use. Follow the manufacturer's instructions and add a few drops of the oil blend into your diffuser. Use the diffuser as instructed in the room that is to be sanitized.

Room Sanitizer # 2

What you need:

- 20 drops lemongrass essential oil
- 20 drops thyme essential oil
- 40 drops eucalyptus essential oil
- 40 drops cinnamon essential oil
- 20 drops citronella essential oil
- Small, dark glass dropper bottle
- Diffuser

Directions:

1. Add all the essential oils into a clean, dark bottle. Tighten the cap of the bottle.
2. Shake the bottle well until the oils are well combined.
3. Store the bottle in a dark and cool place.

How to use:

Shake the bottle well before use. Follow the manufacturer's instructions and add a few drops of the oil blend into your diffuser. Use the diffuser as instructed in the room that is to be sanitized.

Conclusion

Thank you for purchasing the book.

Research suggests you must use sanitizers if you want to prevent germs from entering your body from your hands. Many companies manufacture these products. Since these products are mass-produced, they all have the same proportions of alcohol. Alcohol can make your skin dry. This book will provide some recipes you can use to make these sanitizers at home. The instructions are easy to follow. Since you make these at home, you can add essential oils or tweak the recipes to suit your needs.

I hope you got all the information you are looking for.

Lightning Source UK Ltd.
Milton Keynes UK
UKHW051023040720
365951UK00021B/647

WELLINGTON

THE GEODETIC GIANT

'The whole joy of life is in battle. Not winning.'

Sir Barnes Wallis, CBE, FRS
(1887 – 1979)

WELLINGTON
THE GEODETIC GIANT

Martin Bowman

Airlife
England

First published in the UK in 1989
by Airlife Publishing Ltd
This edition published 1998

British Library Cataloguing-in-Publication Data
   A catalogue record for this book
   is available from the British Library

ISBN 1 84037 006 8

Printed in Hong Kong

Airlife Publishing Ltd

101 Longden Road, Shrewsbury, SY3 9EB, England

Contents

	Acknowledgements	
Chapter 1	Inception and development	1
Chapter 2	Opening gambit	12
Chapter 3	Battle of the Bight	22
Chapter 4	Coastal Command	31
Chapter 5	Night offensive	46
Chapter 6	Bombers' Moon	57
Chapter 7	Millennium	72
Chapter 8	One of our aircraft is missing	80
Chapter 9	Bomber finale	91
Chapter 10	Desert war	106
Chapter 11	Mad dogs and Englishmen	118
Chapter 12	African adventure	127
Chapter 13	Mediterranean missions	138
Chapter 14	Maritime operations	150
	Further Reading	163
	Index	164

Acknowledgements

This work began life over seven years ago. Although it is an account of the Wellington aircraft, it is also a book about people. It could not possibly have been written without the immense help supplied by fellow enthusiasts, researchers, friends and above all, wartime Wellington crewmen and their relatives throughout the world. The following therefore constitutes probably the largest gathering of Wimpy contributors ever assembled in one book. I am most grateful to each and every one.

Many supplied photos from their collections. Some photos will be immediately familiar. I have no hesitation in using them again here for three reasons: they illustrate the story; hitherto they have appeared with inaccurate captions; or they contain additional information to that previously published.

I am particularly grateful to Bob Collis of the Norfolk and Suffolk Aviation Museum for his inspiring and painstaking research on my behalf and for providing me with many contacts. Dr Colin Dring of the Mildenhall Museum also provided much help with photo research and helped track down ex-Wellington men. Mike Bailey also provided welcome advice, as well as his usual expertise in photo-interpretation.

I am most grateful to the following: Les Allington; Wing Commander E. E. M. Angell; Les Aspin, RCAF; Len Aynsley; David K. Brearey; G. Stuart Brown, RCAF; Don Bruce; Jim Burtt-Smith; John Callander; Arthur 'Chan' Chandler; K. Clement; Norman Child; L. W. Collett; A. J. Cook; Gerald F. Cooke; Rupert Cooling; Gary Cooper; E. M. Cox; Noel C. Croppi, AFC; D. Cumming; Eric Day; G. B. Dick; Fred Dorken, RCAF; Huby Fairhead; Henry Fawcett; Harvey Firestone; the late Charles Fox; Dr Paul A. Fox; Malcolm Freestone; Brian French; Peter Frost; Wally Gaul; Michael L. Gibson; Roy Gristwood; Gordon E. Haddock; Les Hallam; B. Hammond; Harold J. Hamnett, RCAF, Retd; Captain T. A. Hampton, AFC; the late Raymond Harding; S. Harle; Flight Lieutenant Keith Haywood, RAF; Robin T. Holmes of the Loch Ness Wellington Project; Johnny Hosford; Alfred Jenner; Arthur Johnson; the late Group Captain Jones; R. Kirk; John O. Lancaster; *Legion* magazine; Tom Leonard, RCAF; Squadron Leader Geoffrey N. W. MacFarlane; Reg Mack; J. A. Ian Mackay, RCAF; Robert G. MacNeil, RCAF; G. H. S. Malcolmson; the late Leslie Marlow; Eric A. Masters; Ian McLachlan; Des Norris; Major Stephen A. Oliphant, USAF; Ernie Payne; Jeremy Petts; Stella Poynton; Charles Ray; A. H. Rawlings; Edward N. Reynolds, RCAF; the RCAF Association; Flight Lieutenant W. 'Rusty' Russell, RAF; Hans-Heiri Stapfer; Terence Mansfield the Lord Sandhurst, DFC; Maurice 'Scats' Satchell; *Sentinel* magazine; Group Captain M. J. A. Shaw, DSO; Squadron Leader R. C. Shepherd, DFC; Leslie Sidwell; Alan G. Smith; Charles Stephens; Reg Thackeray, DFM; Geoff Thomas; J. Tipton; Bryn Watkins; Jack Weekley; Brian Wexham of Vickers Ltd; Group Captain John N. Williams, OBE, DFC; Fred Wingham; James Woodruff.

Martin Bowman   September 1989

Chapter 1
Inception and development

The birth of the British heavy night bomber force began with the introduction of the Vickers Wellington, truly one of the greatest bombers of World War 2. However, this twin-engined machine, famous for its rugged construction, was, like so many aircraft of its generation, born of an Air Ministry specification steeped in 1930's tradition when the bombers of the day were lumbering biplanes like the Handley Page Heyford. Even as the Vickers Type 271 emerged on the drawing board, the firm patriotically suggested the name 'Crecy'. However, this name was not in keeping with the Air Ministry's ambitious new plans for its long-range bomber force and the more famous name of Wellington was later adopted.

It all started in September 1932 with Specification B 9/32 which demanded an experimental twin-engined day bomber capable of carrying a bomb load of 1,000 lb for 720 miles and to possess a range of 1,500 miles. Apart from Vickers, Bristol, Gloster and Handley Page also prepared new designs. In the case of Handley Page, B 9/32 produced the unorthodox HP 52 Hampden which, together with the Armstrong Whitworth Whitley and the Wellington, would shoulder the burden of the early British Bomber campaign.

If the Hampden, with its sleek, long tapered boom and twin tail was considered unconventional for its day, at Vickers R. K. Pierson and his design team applied all that was best in a succession of previous company models. Above all, the Type 271 incorporated geodetics, an ingenious and immensely strong geodetic framework, which was devised and developed by Barnes Wallis for the *R100* airship and later used in the construction of the Type 253 biplane and Wellesley monoplane bomber.

Initially, in March 1933, R. K, Pierson envisaged that the new Type 271 should employ a high wing monoplane design with a fixed undercarriage and be powered by either two Bristol Mercury VIS2 or the Rolls-Royce Goshawk steam-cooled powerplants.

However, by October Pierson had come down in favour of a retractable undercarriage and favoured using geodetic construction throughout. His decision was influenced by the fact that the geodetic latticework construction had reached such a stage by late 1933 that it could be incorporated in the airframes of large aircraft.

The Vickers proposal was accepted and in December 1933 the Air Ministry placed an order for a single prototype Type 271 with Goshawk engines. However, the Goshawk proved to be one of the few Rolls-Royce failures and the more conventional air-cooled 850 hp Bristol Pegasus X was substituted. The prototype finally made its maiden flight at Weybridge on 15 June 1936, with Captain J. 'Mutt' Summers at the controls.

The B.9/32 prototype K4049 with cupola-type turrets. *(Vickers)*

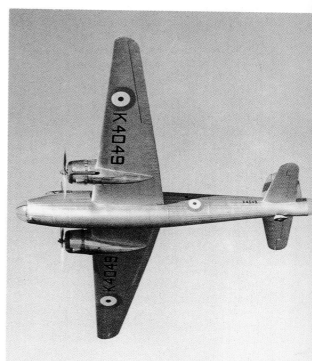

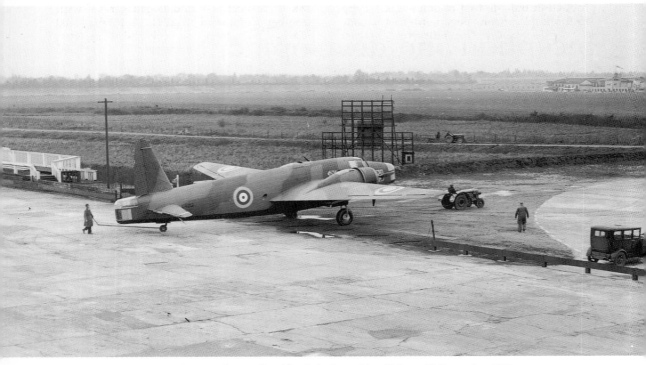

The prototype Wellington I is towed out at Brooklands for its maiden flight on 23 December 1937. *(Vickers)*

Fitted with a Stranraer-type fin and rudder to save on design time, the model bore scant resemblance to later models. Both front and rear gun turrets were glazed over with Plexiglas and no armament was carried. It was successful during a series of trials and was exhibited at the annual RAF display at Hendon. The new aircraft enthralled the RAF and public alike, and the former were particularly impressed with its ability to carry double the bomb load and cover twice the range (3,000 miles) to that originally specified.

In August 1936 the Air Ministry had placed an initial production order for 180 of the Vickers type. On 29 January 1937 Specification 29/36 was issued to cover the first production run of 185 Wellington Mk Is. On 19 April Vickers suffered a setback when the prototype crashed at Waldringfield, 1½ miles east of the A&AEE station at Martlesham Heath, during diving trials. By the end of the year the shape of the proposed production model had altered considerably. The fuselage and tail surfaces were revised and the redesign was incorporated in the first production Type 285 Wellington B Mk I by the time

it made its maiden flight from Brooklands on 23 December 1937.

Other modifications had been made, including the provision of a retractable tailwheel and changes to the bomb bay to enable a much larger bomb load to be carried. Elongated side windows were incorporated in the fuselage, which was increased in length. Wingspan was also extended slightly and the crew positions increased from four to five members. Vickers nose and tail turrets and a Nash and Thompson ventral turret were installed. Subsequent production Wellington Is were fitted with 1,000 hp Pegasus XVIII engines. On 10 October 1938 No 99 Squadron became the first in Bomber Command to receive the Wellington B Mk I.

In 1939, production of 189 examples of the Type 408 B Mk IA began. Both Vickers turrets were replaced by Nash and Thompson and each was equipped with two .303 inch machine-guns (as was the existing ventral position). Various other improvements were made and the crew complement was increased to six.

The Type 409 B Mk IB did not enter

production but the first of some 2,685 Type 415 B Mk IC versions began entering squadron service before the outbreak of war. Several internal improvements were made, not the least of which was to the electrical system. The B Mk IC was easily distinguishable by the addition of a pair of Vickers K machine-guns, installed to fire from each side of the fuselage, in place of the earlier ventral position; and the addition of larger mainwheels which protruded from the engine nacelle when retracted. However, some problems remained. The Wellington IC required tremendous forward pressure on the control column to bring the nose down when going round again with flaps down. A characteristic of the Wellington was to drop its nose during turns.

On 3 March 1939 the Type 298 B Mk II prototype, fitted with 1,145 hp Merlin X engines, flew for the first time, and the Type 299 B Mk III prototype, with twin 1,400 hp Bristol Hercules III powerplants, flew for the first time on 16 May the same year. Both types entered production the following year as the Type 406 B Mk II and the Type 417

Mk III respectively and began service with Bomber Command in 1941. A total of 400 Mk II Wellingtons was built and these were followed by 1,519 Mk III models. A Mk IC fitted with a pair of Pratt and Whitney R1830-S3C4-G Twin-Wasps was redesignated Type 410 to become the Mk IV prototype. A total of 220 production models was built.

To increase Wellington production, Vickers established a new factory at Chester and, later, another factory was producing the type at Squires Gate, Blackpool. Wellingtons were being produced at the rate of 134 a month in September 1940. By the spring of 1941 this had grown to more than double this figure.

Construction techniques

Much has been made of the relative strength of the Wellington airframe but there were several accidents caused by outer mainplanes breaking away. During May 1942 Vickers co-operated with RAE Farnborough in an effort to improve the design of the mainspar, which was prone to fatigue cracks.

Eric Day, who was mostly involved with

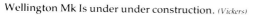

Wellington Mk Is under under construction. *(Vickers)*

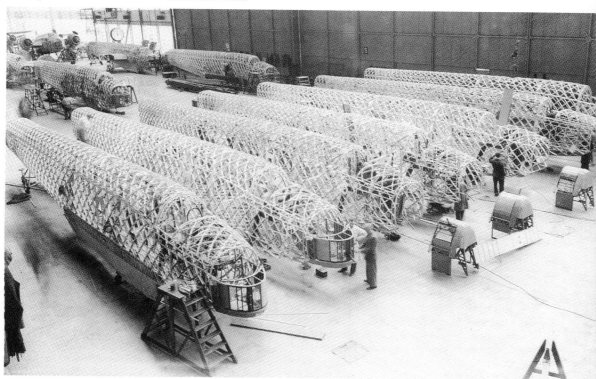

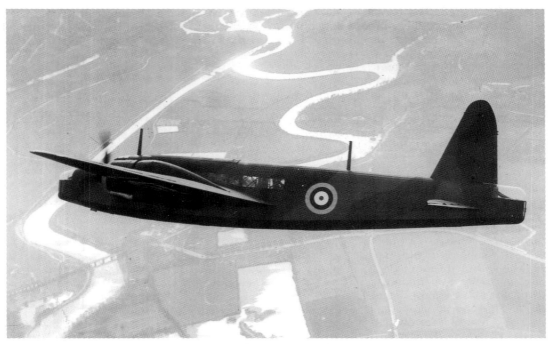

Wellington I L4280 banks over the River Wey during its approach to Weybridge in 1938. It later served with 148 Squadron and on 19 August 1940, while serving with 15 OTU, was destroyed in an air raid at Harwell. *(RAF Museum)*

the Wellington Mk III at 91 Group Servicing Unit, recalls: 'In August 1943 we were suddenly posted to RAF Hemswell, Lincs, which was temporarily closed while runways were being laid. 91 GSU were to be put into a unit of about 300 to work in groups of about seven men under a Corporal and supervised overall by civilians from Vickers on a big new mod, P1303, because of metal fatigue causing cracks in the mainspar at the root of the mainplane where they joined the inner plane in the nacelle. All Wellingtons were to be checked, each OTU sending one aircraft and bringing back another when collecting the former.

'The procedure was as follows: with a Coles crane in attendance the wings were removed. The aircraft was jacked up and the main wheels removed. A hefty beam of timber was bolted on to the oleos where the wheels had been, then the nacelle, complete with engine and propeller, was removed and stood aside, using a specially fabricated tubular metal tripod, which took the weight behind the propeller at the point of the engine reduction gear casing. The whole assembly would stand quite safely until rebuilding began.

'Imagine the amount of work involved in al his as everything had to be disconnected; flying controls, hydraulic, pneumatic, turret hydraulic, fuel pipes, etc, etc. Incidentally, when rebuilding it was sometimes extremely difficult to get all these items to line up and many four letter words were uttered.

'With the aircraft now lying around in very large pieces the Vickers men could examine the root end fixtures of main and inner planes using sophisticated optics and if anything appeared suspect, the wing would be written off and a brand new one fitted. A continuous supply of these were being delivered by the famous sixty feet long "Queen Mary" vehicles.

'In many cases nothing sinister appeared. The mainspar was reinforced with a sleeve and taper pins. Wellington mainspars were based on tubular booms and were not box sectioned as on orthodox aircraft.

'After modification the aircraft was reassembled and pushed out of the hangar six days later. The completed aircraft had to be thoroughly test flown. There was no telling how it would fly with its existing ailerons built into a new port or starboard wing, for example. The entire flying characteristics would be altered. We had Reception and Despatch flights for this purpose and from these the test flying was done. I went on quite a few test flights. We could only take off and land in one direction because of the runway construction. When major adjustments had to be made an aircraft would be test flown a second or even a third time. The entire P1303 job took the best part of a year to complete and this included a move to Upper Heyford when Hemswell became operational for Lancasters.

'When the Wellington was correctly rigged and in a stable flying condition it was a delightful aircraft. The control surfaces were actuated by push-pull rods which ran through roller guides at various stations in their travel. This gave a smooth and positive control, unlike the old method of using 15 cwt steel cable running through fairleads and tensioned by turn-buckles. Of course, the Wellington was something of an oddity, or an in-between, coming as it did between the old Heyfords, Harrows and Hendons and the later, modern Lancasters and Halifaxes. The geodetic build was wonderful for lightness, strength and flexibility but the fabric covering was on a par with aircraft of World War 1. There can be no doubt that stressed skin, monocoque construction, had to prevail for the new generation of aircraft. Nevertheless, the Wellington earned the laurels which it richly deserved.

'Viewed from the ground when in flight, a Wellington looked superb. The high aspect ratio wings gave it a graceful appearance. It was so adaptable it could be made to do almost anything, except tow a glider (for fear of stretching the fuselage like lazy tongs).'

Odds and mods

The Wellington was often called the 'flying mod'. The most weird and wonderful mod of all had to be the high-altitude version. Late in 1939 Vickers produced two high-altitude prototypes in response to Air Ministry specification B 23/39, which called for the development of a high-altitude conversion of the Wellington. The specification stipulated that the type had to be capable of attaining an altitude of 40,000 feet, ie, to put it out of reach of enemy flak and fighters. Both prototypes had a special cigar shaped fuselage with a pressurized cabin in the nose to simulate conditions at 10,000 feet. Originally,

Wellington XVI N2875 served with both 115 and 305 Squadrons and various OTUs before ending its career with CGS on 8 January 1946. *(RAF Museum)*

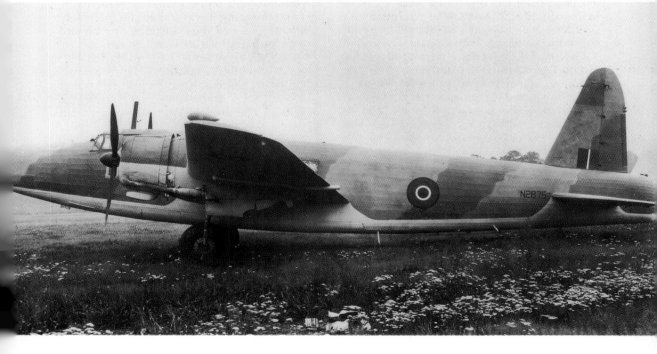

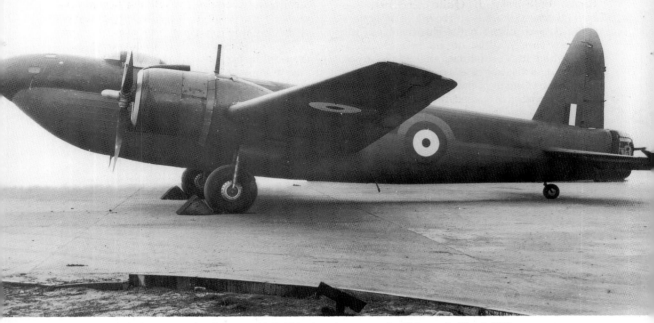

Wellington V R3298 pictured in February 1941. This aircraft was struck off charge in March 1943. *(RAF Hendon)*

it was planned to fit two 1,650 hp Bristol Hercules VIII engines but production difficulties dictated the use of the Hercules III powerplant.

The first of the two Mk V prototypes (*R3298*) made its maiden flight in September 1940 and achieved a height of 30,000 feet. Only one Mk V model (the second off the production lines) was completed and nineteen more were finished to Mk VI standard. Meanwhile, the first production aircraft was re-designed the Mk VI prototype and as such, fitted with two 1,600 hp Rolls-Royce Merlin 60 RM6SM engines. In April 1941 this engine was bench tested with a two-stage supercharger. Without such a device, the Wellington had no chance of reaching the prescribed 40,000 feet.

On 19 August 1941 a further 100 Mk VIs were ordered, although 56 were later cancelled. The majority of the survivors became Mk VIs equipped with Gee navigational systems. Late in March 1942 No 109 Squadron at Tempsford received four Wellington Mk VIs — *W5801, W5802, DR481* and *DR285* — for commencement of trials with the Oboe radar blind bombing device.

Geoffrey MacFarlane, a wireless operator and 109 Squadron's first Signals Leader, flew with Squadron Leader Bufton in *W5801* on its first squadron air test on 30 March. He recalls: 'Flying in the Mk VI was quite an experience in itself. It had a pressure chamber up forward, resembling a large boiler about five feet in diameter with a large valve at the front which had to be closed after the pilot, navigator and wireless operator (no gunner, naturally) had squeezed in through a just-large-enough, if we bent double, circular "door" which had to be clamped closed with four very large and solid steel clips. Finally, a large wheel in the centre of the locking contraption had to be turned many times to close the main valve and so make the chamber airtight. Then pressure could be built up to a comfortable level.

'There was also a low cupola above the pilot's head out of which he only could just see — when the tail was down, so that taxying was a rather "hit or miss" affair. Getting out of the contraption in a hurry was seldom performed in less than 1½ minutes; then there was a forty-foot trot to the rear exit

— hardly calculated to give one confidence in survival if the worst happened.

'Although the Oboe blind bombing system was extraordinarily accurate it had two drawbacks, both related. Quite obviously the aircraft carrying the airborne component must be able to reach the Ruhr at least if it was able to be used to its full potential. Because of the frequencies on which it was operated and with the controlling ground stations in England (not until after D-Day could specially prepared mobile stations be deployed in Europe) a target range of at least 270 miles was a "must". High flying aircraft which could reach 30,000 feet plus were a minimum requirement.

'It was alleged that the Mk VI was capable of reaching 35,000 feet with a load sufficient for our needs, cruising at 280 mph. (The Mk VI underwent many changes and only by extending the wing by twelve feet was the Mk VI finally able to reach the magic 40,000 feet.) My log book shows no record of any height reached in one above 30,000 feet, though I do have a vague recollection of once just making 32,000 feet.

'Our Wellingtons were fitted with the embryo airborne part of the Oboe system (nicknamed "Broody Hen") thereby carrying out the initial trials of what later became the most accurate British blind bombing system of World War 2 when it was fitted to Pathfinder Mosquitos of our squadron and 106 Squadron. Fortunately for us, and for the two Oboe squadrons, a week before it was almost decided to use the Mk VI operationally, it was rejected in favour of the Mosquito. The Mk VI had proved too slow and had other disadvantages which made it unsuitable for use in the Oboe squadrons.'

Radio-intercept Wellingtons

During 1941 and 1942 No 109 Squadron (formerly the Wireless Intelligence Development Unit) was designated the Wireless Intelligence Special Duty Squadron. It had a number of different types of aircraft, all fitted with special radio intercept equipment. Wellingtons had been introduced in January 1941 and were used especially on the longer distance flights, both by day and by night.

This Wellington VI W5795 dived into the ground from high altitude four miles north-east of Derby on 12 July 1942. *(RAF Museum)*

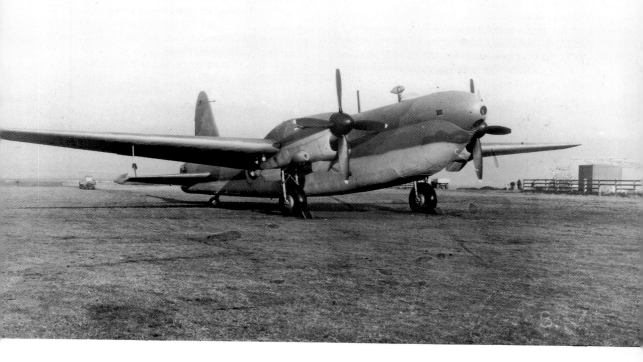

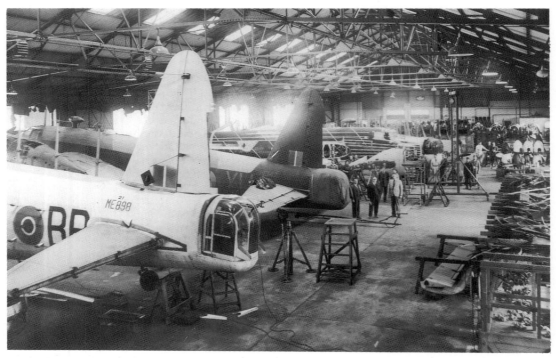

Wellington XIIIs at Sywell, Northamptonshire in 1945. Nearest aircraft is ME898. Sywell was formerly 6 OTU/18 OTU. *(RAF Museum)*

Geoffrey MacFarlane recalls: 'Wellingtons were invaluable in the radio-intercept role. These and Ansons were the main "workhorses" of our squadron, which was the airborne unit initially tasked with finding and pinpointing German radio beams used in their blind bombing systems, and other radio intercept duties which devolved upon us.

'On 8 May 1941 we were able to prove the existence of nine sites along the French coast of an advanced type of Fighter Control radar, capable of much greater accuracy than earlier models. This resulted in one, the site at Bruneval, being raided and dismantled by Combined Operations forces in 1942. We were also used in the interception of the German battleship *Bismark* on 27 May 1941.

'Because the Wellington was such a rugged aircraft we were able to operate it in the radio countermeasures role, from late June 1941, for a few months in the Middle East with only one rigger as ground crew. Despite our best maintenance efforts, our port engine became so temperamental that we made several flights to Crete, Malta, Sicily and Gibraltar with the engine only about 25 per

cent serviceable. On leaving Gibraltar for the UK when our detachment was over it became completely unserviceable but in spite of this we were able to fly for seven hours to Land's End on the other engine and were, I believe, the first Wellington to do this.'

Into service with Coastal Command

In the spring of 1942 the first Wellington GR Mk VIIIs entered service with Coastal Command. Just over two years earlier, Mk ICs had taken part in maritime operations for the first time when Wellington DWIs, fitted with 48 feet diameter dural hoops, had been employed in exploding enemy magnetic mines at sea. Altogether, some 394 GR Mk VIIIs were built. As on the Mk IC the type was fitted with the Bristol Pegasus XVIII powerplant. The GR Mk VIII differed from the Mk IC in being the first to be equipped with ASV Mk II radar and fitted with radar masts on top of the fuselage. Some versions also carried Leigh Lights.

The GR Mk VIII was subsequently joined

in Coastal Command service by a series of more advanced marks of Wellington. Some 180 Mk XIs, built at Squires Gate, were followed on the production lines by 843 Mk XIII models. Meanwhile, 58 Mk XII versions were produced at Chester and Weybridge. Squires Gate and Chester turned out a further 841 Mk XIVs. Altogether, some 3,406 Wellingtons were built at Blackpool, with the last leaving the production lines on 13 October 1945.

Both the XI and XII versions were powered by Hercules VI or XVI powerplants and carried no nose turret or radar masts on top of the fuselage. An ASV Mk III radar was housed in a chin radome beneath the nose. Beneath the wing provision was made for two eighteen inch torpedoes, and a retractable Leigh Light was installed in the bomb bay. ASV II radar and masts and the nose turret were re-introduced on the Mk XIII which was fitted with two Bristol Hercules XVII engines. The final general reconnaissance version, the Mk XIV, differed little from the Mk XII but was powered by Hercules XVII engines. Some Coastal Command Wellingtons served as 'flying classrooms' after conversion to T XVII and T XVIII standard.

Middle East and Far East service

As early as December 1941 Wellington Mk ICs were converted for mine laying and torpedo bombing operations in the Mediterranean. Wellingtons flew anti-submarine operations in Europe and the Far East until the end of the war. Two Wellington bomber squadrons — Nos 99 and 215 — also served in the Far East.

The climate affected both airmen and aircraft alike as Charles Fox, a pilot in No 215 Squadron based at Pandeveswar, a fair weather strip twenty miles from Asansol, recalls: 'The flying conditions were something we had never experienced before. Taking off with a bomb load in the heat of the day was sometimes frightening. Plus the storms day and night. Clouds rising to 20,000 feet had to be flown through. We just could not get above them and they covered such an area we hadn't time to go around. The air currents in these storms were such that even with the stick forward we were still

Rare photo of the only known Wellington which 'flew the Hump' (Himalayas) seen here at the end of its fourth trip coming to grief at Kunming after flying in from SEAC HQ Columbo via India and Chunking with Lt General Carton-De-Wiarte, Prime Minister Winston Churchill's personal liaison to General Chiang Kai-shek, whose government sat in Chunking at the time. *(K C Clement)*

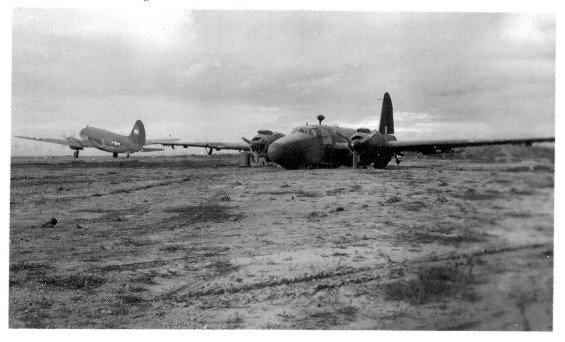

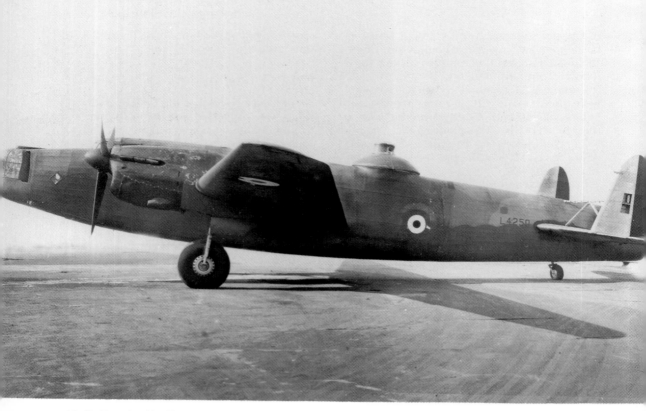

Merlin X engined Wellington II L4250 with dorsal cannon and twin-fin tailplane modified from the original single-fin layout. *(via Hans-Heira Stapfer)*

climbing and vice versa. I was lucky in having such a great pilot. He didn't show any fear but I'm sure that he must have felt something. His comment was "if this f------ aircraft flaps her wings any further, we won't need engines!"

'The squadron stayed at Pandeveswar from May 1942 to August 1942, when we were posted to south-east India. During those months, operations were carried out, both day and night, against the Japs. Our crew took part in two daylight raids on Akyab airfield within three days. Surprisingly, we had no opposition, although two twin-engined aircraft were sighted taking off and heading south towards Rangoon. We then went in and dropped our load in two runs. Although we had one 250 lb bomb hang up we carried on and strafed everything in sight. There were some Blenheims on the ground and as we left I noticed one Hudson on fire. I presume these had been unserviceable when the Japs took the airfield.

'Some of the operations we flew were supply drops to both troops and civilians making their way to India from Burma. The most notable to me was trying to drop medical supplies to a group of civilians in the Naga hills on the Indo-Burma border.'

The Wellington X, which entered service with RAF Bomber Command in 1943, was the final bomber version to see service in World War 2. An improved version of the B Mk III, it was powered by two Bristol Hercules XVI engines and some 3,804 examples were built. At one stage the Wellington X equipped some 25 OTUs (Operational Training Units) and the type saw widespread service in the Middle East.

Both Nos 99 and 215 Squadron in India operated the Wellington X against Japanese targets, and during the battle of Imphal in April-May 1944 they ferried much needed bombs to Hurricane fighter-bomber squadrons on the Imphal Plain. During August and September 1944, Nos 99 and 215 Squadrons converted to the Liberator.

In 2nd Tactical Air Force No 69 Squadron was unique in that it used Wellingtons for photo-reconnaissance at night. One cannot complete the Wellington's diversity of wartime operations without a mention of the role played by the Mk XV and XVI (most of which were converted from Mk ICs) in Transport Command. Their bomb bays were sealed and none carried armament.

The Wellington, then, enjoyed a highly successful career spanning many roles in every theatre of war. However, it could have been so different. The early use of the Wellington was less than auspicious and many could have been forgiven, in the fateful months of 1939, for thinking that the Wellington had a limited future as a bomber in the face of such strong Luftwaffe opposition. They were almost proved right . . .

Chapter 2
Opening gambit

During the evening of Wednesday, 23 August 1939, RAF units in Great Britain and abroad were secretly placed on a war footing and mobilization of the Auxiliary Air Force and 3,000 members of the Volunteer Reserve was begun. The British public, probably aware they were enjoying the last days of an August at peace for some time to come, went about their business knowing they too would soon be called into the Services.

The fragile peace was quickly shattered during the early hours of 1 September. Poland was invaded by German armoured divisions supported by the Luftwaffe employing Blitzkrieg ('lightning war') tactics developed from experience gained during the Spanish Civil War. In Britain full mobilization followed while units of Coastal Command began flying patrols over the North Sea. At bomber bases camouflage was liberally applied to buildings and aircraft alike and brown tape was stuck over every pane of glass in criss-cross patterns.

At the outbreak of war the overall strength of Bomber Command stood at 55 squadrons. On paper this sounds a respectable figure but by the end of September it had been pared down to 23 home-based first-line squadrons. These consisted of six squadrons of Bristol Blenheim IV light bombers of No 2 Group and six squadrons of Wellington Is and IAs of No 3 Group (with two in reserve) stationed in East Anglia. The rest of the force comprised five squadrons of Whitleys of No 4 Group based in Yorkshire and six squadrons of Handley Page Hampdens of No 5 Group in Lincolnshire.

Altogether, the Wellington was first-line

The only known photograph of L4215, the first Wellington I to enter RAF service, seen here circling Mildenhall on 10 October 1938 for acceptance by 99 Squadron. *(via Dr Colin Dring)*

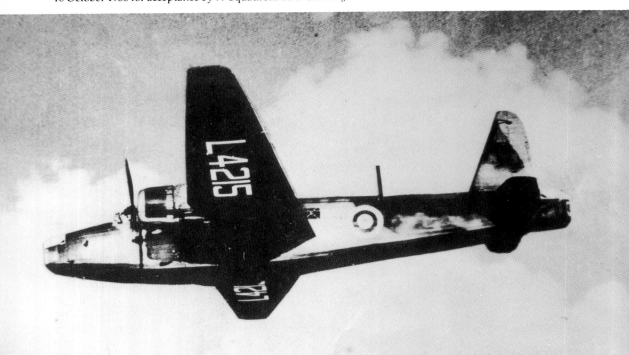

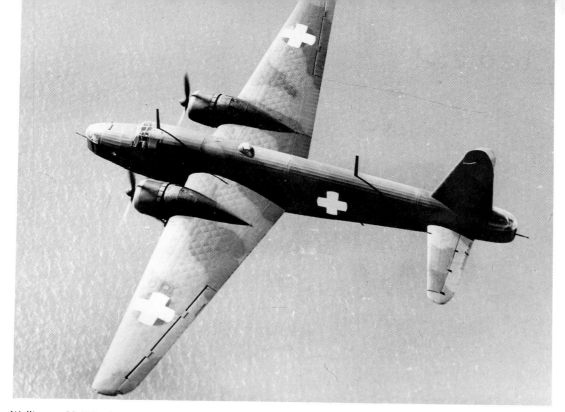

Wellington I L4367 of 75 Squadron from Stradishall, Suffolk in the markings of 'Westland' during the annual air exercises held during August 1939. This aircraft later served with 20 OTU was retired in October 1942. *(Rupert Cooling)*

equipment for No 9 Squadron at Honington, Suffolk; No 37 Squadron at Feltwell, Norfolk; Nos 99 and 149 Squadrons at Mildenhall and Newmarket, Suffolk, respectively; and Nos 38 and 115 Squadrons, at Marham, Norfolk; while Nos 214 and 215 (at Methwold) were similarly equipped in Reserve. On 1 June 1939 No 1 RNZAF Unit had begun forming at Marham to fly Wellingtons. A decision had been taken early in 1937 that the New Zealanders would have a complement of thirty Wellingtons, of which six would be ready to leave for the antipodes in August 1939. When war clouds had gathered the unit was put at the disposal fo the RAF and the unit moved to RAF Harwell where it became No 15 OTU.

Under the RAF Bomber Command 'Scatter' plan, the majority of bomber squadrons were immediately dispersed to satellite bases. For instance, Wellingtons of No 115 Squadron, which had been based at RAF Marham, Norfolk, since converting from Handley Page Harrows in April 1939, were sent to the satellite airfield at Barton Bendish. At Mildenhall, Wellingtons of No 149 Squadron

were at first dispersed around the airfield and on the south side by Mons Wood. By 2 September all of No 149 Squadron's bombers had been moved to the famous Rowley Mile racecourse on Newmarket Heath. Although long and flat, crews had to remember to hurdle the twenty foot high Devil's Dyke running along one boundary.

On the afternoon of 2 September ten squadrons of Fairey Battles flew to France to take up their position as part of the Advanced Air Striking Force. It was a sombre Neville Chamberlain, the British Prime Minister, who announced his country's declaration of war over the air on the BBC the following morning, 3 September. His resigned tones had barely vanished into the ether when reconnaissance revealed German warships leaving Wilhelmshaven. At 17:00 hours an order was sent to RAF Mildenhall for twelve Wellingtons of No 99 Squadron to be made ready to attack them. The squadron had received its first three Wellington IAs on 1 September and a fourth had arrived during the day. No Wellingtons could be airborne until 18:30 hours and then only three aircraft were operational. They took off but bad weather and oncoming darkness forced them to abort. They returned to Suffolk after jettisoning their bomb loads in the North Sea.

It was evident that the RAF was not fully prepared for an immediate strike at the enemy. There were other problems too. The policy of sending aircraft westwards beyond the range of German raids was all well and good, but problems occurred when some had to be sent back to their original bases for repairs. For instance, on 3 September, Frank Petts, a Sergeant Pilot in No 38 Squadron, had flown his Wellington I from Barton Bendish to South Cerney only to have to return to the main base at Marham to have a suspect engine changed.

Meanwhile, the President of the United States, Franklin D. Roosevelt, had appealed to the belligerent nations to refrain from unrestricted aerial bombardment of civilians. The British heeded this request while the French Armée de l'Air had precious few modern bombers to mount an offensive. In any event, the RAF was prevented from using a direct passage to the German indus-

trial heartland because of the strict neutrality of both Holland and Belgium, while France requested that Bomber Command did not attack land targets in Germany for fear of reprisal raids on French cities which her bombers could not deter nor her fighters protect.

The only way to carry the war to Germany, then, was to make attacks on German capital ships. The task of bombing the German Fleet fell, therefore, to the Blenheims of No 2 Group and Wellingtons of No 3 Group in East Anglia, which were ideally placed to attack installations in the Heligoland Bight. However, British War Cabinet policy decreed that no civilian casualties were to be caused as a direct result of the bombing. RAF Bomber Command could strike at ships at sea or underway but vessels moored in harbours were not to be bombed for fear of injuring 'innocent' civilians.

This policy was a carry over from the days of British 'gunboat diplomacy' throughout the Empire before the war when it was the practise to warn warring tribes before their forts were to be destroyed by RAF biplanes. Even at the time of the Munich Crisis of 1938

The port of Brunsbüttel, target for the Wellingtons on 4 September 1939. *(RAF Honington)*

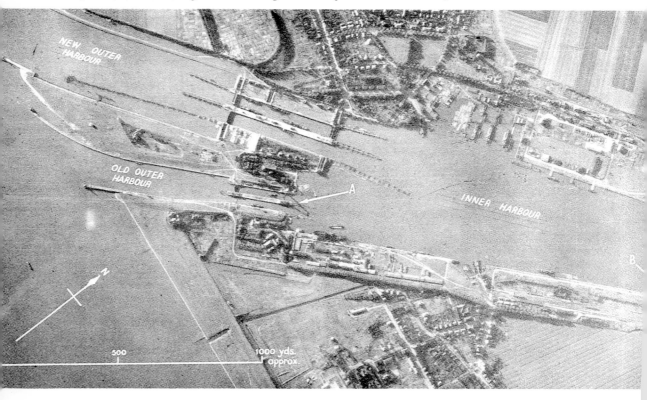

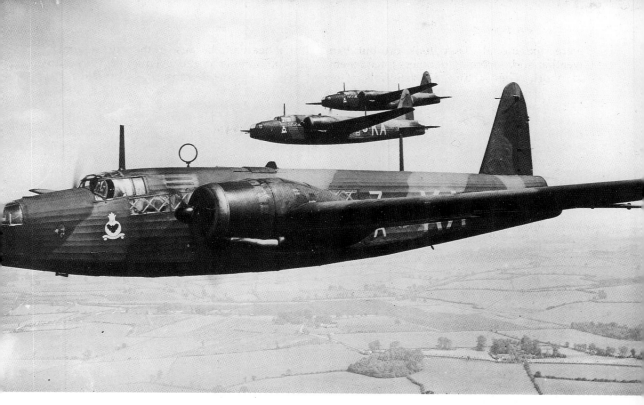

9 Squadron Wellington Is photographed in formation in 1939. KA-ZA L4288 (nearest the camera). The squadron emblem of a green bat is derived from the official motto *Per noctem volamus* ('Throughout the night we fly'). Ironically, early heavy losses occurred during daylight operations, which, like the badge itself, were soon discarded. *(IWM)*

this colonial dictum was apparently still in force. Incredibly, the RAF had been tasked to drop leaflets giving the Germans in the Ruhr advanced warning that heavy bombers would strike within the next 24 hours! Fortunately, the crisis had abated and the need never arose.

Plans were laid for the first RAF raid of the war to take place during the afternoon of 4 September. While fifteen unescorted Blenheims took off for a strike on the *Admiral von Scheer* at Wilhelmshaven, eight Wellingtons of No 9 Squadron and six Wellingtons of No 149 Squadron, also without escort, flew on over the North Sea towards Brunsbüttel. Their targets were the battle cruisers *Scharnhorst* and *Gneisenau* which had earlier been spotted by a Blenheim reconnaissance aircraft from RAF Wyton.

Squadron Leader Paul Harris was leading No 149 Squadron this day. En route Harris ordered his gunners to test fire their Brownings. He was startled to discover that not one gun was in working order! However, not wishing to miss the first action of the war,

he decided to press on to the target. Unfortunately, bad weather added to the problems beset by the crews and five of his squadron were forced to return early. Harris lost sight of the two remaining aircraft in thick cloud. As he flew over Tonning, his Wellington took a direct flak hit. Harris' bomb aimer aimed his bombs at a bridge over the Eder and turned for home. Harris nursed the ailing aircraft the 300 miles back to England and landed at Mildenhall six and a quarter hours after taking off.

Meanwhile, No 9 Squadron had fared little better. Three Wellingtons, led by Flight Lieutenant Peter Grant, managed to reach the German battleships amid fierce anti-aircraft fire but, although they succeeded in dropping their bombs, none struck the ships. A further three Wellingtons which succeeded in penetrating the harbour were attacked by Messerschmitt Bf 109s and two of the bombers were shot down. The day's losses reached seven when five Blenheims failed to return.

Debriefing revealed that some aircraft had

failed to find the warships. One aircraft mistook the River Elbe for the Kiel Canal and one even dropped two bombs on Esbjerg. Crews that had scored hits on the vessels had discovered to their dismay that the general purpose bombs, fuzed for eleven seconds delay, had simply bounced off the armoured decks and fell into the sea without exploding. The only casualties suffered by the German Navy occurred when a stricken Blenheim crashed into the bows of the cruiser *Enden*.

Despite the losses, No 3 Group prepared for another shipping attack the following day, 5 September. Plans were quickly scrapped, however, when it was feared that the Luftwaffe was about to launch an all-out attack on British bomber stations in East Anglia. The 'Blackout Scheme' was put into effect and squadrons were sent to safety further afield. No 149 Squadron, for instance, flew their Wellingtons to Netheravon in Wiltshire and did not return to East Anglia until 15 September.

Meanwhile, like others, Frank Petts was temporarily residing at South Cerney. 'On 5 September I was posted to No 9 Squadron. I took *L4391* to Marham in company with Flying Officer Buckley (later killed after the mass escape from Stalag Luft III). In No 38 Squadron orderly room I was told that No 9 Squadron was at Stradishall, so after collecting the rest of my kit from Fincham village I set off by car, with blacked-out headlights. I soon found that No 9 Squadron had moved to Honington some weeks previously so off I went in the blackout and eventually got to bed on the right station.

'Next morning at breakfast in the Sergeants' Mess there was a call for all aircrew to report to the Flights. I called first on the Squadron Commander, Wing Commander Hugh Pugh Lloyd (later AOC Malta) and was assigned to "A" Flight. From Flight Commander "A" Flight there was a brief greeting followed by instruction to take *L4273* from the far side of the aerodrome, complete with any ground crew I could find, to Boscombe Down. Boscombe Down was being used as a staging post from which aircraft, including at least one HP 42, were ferrying to France. We stayed at Boscombe Down until 15 September with, in the intervening days, some formation practice,

9 Squadron Wellingtons in formation. KA-A L4274 (nearest the camera) piloted by Squadron Leader Lennox Lamb RNZAF, was destroyed in a mid-air collision on 30 October 1939.

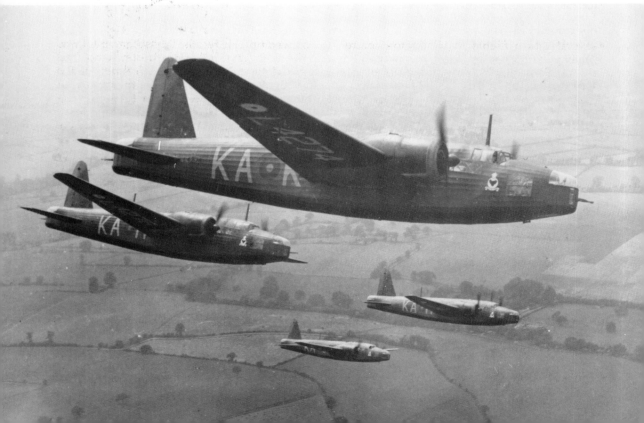

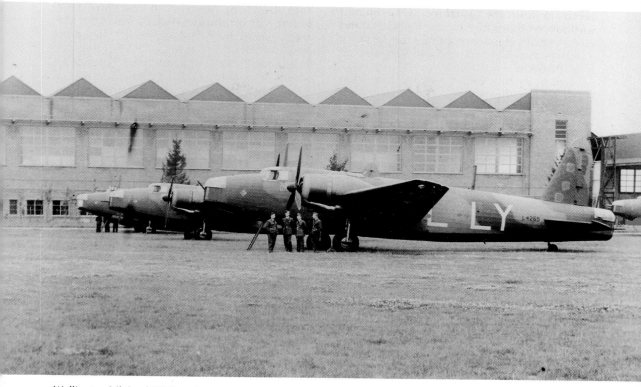

Wellington Mk Is of 149 Squadron which fully converted to the type from obsolete Heyfords by June 1939. Nearest aircraft is L4265 which served later with 15 OTU where, on 18 March 1942, it crashed on take off from Mount Farm. *(via Dr Colin Dring)*

several return flights to Honington for re-fuelling, as Boscombe Down had no fuel for us, and some bombing and firing at Berner's Heath.

'One emergency modification made at this time to our Wellington Is is worthy of mention. The ammunition feeds to the front and rear guns were found to be quite unsatisfactory so they were ripped out and replaced with canvas trays from which the ammunition went straight to the guns.

'At first we made the cross-country flights with undercarriage down as, although we carried two colour Very cartridges of the "colour of the day", we wanted to leave RAF fighters in no doubt of our nationality. During one of the sorties to Berner's Heath one aircraft hit a tree whilst low flying and crashed and burned. For the rest of our stay at Boscombe Down we had little to do except play snooker and be first in for meals as there were suggestions that the mess had not got rations for the large numbers using it.'

Sergeant Petts returned to Honington and

'crewed up'. He recalls: 'My second pilot was Pilot Officer G. C. Heathcote, who had arrived from 148 Squadron. In spite of the difference in rank I was made the captain of the crew as I had the greater total of flying hours and in particular, more experience on Wellingtons. My other crew members were Sergeant (Observer) Robertson, who although qualified to navigate, was used mostly as rear gunner, Leading Aircraftsman Balch as front gunner and Leading Aircraftsman Kemp as Wireless Operator/Gunner on the set.

'During these early days in 9 Squadorn I heard from other NCO aircrew their stories of the squadron's first operation on 4 September to Brunsbüttel on which my new Flight Commander (Squadron Leader Lennox Lamb, a New Zealander) had led a section of Wellingtons and had lost numbers 2 and 3 to Bf 109s. Sergeants Purdy, Kitson and Ramshawe were especially bitter about the loss of the two crews, the captains of which were very experienced Flight Sergeants

(Borley and Turner). I also heard from Lamb a different version of the same story and later an account of the interview he and the other surviving captains had with HM King George VI at Buckingham Palace.'

During a temporary respite from the shooting war the Wellington crews of No 9 and 149 Squadrons licked their wounds while others carried the war, albeit tentatively, to the enemy. On the night of 8 September No 99 Squadron had flown its first operation when three of its Wellingtons were despatched to drop propaganda leaflets over Hannover. One aircraft was forced to abort but the other two successfully completed the operation.

The Wellington and Blenheim crews were rested while Hampden squadrons bore the brunt of bombing raids in East Anglia. Ground crews used the time to iron out the bugs and eliminate teething troubles inherent in the Wellington IA, which had been introduced almost overnight into squadron service. Sergeant Petts recalls: '9 Squadron's first Wellington IA (N2871) with front, rear and dustbin turrets, arrived before our return

from Boscombe Down. No 1 section had the first three; as my aircraft I had N2873.'

On 19 September trials were conducted by No 149 Squadron using a Wellington IA filled with 1,500 lb of bombs and 720 gallons of fuel. The heavily laden bomber required a 1,080 yard run to become airborne which left little margin for error at Mildenhall. Operations would have to be conducted from the Rowley Mile strip, the longest of its kind in Britain, where a Wellington IA could operate carrying some 2,000 lb of bombs. Bomber Command, however, decreed that the Wellington must not carry more than 1,500 lb of bombs.

Squadrons were delayed from using their new Wellington IAs by a combination of bad weather and the lack of suitable targets as dictated by War Cabinet policy. Sergeant Petts recalls: 'During the next few weeks sections stood by in turn and on several occasions aircraft took part in sweeps over the North Sea. Otherwise, we were mainly occupied in bombing and firing practice and formation exercises, some of them in co-operation with fighter squadrons.

Wellington I L4213 served with AAEE before becoming an instructional airframe in December 1940. *(Vickers)*

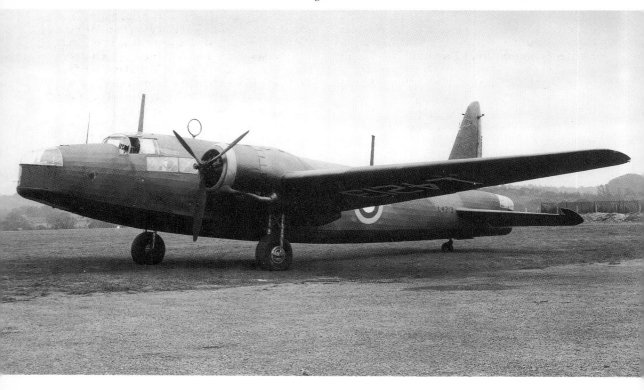

'In 1939 the officially accepted theory was that fighters had such a small speed advantage over the "modern" bomber that any attack must become a stern chase. It was also accepted that fighters attacking a section of three bombers flying in "Vic" would attack in "Vic" formation.

'The Air Fighting Development Establishment, with which No 38 Squadron had worked in the summer of 1939, had developed techniques for use by bombers attacked in this way. They consisted of various manoeuvres involving changes of formation, sometimes followed, when the fighters were committed to the attack, by sudden throttling back. One such manoeuvre was "Rotate" in which numbers 2 and 3 of the section, or numbers 2, 3, 4 and 5 in a "Vic" of 5, rotated clockwise or anti-clockwise about the line of flights of the leader. Another defensive manoeuvre was "Scissors", which started like a "Rotate" but halfway round, reversed to bring numbers 2 and 3 back to their original position.

'An alternative to the evasive manoeuvres developed by the Air Fighting Development Establishment was devised by Squadron Leader Lamb for use by his own (No 1) Section — the other sections would not touch it, holding it to be unsound and dangerous. The new tactic was tried on 27 October during co-operation with No 66 Fighter Squadron from Duxford. We flew in a "Vic" of three; I was in the No 3 position as usual. As the fighters, in "Vic", turned in to attack, our No 2 slid beneath No 1 and I slid beneath No 2. As the fighter leader closed in, Nos 2 and 3 probably having broken away as their targets changed position, we, on command from our leader, throttled right back.

'Sudden throttling back, to increase the closure rate and upset the attacking fighter pilot, was a sound tactic in the right circumstances but not with three Wellingtons in close formation stepped down vertically, as at the reduced speed there was inadequate control for such a formation. We tried this manoeuvre on 27 October; No 2 dropped towards me and I immediately put my nose down, at the same time applying full power in such a violent manoeuvre that Sergeant Robertson, as rear gunner, was knocked unconscious as he hit the top of the turret, and Kemp, who was in the dustbin turret, was thrown out of it into the fuselage.

'We tried this questionable evasive tactic next on 30 October, flying near Honington at a height of 800 feet, just below the cloud base.' At the controls of the leading Wellington I was Squadron Leader Lamb. The second Wellington was flown by Flying Officer John Chandler.

The flight proceeded without incident until, at 10:15 hours, the three bombers were observed running in towards Honington. At this point the two wingmen were apparently instructed to carry out a formation crossover, the aircraft on the left losing height and passing beneath the leader in a right-hand turn, whilst the other climbed up and over in a turn to the left. Petts continues: 'As on the previous occasion, we changed from "Vic" to a formation stepped down vertically 1, 2 and 3, and then throttled back suddenly. My attention was switched quickly backwards and forwards between my Airspeed Indicator and the aircraft just above me, until on looking upwards again, I saw No 2 hit with his fin behind No 1's starboard engine and start to loop into No 1.'

It can only be assumed that Squadron Leader Lamb failed to gun up his engines immediately after giving the command 'Attack over' and that Chandler's aircraft climbed into his from behind and below before any evasive action could be taken. The propellers of Lamb's Wellington tore through the rear fuselage of the aircraft below, completely severing the tail unit, which spun away like a falling leaf. Chandler's tail-less Wellington then reared up into a steep climb, turned over onto its back and struck the leader's Wellington again with its port wing.

Petts' instantaneous reaction had been 'nose down hard, full throttle and full revs on the propeller controls. I pulled out of the dive below tree-top level and was reassured by my rear gunner's "They've missed us!" Later, he said that Nos 1 and 2 had dropped, locked together and were breaking up.' Both aircraft plunged earthwards. Chandler's Wellington crashed against a large tree and caught fire on impact while Lamb's machine dived nose first into a dyke and completely disintegrated. Both landed less than fifty feet apart in marshy ground near Sapiston Water Mill, only three quarters of a mile from the Honington runway.

All nine airmen from the two Wellingtons were killed in the tragedy. However, one man had cheated death. Petts concludes: 'Later, sitting in the Mess with a large brandy and talking of what had happened, I suddenly realised that sitting next to me was Sergeant Smith, whom I had seen get into Lamb's aircraft! Recovering from the shock, I asked him, "And how did you get out of that?" In reply, he explained that he had taken his usual place in the rear turret but Flying Officer Torkington-Leech had come back and said that he would be rear gunner for the exercise. Smith had decided that if he could not be rear gunner he would not fly at all and promptly got out of the aircraft and returned to the crewroom.

'Our new Flight Commander was Squadron Leader Guthrie. I had known him at Marham where he had been in 115 Squadron when I was a Sergeant in 38 Squadron.'

Sergeant E. T. 'Slim' Summers at Slitting Mill, Rugeley, Staffs in 1937. *(via Bob Collis)*

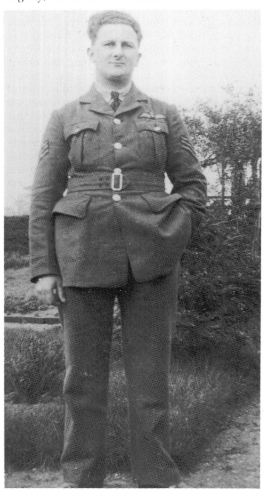

Tragedy continued to dog the Wellington units when, on the afternoon of 5 November, a Wellington I of No 38 Squadron, flown by thirty year-old Sergeant E. T. 'Slim' Summers, AFM, an instructor, crashed while being ferried from Marham to the satellite airfield at Barton Bendish. Summers was one of the most experienced pilots in the squadron, having accumulated 1,102 flying hours, of which 167 hours were on Wellingtons.

'Slim' was a very colourful and ebullient character and had earned his Air Force Medal earlier that year, on 2 January 1939. On 15 May he had saved the life of his rear gunner during a low-level bombing exercise in a Wellington. The starboard engine had failed and 'Slim' was unable to turn the aircraft against the port engine. A fire broke out between the tail and centre section and the aircraft was landed in a field near RAF Marham, on the port engine. A normal landing would have blown the flames into the area of the rear turret. After touchdown the bomber ran into a hedge and the undercarriage collapsed. The crew quickly vacated the aircraft, which was still burning but 'Slim', who was wearing an old style aircraft harness, became caught up in the side window. He extricated himself by releasing the harness and though the aircraft was burnt out, the crew escaped serious injury.

'Slim's' fame spread and he was known locally, for when he was not on duty Summers lived at the Whitington 'Bell', near the Marham base, with his wife. On 8 August 1939 he was asked if he would fly a Wellington out of a field at Roudham Heath near Thetford after it had crash-landed with the undercarriage retracted during a night exercise. The daredevil Summers successfully got the Welllington off and flew it back to Marham.

On the fateful day of 5 November he was not so lucky. On board Summers' Wellington were six ground crew — riggers and fitters who would maintain the aircraft when it arrived at Barton Bendish. 'Slim' Summers attempted a very dangerous manoeuvre near the ground (it is thought he was trying to fly wingtip low between two trees). It must be assumed that he did not allow for the keel action of a heavy aircraft in a steep turn; also he failed to judge the height of the trees. The aircraft crashed inverted at Boughton killing all seven on board.

Meanwhile, the Air Ministry planners

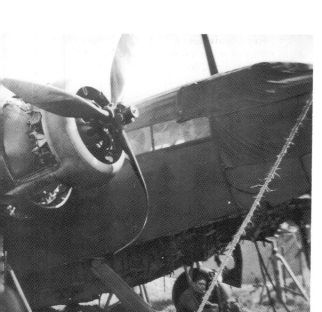

On 8 August 1939 'Slim' Summers flew a repaired L4235 of 38 Squadron off a meadow near Marham after Sgt McGregor had force landed in a nearby plantation of young trees following an engine failure during a night exercise. *(via Bob Collis)*

were still of the opinion that close-knit formations of Wellingtons, with their healthy defensive armament, could survive everything the enemy could throw at them and penetrate heavily defended targets. Recent heavy losses in British merchant shipping and pressure, from Winston Churchill, the First Lord of the Admiralty, in particular, prompted the War Cabinet to order Bomber Command to mount, as soon as possible, 'a major operation with the object of destroying an enemy battlecruiser or pocket battleship'. However, the directive added, 'no bombs are to be aimed at warships in dock or berthed alongside the quays'. The War Cabinet wanted no German civilian casualties.

During the late afternoon of 2 December 1939, Nos. 115 and 149 Squadrons at Marham and Mildenhall were alerted that a strike would be mounted against two German cruisers moored off Heligoland. Immediately, 24 of the RAF's latest Wellington 1As were bombed up with four 500 lb SAP (Semi-Armour Piercing) bombs and 620 gallons of fuel, ready for a strike early the following morning.

Leading the attack would be Wing Commander Richard Kellett, AFC, the Commanding Officer of No 149 Squadron. Kellett was one of the better known pilots in the RAF. In November 1938 as Squadron Leader he had been one of the airmen who had established a new long-distance record-breaking flight in one of two Wellesleys from Ismailia to Darwin, Australia.

On the morning of 3 December the weather had improved and at 09:00 hours Wing Commander Kellett led his twelve Wellingtons off in four flights of three. Kellett rendezvoused with twelve Wellingtons from Nos 38 and 115 Squadrons from Marham and the force flew out over the North Sea towards Heligoland. At the head of the bomber force Kellett positioned his section well out in front. Following some distance behind and leading the remainder was Squadron Leader Paul Harris. Off to his right and a little way behind and leading the remainder flew the third section led by a young Canadian, Flight Lieutenant J. B. Stewart. The fourth section, led by Flight Lieutenant A. G. Duguid, flew directly behind Stewart.

Two cruisers were spotted at anchor in the roads between the two tiny rock outcrops that are Heligoland in the German Bight. Kellett prepared to attack from up sun. As a result of the early losses, the bombing altitude had been raised to 7,000 feet (considered 'high level' bombing altitude at this time). Squadron Leader Harris claimed hits on one of the warships and Flight Lieutenant Stewart attacked a large merchantman anchored outside the harbour but a cloud obscured the targets and results were unconfirmed.

Although radar had warned the German gunners of the impending raid the thick cloud at their bombing altitude had fortunately hid the Wellingtons from view. Four Bf 109s climbed and intercepted the bombers but their aim was spoiled by cloudy conditions. One RAF gunner did, however, manage to destroy one of the Messerschmitts with a well aimed burst of fire from his rear turret guns.

Again the bombs were to fail miserably, although an enemy minesweeper was sunk when one bomb went clean through the bottom of the vessel without exploding.

Back at the British bases hopes ran high now that the RAF had penetrated enemy air space, duelled with the Luftwaffe and escaped unscathed. These hopes were to be shortlived.

Chapter 3
Battle of the Bight

'Up periscope!' Running silent and deep the Royal Navy submarine HMS *Salmon* spotted the German cruisers *Nürnberg* and *Leipzig* in the cold waters of the North Sea. It was 13 December, ten days after the disastrous RAF raid on Heligoland. *Salmon* stalked its prey and fired a salvo of torpedoes, hitting the two cruisers. The submarine scurried away leaving the German ships to limp back to Wilhelmshaven. Coastal Command contacted Bomber Command to send bombers to finish them off.

Flares were loaded into the Wellingtons for a night attack but this was later cancelled. By dawn the following day a force of Hampdens had taken off to intercept the battle squadron but they returned to base without having spotted the enemy. An armed reconnaissance by twelve Wellingtons of No 99 Squadron was ordered. Each aircraft carried three 500 lb semi-armour piercing bombs and any large battle cruisers or cruisers seen were to be bombed if the weather allowed the aircraft to reach a height of 2,000 feet. Leading the formation were Squadron Leader (later Air Marshal, Sir,) Andrew 'Square' McKee, the pilot, and Wing Commander J. F. Griffiths, the CO. The formation, which consisted of four sections of three aircraft each, took off from Newmarket at 11:43 and set course for Great Yarmouth. There the visibility was down to two miles just below 10/10ths cloud and crews peered into the thick sea haze in a vain search for a horizon.

The weather deteriorated even further and at 13:05 hours, when the formation reached the Dutch coast, the Wellingtons were flying at 600 feet in fine rain. Behind No 1 Section came No 2 Section, led by Flight Lieutenant J. F. Brough, flying in line astern, and Nos 3 and 4 Sections, led by Squadron Leader R. G. E. Catt and Flight Lieutenant E. J. Hetherington respectively, flying in the same formation, but echeloned to the right of Nos 1 and 2 Sections.

Griffiths altered course in the direction of Heligoland in order to give the enemy flak ships the impression that Heligoland was the objective. The weather continued to worsen and the formation was now down to just 300 feet. At 13:47 hours course was altered for the Schillig Roads near Wilhelmshaven. Visibility was down to half a mile and the Wellingtons were now flying at only 200 feet.

Despite the weather conditions the aircraft maintained a good formation and they flew on towards Wangerooge island. They were spotted by five stationary trawlers, one of which fired off a red signal flare. Shortly afterwards a submarine was sighted and also fired a red flare. The leader replied by firing two red signal cartridges in rapid succession on the offchance that this might be the recognition signal. The submarine immediately did a crash dive and the formation turned on a north easterly course.

At 14:25 hours the *Leipzig* and *Nürnburg* were sighted. Griffiths attempted to carry out an examination to assess any possible torpedo damage but the fast closing speeds made this impossible. Griffiths swung the formation around and was about to try again when eight cargo boats were sighted. Immediately, they opened fire on the Wellingtons. A minute later three destroyers steamed up directly under Griffiths' bomber and opened fire. The Wellingtons were only 200 feet off the water and crews were buffeted by a barrage of light anti-aircraft fire from the ships below. Five minutes after the destroyers had opened fire, the *Leipzig* and *Nürnburg* added their pom-poms and other anti-aircraft firepower to the battle.

Griffiths turned the formation away and shortly afterwards a formation of three single-engined fighters were sighted approaching the bombers from Wangerooge, which came up out of the mist. The fighters closed and the RAF gunners responded with rapid firing. The first attacks were made on Nos 3 and 4 Sections by fighters approaching in line astern from sea level. One enemy fighter was shot down and was seen to dive into the sea. Flying Officer Cooper's Wellington of No 4 Section was seen to break away and enter the clouds. It was last seen heading towards the German coast with its under-carriage down, apparently under control.

Bf 110s badly damaged Flight Lieutenant Hetherington's Wellington and the No 4 Section leader was forced to jettison his bombs into the sea. He went into the clouds and was able to nurse his ailing Wellington back across the North Sea with petrol pouring from its tanks (the Wellingtons did not yet have self-sealing fuel tanks). Almost home, the machine crash landed in a field near Newmarket racecourse. The aircraft was a write-off and Hetherington and two of his crew were killed. The injured were removed to Newmarket hospital.

Of the five Wellingtons which failed to return, Sergeant Healey's aircraft, which was seen to go down with the fabric on the underside of the fuselage torn away and the geodetic members exposed, was lost before any enemy fighters were seen to be attacking. This was observed by several members of crews 'who are of the opinion that he was struck by AA shell'. Pilot Officer Lewis' and Flight Sergeant Downey's Wellingtons collided, which 'may have been due to ack-ack fire'.

So disastrous were the losses on this raid that Air Vice-Marshal 'Jackie' Baldwin, AOC No 3 Group, was compelled to compare it to the Charge of the Light Brigade. Despite the losses Bomber Command opined that the Wellingtons had survived repeated fighter attacks and faith in the old adage that 'the bomber will always get through' seemed as unshakeable as ever. Indeed, the debriefing report was to state later, 'After careful analysis of individual reports by all members of crews, it seems almost possible to assume that none of our aircraft were brought down by fire from the Messerschmitts'.

At Bomber Command the consensus was that in future, concealment was more import-ant than defensive firepower. Henceforth bomber formations would fly at 10,000 feet and crews were urged to seek the safety of cloud cover whenever possible.

In his report of the events of 14 December, the Senior Air Staff Officer at Bomber Command Headquarters, Air Commodore Norman Bottomley, wrote: 'It is now by no means certain that enemy fighters did in fact succeed in shooting down any of the Welling-tons. . . the failure of the enemy must be ascribed to good formation flying. The main-tenance of tight, unshaken formations in the

face of the most powerful enemy action is the test of bomber force fighting efficiency and morale. In our service it is the equivalent of the old "Thin Red Line" or the "Shoulder to Shoulder" of Cromwell's Ironsides. . . Had it not been for that good leadership, losses from enemy aircraft might have been heavy.'

On the other side of the North Sea the reaction was in complete contrast to the British version of the events. The Luftwaffe report stated 'German pilots registered five kills, plus one probable but unconfirmed kill. One German fighter shot down.' The German naval gunners did not submit a single claim for any Wellingtons shot down.

On the evening of 17 December Wing Commander Kellett and Squadron Leader Harris of No 149 Squadron were summoned to Group Headquarters at Mildenhall, along with the squadron commanders and section leaders of Nos 9 and 37 Squadrons for a briefing on another raid on Wilhelmshaven the following morning. Unfortunately, there would be little cloud cover for the weather forecast for 18 December predicted clear conditions. Harris was informed that Flight Lieutenant Peter Grant would be flying with him, together with three of No 9 Squadron's aircraft. This was the first time they had ever flown together and, as they strolled away from the briefing, Paul Harris put his hand on Peter Grant's shoulder and said, 'Stay close to me whatever happens'.

At Honington crews knew 'something was up'. Sergeant Frank Petts recalls: 'On a number of previous occasions reconnaissance Blenheims had found German warships off the German coast in the Heligoland area and had been followed by a bomber striking force. In the short days of mid-December it was decided to dispense with the preliminary reconnaissance and to despatch a bomber force in the morning to search for and attack German warships. It was established sub-sequently that security about the proposed operation on 18 December was extremely poor; certainly on the evening of 17 December it was widely known in Bury St Edmunds that No 9 Squadron crews had been recalled because of an operation planned for early the next day.

'On reporting to the Flights at 07:30 hours on 18 December we learned that No 9 Squadron was to supply nine aircraft for a force of 24, with nine from No 149 Squadron and six from No 37 Squadron at Feltwell. There were to be four groups of six aircraft: three of No 149 and three of No 9 in front, six of No 149 to starboard, six of No 9 to port and six of No 37 in the rear. Targets were to be any German warships in the area of Heligoland or the Schillig Roads. Bomb loads were four 500 lb General Purpose bombs per aircraft.'

No 9 Squadron was airborne from Honington at 90:00 hours. At 10:00 hours nine Wellingtons of No 149 Squadron, led by Squadron Leader R. Kellett, took off from Newmarket Heath and rendezvoused over King's Lynn with the nine Wellingtons of No 9 Squadron. The six Wellingtons of No 37 Squadron took off from Feltwell and flew straight across north Norfolk, falling in behind the rear elements of the formation while over the North Sea.

Sergeant Petts recalls: 'I was outside left of the whole formation, flying No 3 in a "Vic" of three. We climbed on course to 15,000 feet. Halfway across the North Sea we left all cloud cover behind; soon all aircraft manned and lowered their dustbin turrets'.

The formation flew a dog leg course over the North Sea, first flying northwards and then at latitude 55° North, headed due east for the German island of Sylt. After fifteen minutes on this new heading Flight Lieutenant Duguid, who was leading the second 'Vic' behind Kellett, began to have trouble with one of his engines. As he lost speed and dropped back, he signalled by Aldis lamp to his two wingmen to close up on Kellett's vic. Riddlesworth, his No 3, obeyed but Kelly, his No 2, apparently failed to pick up the Aldis signal. Kelly peeled away from the formation, followed his leader down and headed for home as well.

At 12:30 hours Kellett sighted Sylt about fifty miles ahead. The formation was still at 15,000 feet and there was not a cloud in the sky. Sergeant Petts observed the coast and the low-lying land beyond and was puzzled. 'I was not sure how large a navigational error was involved but I was surprised that we were so far north'. In fact the course northwards had been planned to take the Wellingtons as far as possible from the concentration of enemy flak ships among the Frisian Islands.

However, the clear skies were an open invitation for enemy fighters. Petts recalls: 'We left Sylt to port and shortly afterwards turned left towards the Schillig Roads where we had been told at briefing there were likely to be warship targets. We saw none but continued on a south-westerly course and I remember wondering how far we were going in search of battleships and cruisers.' As the Wellingtons approached the German coast near Cuxhaven, Bf 109 and Bf 110 fighters of Jagdgeschwader 1, guided by radar plots of the incoming formation made by the experimental 'Freya' early warning radar installation at Wangerooge, and directed by ground control, were waiting.

Petts continues: 'My rear gunner called, "There's a fighter attacking behind — they've got him!" Then to starboard I saw a Bf 109, with smoke pouring from it, change from level flight to a near vertical dive so abruptly that the pilot could hardly have been alive and conscious after the change of direction. I

Sergeant Pilot Frank Petts. *(Jeremy Petts)*

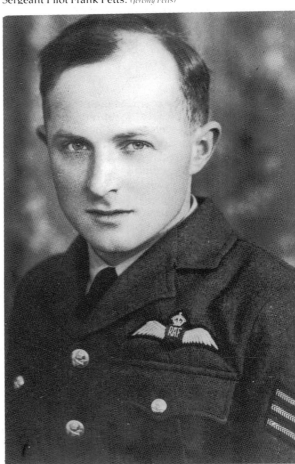

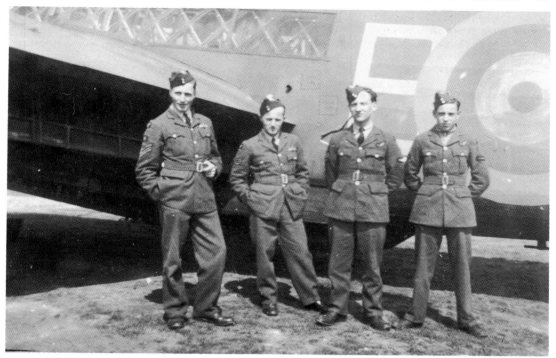

Left to right: Sgt Lawson; Sgt Pilot Frank Petts; Whitham; and Balch, who claimed two enemy fighters shot down on 18 December 1939 raid. *(Jeremy Petts)*

remember that at this stage I thought, rather prematurely, that encounters with German fighters were "easy".'

The Wellingtons flew on past Bremerhaven, then came a wide turn to starboard to take the formation over Jade Bay to Wilhelmshaven. Petts in his position at outside left of the whole formation found it increasingly difficult to maintain his position. 'Repeated calls to my Section Leader to ask him to slow down brought no reply and in spite of opening up to full boost and increasing propeller revs to maximum, I still could not keep up.'

'Over Wilhelmshaven we flew into intense Ack-Ack fire (joined by the anti-aircraft guns mounted on the battleships *Scharnhorst* and *Gneisenau*) and in trying to work out whether evasive manoeuvres were any use against the black puffs bursting all around I was for a while less pre-occupied with the problem of staying in formation. Quite suddenly the black puffs stopped and there in front were the fighters (thinking things over next day I decided that there must have been about forty of them) and still in spite of full throttle and full revs, I was lagging behind.'

Kellett led the formation through the flak-stained sky over Wilhelmshaven and each bomb aimer prepared to drop his three bombs on the ships below. Suddenly, Kellett gave the order not to bomb. All the battleships and cruisers were berthed alongside quays and harbour walls. Kellett's orders were precise: he was not to risk German civilian casualties. Bomb doors were opened but no bombs fell.

Moored in the middle of the harbour were four large ships that appeared to be merchantmen. Heavy anti-aircraft fire was coming from them. It was all the encouragement Paul Harris needed. They appeared to be fleet auxiliaries so he dropped his bomb load on them. Another Wellington in his section did the same but the results were obscured by cloud.

Kellett's formation had become strung out and disjointed. No 9 Squadron on the left of the 'Big Diamond' and No 37 Squadron, bringing up the rear, had become detached and had fanned out in the face of heavy barrage.

The Wellingtons were easy pickings for the Luftwaffe which had been patiently waiting for them. The RAF crews were caught cold as the cunning fighter pilots made beam attacks from above. Previously, attacks had been made from the rear but now the German pilots tore into the bombers safe in the knowledge that the ventral gun was powerless at this angle of attack. They knew too that the front and rear turrets could not traverse sufficiently to draw a bead on them.

Petts dumped his bombs, hoping it would gain him a little extra speed. 'About this time Balch on the front guns got his first fighter. A Bf 109 away to port was turning in a wide sweep, possibly to attack the sections in front. I saw the tracer in Balch's first burst hit in the cockpit area and the canopy or part of it, fly off; the second burst also hit and the '109 immediately went into a catastrophic dive with white smoke pouring from it.

'At this period I decided that in spite of my full throttle and full revs I should never keep up. Ginger Heathcote pointed out the 37 Squadron six forming the rear of the formation, and suggested that I drop back to them. It was as well that I did not. 37 Squadron were flying in their own formation of three pairs stepped up in line astern. As the attacks developed, one of the six [Flying Officer "Cheese" Lemon] went to dump his bombs. To open the bomb doors he first selected master hydraulic cock "on", not realising that he had flaps selected down. The result was sudden lowering of full flap leading to a sudden gain of considerable extra height. Enemy fighters left this aircraft alone but shot down the other five of 37 Squadron.

'Having decided that I could not catch up with my Section Leader, I turned about 40° to starboard, put my nose hard down and with the dustbin turret still in the lowered position, screamed down to sea level. All the way down from 15,000 feet and then for some time just above the water I kept full throttle and full revs except when I reduced power for short periods in an evasive manoeuvre as fighters lined up to attack.

'During the dive I was too pre-occupied with what was going on outside to pay much attention to my instruments. I did, however, notice my ASI reaching the 1 o'clock position, second time round. It was not until we returned to the aircraft next morning that I looked to see what that meant in terms of indicated airspeed — it was 300 mph! This was about twice normal cruising IAS and I

Wellington IA WS-B N2873, Frank Petts' aircraft, pictured at Honington. The yellow ring has recently been applied to the roundel. *(Jeremy Petts)*

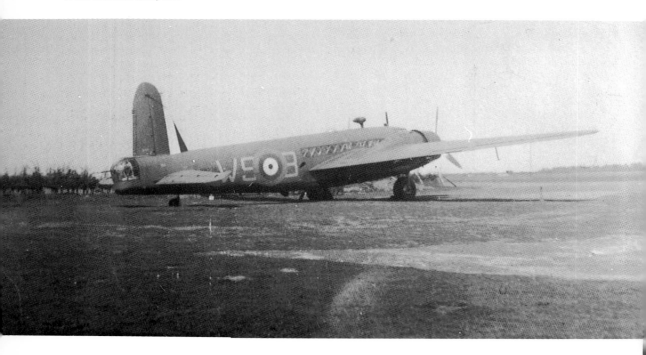

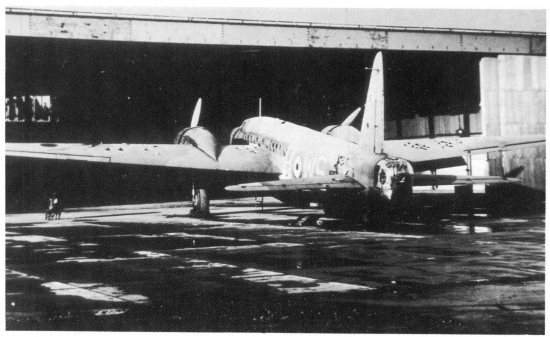

The heavily damaged Wellington IA N2871 WS-B which F/O Macrae of 9 Squadron managed to land at North Coates at 1600 hours, following the disastrous raid on 18 December 1939. *(Rupert Cooling)*

could not help wondering how much faster I could have gone before something broke.

'I cannot remember just how many fighter attacks there were; the first came before I left cruising altitude, there were more on the way down with Me 110s passing us as they broke away, and finally we were chased along the water by three '110s. Robertson on the rear guns kept me informed as each attack developed and there were commentaries from the other two gunners.

'We met each stern attack with a drill that we had agreed as a result of experience gained in fighter co-operation exercises. The usual sequence ran: "There's one coming in, he's coming in. Get ready, get ready. Back, back." Throttles slammed shut and pitch levers to full coarse. Bursts from our guns and enemy tracer passed the windows. "OK, he's gone." Open up again to full throttle and full revs.

'Mostly the tracer was on the starboard side and it was not until some weeks later when we started taking aircraft back to Brooklands to have armour plate fitted behind the port wing tanks that I realised that previously we had enjoyed this protection only on the starboard side.

'Altogether that day my gunners claimed three '110s and two '109s. I saw Balch's first '109 before we left formation and a '110 which also was his and I have a clear recollection of Robertson's jubilant shout as he got the last '110. For the other two I could not offer much in confirmation even later the same day and there may have been some duplication of claims from other crews over hits before we started the descent.

'Balch's '110 deserves a mention. The attack developed in the same way as others but immediately the tracer ceased there was a shout from Robertson, the '110 came past close to our starboard wing, next there was a burst from my front guns and the '110 was gone. This was a fine example of the effectiveness of sudden throttling back at the right moment in causing a fighter to close more quickly than he intended to. Robertson said that he had fired without apparent effect on this '110 as it closed and then as it overshot and passed beyond his reach the enemy rear gunner put his fingers to his nose at Robertson before opening fire. At that moment Robertson saw Balch's tracer and that was that.

'I believe the first of the three '110s which

followed us down was hit by both Robertson and Kemp. The drill had proceeded as before but Robertson's "Get ready, get ready; back" was followed by a jubilant "I've got him; he's gone in!" The '110 had, of course, been obliged to get down to our level just above the water for his stern attack and there was no height in which to recover any loss of control. Robertson's next comment was, "The other one's going home; he's had enough!"

'There had already been calls from Kemp and Balch that they had been hit and Heathcote had gone back to Kemp. Whilst I started checking at my end he helped Kemp (who was losing a lot of blood from a thigh wound) out of the dustbin and onto the rest bunk. Kemp in full kit was a tight fit in the dustbin and this move must have called for quite an effort from both. Heathcote next let Balch out of the front turret and went aft again. Balch had been hit in the sole of one foot but he was not in urgent need of attention.

'Robertson reported that he had emptied his guns into the last '110 and Kemp had called that the centre guns were out of action. Heathcote reported that there appeared to be no major damage to the aircraft, although it was a bit draughty as there were plenty of holes.

'For my part I eased back to normal cruising throttle and propeller settings and checking round was shaken to find the starboard oil pressure guage reading zero. The propellers on Wellington 1As did not feather so I had to be content with pulling the starboard engine right back as with that setting it would give less drag than if switched off and if it did not seize it might be of some use if I wanted it. I opened up the port engine to "climb power" and found that I was able to climb gently to 1,000 feet or so. During this time I had turned onto a course of 270°. When Heathcote came forward again he agreed that 270° was as good as any because we did not know where we were and steering due west ought to hit England somewhere.'

For almost half an hour 44 Luftwaffe fighters had torn into the Wellingtons. Fighter

Frank Petts' rear gunner, Sgt Kemp (centre) recovering at RAF Hospital, Littleport, following wounds sustained during the Heligoland raid of 18 December 1939. *(Jeremy Petts)*

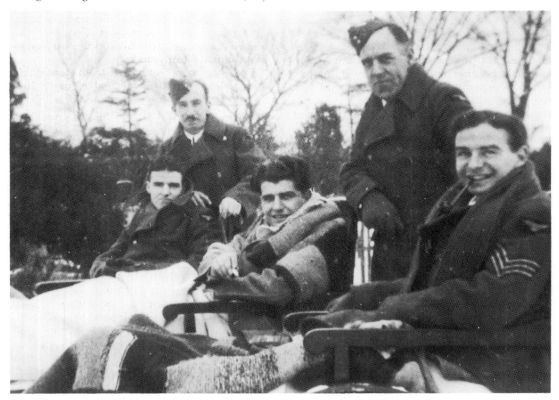

attacks continued until the bombers were only eighty miles from home. In the lead, Wing Commander Kellett remembered Paul Harris' suggestion after the 3 December raid and 'flew a little slower' to allow the stragglers to keep up. Off to his right Flight Lieutenant Peter Grant obediently stuck rigidly to Squadron Leader Harris' Wellington. This tightly knit formation of ten aircraft fought their way through with only one casualty. 'B-Beer', piloted by Flying Officer J. H. C. Spiers, was shot down during a beam attack by a Bf 110. There were no survivors.

In all, seven bombers had been shot down during the intense battle, for the loss of only two German fighters. Three Wellingtons crash-landed in England. The one survivor from No 37 Squadron, Flying Officer Lemon, landed at RAF Feltwell. Two more aircraft were forced to ditch. The first, 'P-Peter', piloted by Flying Officer Briden of No 149 Squadron, ditched near Cromer Knoll. Squadron Leader Harris circled the scene of the crash and attempted to drop a dinghy to the stricken crew but its attached rope snagged the tail of his Wellington and Harris was forced to land on the fighter airfield at Coltishall, near Norwich, which was still under construction. All of Briden's crew perished. This brought No 149 Squadron's losses to two.

Sergeant John Ramshawe of No 9 Squadron also failed to make it back across the North Sea. His bomber had been badly damaged when attacked by several Bf 110s and his rear-gunner, Leading Aircraftsman Walter Lilley, killed. The fuel tanks were holed but Ramshawe managed to nurse the ailing Wellington to the coast of Lincolnshire, where he ditched. Four of the crew were picked up by a Grimsby trawler 100 miles from the Wash.

Altogether, No 9 Squadron lost five aircraft from the nine despatched. Sergeant Petts was lucky. 'Towards the western side of the North Sea we encountered some broken cloud which on first sighting raised false hopes that we were reaching land. We were finally sure that we were seeing land when we made out the shape of a Butlin's holiday camp ahead and knew that we were approaching Clacton or Skegness. I had seen Skegness some months previously and when we reached the coast I was able to confirm that this was it.

'I turned south-west to skirt the Wash as there was no point in crossing additional water on one engine. I first intended to carry on to Honington but in view of Kemp's condition and deteriorating weather ahead I decided instead to land at Sutton Bridge. Preliminary gentle checks of undercarriage and flaps, a slow approach and smooth landing and we stopped after a very short landing run — our damage included a burst starboard tyre. It was just 4 o'clock; we had been airborne for seven hours.

'My first concern was for an ambulance for our two wounded. Next, a call to Honington — but no transport was available until morning — a preliminary debriefing and then something to eat. Next morning we went back to the aircraft to survey the damage and to collect various loose articles that we had left inside. The damage was mostly down the starboard side of the fuselage and on the starboard wing — the lost oil pressure had resulted from a holed oil tank. As a souvenir I took only a piece of wing fabric complete with a cannon shell hole.

'The operation of 18 December, carrying, in search of warships, bombs quite unsuitable for such targets, cost twelve Wellingtons, eleven complete crews and several wounded. Among the 9 Squadron casualties was my Flight Commander and Section Leader, Squadron Leader Archibald Guthrie. His name is now one of the first on the Air Forces Memorial at Runnymede".

The survivors returned from ten day's special leave to discover that changes had been made. At Honington a new Flight Commander, Squadron Leader (later Air Commodore) L. E. Jarman joined No 9 Squadron from Training Command. 'Shortly afterwards,' recalls Frank Petts, 'a new CO, Wing Commander McKee (later C-in-C Transport Command) arrived from No 99 Squadron. There was a feeling, voiced mostly by the Sergeant captains, that we knew more about the war than either of them.

'My crew was reorganised with Sergeant Robertson taking up his proper job as navigator, Balch, whose foot wound had been slight, as rear gunner, Aircraftsman Whitham on the set and centre guns and Aircraftsman Fraser as front gunner. By the end of January 1940 Pilot Officer Heathcote got his own crew and Sergeant Chris Lawson joined mine as second pilot.'

The RAF post-mortem into the disastrous raid on Wilhelmshaven had concluded that its

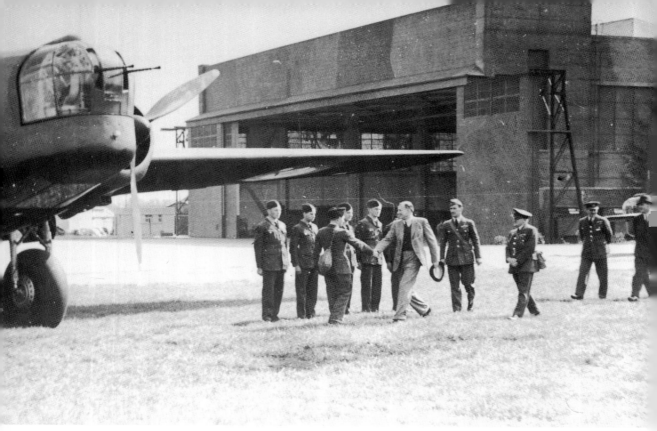

Frank Petts shakes hands with Captain H. H. Balfour, Under Secretary of State for Air, who is followed by Squadron Leader L. E. Jarman and Wing Commander 'Square' McKee. Honington, May 1940. *(Jeremy Petts)*

Wellingtons and Hampdens could no longer cross German territory in daylight and expect to survive against Luftwaffe opposition. From thenceforth Blenheims, whose losses had been lower, were despatched singly or in pairs, to overfly the German North Sea bases. However, a few daylight bomber sweeps were flown over the North Sea. On 2 January 1940 three Wellingtons of No 149 Squadron were attacked by twelve Bf 110s. Two of the bombers were shot down and a third had a lucky escape.

Meanwhile, RAF ground crews at the Wellington and Hampden bases installed armour plate and applied self-sealing covering to fuel tanks. Frank Petts wrote: 'The first three months of 1940 were comparatively uneventful. No 9 Squadron carried out a number of sweeps over the North Sea but they were without incident.' Although he was not yet aware of it, No 9 Squadron was being prepared for a new role, one it had not been trained to carry out.

Chapter 4
Coastal Command

Until the spring of 1940 the war at sea had gone steadily in Britain's favour. Even the Germans' victorious campaign had cost the Kriegsmarine one-third of its cruisers and almost half its destroyers. However, in April the sea war flared up again. Units of Bomber Command found themselves called upon to bolster No 18 Group Coastal Command, which was responsible for Britain's Northern Approaches.

On 2 April No 9 Squadron was despatched to Lossiemouth. The move came none too soon. In total secrecy, on 3 April, Germany mounted 'Weserubung Nord' and supply ships sailed for the invasion of Norway. The British and French, not least the neutral Norwegians and Danes, were caught off balance. The Wellingtons were finally brought into action on 7 April, as Sergeant Petts recalls 'Accompanied by some aircraft from 115 Squadron operating from Kinloss — there were six aircraft from each squadron — we searched off the Danish coast for heavy German naval units. We did not find them but on the way home flying close to broken cloud, 115 Squadron were jumped by Bf 110s.

'It happened as quickly as my rear gunner could tell me about it. "Fighters attacking behind — they've got one of 115 — he's on fire — they're baling out — they're shooting them up on the way down — they've gone!" The practice of shooting baled-out crew members received no publicity until much later in the war. In this case it is unlikely that the 115 crew would have survived a drop into the sea as we did not have individual dinghies and our last sighting of a ship — a small vessel which I took to be a fishing boat — had been twenty minutes earlier.

'From Lossiemouth our offensive armament consisted mostly of "B" bombs which I always felt must have been invented by some small boy whilst playing in his bath. A "B" bomb was larger than two ten-gallon oil drums laid end to end but weighed only some 220 lbs. Its secret was that it floated in water. To be used successfully it had to be dropped just ahead of a ship so that as it bobbed up to the surface it would hit the bottom of the ship which had obligingly moved over it. It could not be dropped successfully from above 11,000 feet as from a higher altitude it would break up on impact with the water.

'The "B" bomb was a "humane" weapon, unlike the mines sown from aircraft later in the war, as it was designed to be a danger only to the ship at which it was aimed. This selectivity was only achieved by the use of soft soap. Literally, soft soap held the nose cone in place and figuratively it summed up this particular weapon. The idea was that if no ship hit the bomb the soft soap would dissolve and after about twenty minutes the nose cone would come adrift and the bomb would fill with water and sink.

'To start with we carried only four "B" bombs each; there was room for more in the bomb bay but Lossiemouth was not a very large aerodrome and in 1940 large patches of it were partly waterlogged. I argued with the CO that I could get out of Lossiemouth with six "B" bombs even if no-one else could and if we were going to carry such things all the way to Norway we might as well increase by fifty per cent the chances of an attack being successful by dropping a stick of six instead of only four.

'Some sorties were flown from Lossiemouth without my sections as on 7 April when we carried "B" bombs again. I had only just got back to the Sergeants' Mess when there was a call from the CO that he wanted to see me at my aircraft which I had left in dispersal at the far side of the aerodrome. He refused to send transport and quite obviously he was annoyed. When I reached my aircraft, there with its nose protruding from between the bomb bay doors to within a few inches of the ground was one of those damned "B" bombs.

'To load bombs onto a Wellington each release was pulled down on its cable and engaged with the bomb. By means of a cranked handle each bomb in turn was then wound up on its cable until the release unit

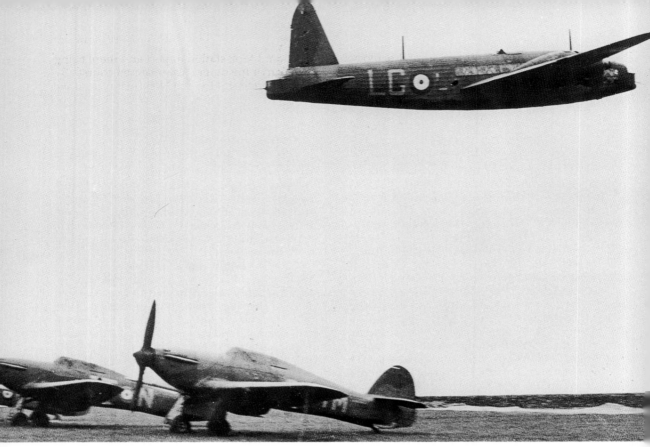

Wellington I L4387 LG-L of 215 Squadron on detachment with Coastal Command in April 1940. This aircraft was on loan to a crew of 75 Squadron who used it for a daylight reconnaissance of Narvik. *(RAF Honington)*

clicked home. Clearly in this case the unit had not clicked home properly and the bomb had gradually dropped although it could not have dropped clear as the release unit holding it was restrained by the cable. Fortunately, the landing on return to base had been one of my smoother ones. The CO's argument was that I should have seen that my bombs were loaded properly; mine was that armourers were paid to do just that. I suppose that on balance I lost because I had to walk back to the Mess.'

For three days, starting on 9 April, Coastal Command flew over a wide expanse of the North Sea and the Norwegian coast, trying to spot the large German cruisers which had orders to return to their home ports after they had discharged troops and supplies. On 10 April Sergeant Petts and his fellow Wellington pilots set out once again in search of German warships. 'Some 45 minutes from base we received a three-letter code group which we could not decipher. Fortunately, a naval observer was flying with the CO and he happened to know it was "Return to

base" in Naval code. 18 Group used Naval code but we from 3 Group were Bomber Command and did not.

'On 11 April in two sections of three aircraft we set out to intercept a German supply ship which the previous evening had been seen slipping southwards down the Norwegian coast. We were to search the coastal waters and fjords just north of Bergen. It was before taking off on this particular operation that there occurred one of the brushes with the CO which appeared to be the special preserve of the Sergeant captains. We still felt that we knew more about the enemy than he did and we knew that the 99 Squadron operation after which he had been awarded the DFC was a picnic compared with ours on 18 December.

'As a final word at the end of the briefing the CO, who was not coming on the sortie, asked "And have the captains worked out how they are going to attack any German aircraft that you see?"

'I voiced the general sentiments, "Sir, we do not attack German aircraft, we run away from 'em!'' There followed a mild explosion and then a dissertation on how easily Wellingtons could dispose of German fighters.

' ''Sir, and how would you deal with a '110 that sits back out of range of your guns and uses his cannon on you?''

' ''Nonsense, they can't do that.''

' ''They can, Sir; they did it to me. And what about the beam attacks from above, and what happens if a '110 sits on top of you, where you can't get him and uses his rear guns?''

' ''You're imagining these things.''

' ''Well, it's true they didn't use that one on me but ask Sergeant Ramshawe; they did it to him. The net result was probably a draw but the CO had the last word on the lines that we would never win the war with that sort of spirit.''

'Running into cloud halfway across the North Sea we followed our established drill, first fanning out and then resuming the same course as the leader. After some fifteen minutes I emerged into broken cloud hoping to see the other five aircraft. Away to starboard was one Wellington. I turned to intercept it and soon found it was No 2 of my

section. I took station to port and there being no sign of the others, we resumed course. By the time we sighted the Norwegian coast we were flying round and below broken cloud, the base of which varied from below 500 feet to about 2,000 feet; inland the cloud was solid on the mountains.

'We flew north, skirting the coast, but found no ship. Any search up fjords was out of the question and we turned south again. We circled the lighthouse at Haugesund and waved back to the keepers who came out onto the balcony. We flew south again and after a while turned away from the coast. Suddenly, I realised that without warning my leader was climbing steeply, obviously having increased power. I increased power myself and tried, without success, to call him on the RT — he was probably trying to call me at the same time. Almost immediately I knew what was wrong. Balch from the rear turret reported aircraft approaching on the starboard quarter and said he thought they were Me 110s.

'By this time Robertson was back in the astrodome position; he called, ''The leader's signalling — he's not sure — he's flashing

Wellington IAs, N2912 in foreground, at 11 OTU (still wearing their 215 Squadron codes) in the summer of 1940.
(RAF Honington)

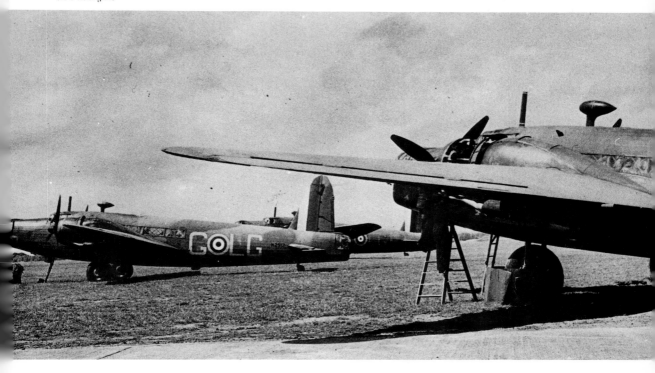

ident letters." I replied, "Get the Aldis and give him something; anything will do." I was now at full power climbing steeply towards cloud and overhauling my leader. Balch called, "It's not stopping 'em; the leader's turning in, he's coming in." I had regained position and just in time we reached cloud. As soon as we were right into the cloud the leader changed course. After a minute or two we turned again onto a westerly course and held it until some ten minutes later we emerged to find we were among broken cumulus. There was no sign of enemy aircraft and we breathed more freely.

'A few minutes later, below us and away to starboard, a twin-engined aircraft with twin rudders broke cloud on an easterly course. "Me 110? One of them still looking for us? No, looks like a Hudson; it is a Hudson. Must be on a recce; hope they don't see him." The remainder of the flight was uneventful. The other four aircraft had returned without seeing the ship or an enemy aircraft.

'Intelligence appeared not to believe our account of what we had seen because "There were no '110s as far north as that". I remember countering that both Balch and Robertson knew a '110 when they saw one as they had seen enough of them on 18 December.

'On 12 April we were out again looking for ships — the largest of them the *Scharnhorst*, which was supposed to be limping back to Germany after an encounter with HMS *Renown*. We flew a square search in a clear sky and within sight of the Danish coast but saw no ships or enemy aircraft; only a squadron of Hampdens presumably searching for the same targets as we were. Our failure was in spite of the fact that at the time we were searching, a London of Coastal Command was still shadowing the German ships and sending back position reports — but he was Coastal Command and we were Bomber, and the two did not often meet.

'After we had been some time in the search area there was a feeble call on the intercom from the navigator asking the second pilot to go back to him. Lawson went back and found Robertson collapsed over his chart table. He helped him to the rest bunk, covered him up with his spare flying clothing and came forward again to tell me what had happened.

'At first we thought that by not discussing the matter on the intercom we could keep it from the front and rear gunners who were already subject to considerable nervous strain as we were still only minutes from enemy-occupied coast and it was likely that enemy fighters would appear at any moment. It was, however, impossible to keep our casualty secret as after a minute or two he himself called on the intercom. He was obviously very distressed and kept saying he could not stand any more and then plaintively, "Are we going home yet?" I assured him that we were although there was in fact no indication that the CO had decided to abandon the search.

'A few minutes later we turned east again on the first leg of another square. Lawson in the meantime prepared to take over the navigation, expecting to find an airplot starting from the time we left the Scottish coast; he found instead a blank chart. Each navigator in the formation was, of course, expected to keep his own plot in case he had to take over the active navigation. When later we checked on the navigation logs and charts for our previous sorties from Lossiemouth we found more blanks; obviously the navigator had not been in a fit state to fly on any of these operations but he had managed to conceal the fact from everyone until the final breakdown.

'Return to base was uneventful. As soon as we got back to Lossiemouth I called an ambulance and when it arrived we carried our casualty from the rest bunk and handed him through the exit hatch to the medical attendants and he was off to hospital.

'On 14 April No 9 Squadron returned to Honington. Since the outbreak of war 9 Squadron had flown a fair number of sorties, had lost, by accident or enemy action, nine or ten aircraft and forty or fifty experienced crew members but could claim no offensive successes. There was obviously something wrong with the way this war was being fought and as far as we were concerned we were being used in a role for which we had never been trained. In the two years between my joining 38 Squadron and the outbreak of war the emphasis in 3 Group had been on training for night bombing; there were no naval co-operation exercises and we were not concerned with ship recognition. As soon as war started we were given postcard size books of silhouettes which said, in effect, "This is the *Hood*, leave it alone."

"This one, which is much the same size, is the *Scharnhorst* and you attack on sight!"

'During April there was one break in the ship routine. On the night of the 20th a number of 9 Squadron aircraft flew from Honington to attack the enemy-occupied aerodrome at Stavanger. We had strict orders not to attack without positive identification of the target: we had of course no aids to help in this identification. Our only en-route navigation aid was Radio Luxembourg, which, unlike Allied or enemy broadcasting stations, was good for loop bearings, but we made our landfall a few miles north of Stavanger, having broken cloud well out to sea.

'We could not afford to overshoot before descending or we might have finished up in the mountains. At one point the coast was clear of cloud but southwards stretched a solid sheet of low stratus. We tried from several directions but could not find a break and the cloud base was too low for us to creep in beneath it so we brought our bombs back. Several other crews had the same experience but the last to arrive found a break and were able to bomb.

'There was much cloud over the North Sea and Flying Officer Heathcote, who had previously been my second pilot, was involved in what afterwards passed for an amusing incident. They were on the way home, flying between cloud layers and with only a vague idea of their position when, without warning, there, right in front of them, were mountains. There was a violent heave back on the control column and the Wellington performed some unusual manoeuvres. Subsequently, there was some argument among members of the crew as to how much of a loop they had carried out; it was in fact probably only the first quarter with a violent recovery. Certainly at some stage heavy wooden boxes full of spare ammunition jumped clean over the main spar which was about three feet high. It turned out that the "mountains" were in fact just another bank of cloud.

'Towards the end of April I decided that instead of chasing ships I wanted to go to one of the Training Squadrons, or Operational Training Units, as they had been renamed. I tackled the CO and he promised to fix it. On 9 May I was posted to 11 OTU at Bassingbourn.'

Germany's occupation of Norway, the subsequent overrunning of France and the Low Countries, and Italy's intervention in the war had changed the situation in the war at sea radically. U-boats and E-boats began operating with deadly effect from French Atlantic bases. Soon aircraft such as the four-engined Focke Wulf 200, an adapted commercial transport with a range of 2,000 miles, began to menace Britain's Western Approaches and reach out into mid-Atlantic waters previously immune from German intervention.

RAF Coastal Command was at once confronted with a series of fresh problems ranging from anti-invasion patrols to long-range escort duties. In June 1940 Air Chief Marshal Sir Frederick Bowhill could only call upon 500 aircraft for such diverse tasks and only 34 of these, the Sunderlands, could only operate beyond 500 miles from Britain's shores. At first the U-boats attacked shipping in the South-West Approaches but by August they became bolder, following up on the surface during the day and delaying closing in on convoys until nightfall. To escape detection by the Asdics they remained on the surface and attacked under cover of darkness. Coastal Command did not have an answer to such tactics and from the beginning of June to the end of 1940 over 300 million tons of Allied and neutral shipping was sunk.

The only salvation available to RAF crews was ASV (Air to Surface Vessel) radar. Relatively few aircraft in Coastal Command were fitted with the device and those that were did not always perform as efficiently as crews would like. Ideally, a U-boat had to be fully surfaced and no more than three miles distant for ASV to be effective.

On 21 November 1940 No 221 Squadron re-formed at Bircham Newton, Norfolk, equipped with Wellington 1s. Early in 1941 ASV sets were installed and in March 1941 the squadron began replacing its Mark 1s and 1Cs with Mark VIII 'Stickleback' Wellingtons, nicknamed, 'Goofingtons'.

By May 1941 the U-boats were largely reduced to operating off West Africa or in the central Atlantic, the latter being beyond the range of Coastal Command aircraft. In June 1941 Bowhill was posted to form Ferry Command while Air Marshal Sir Philip Joubert took over Coastal Command. Joubert inherited a force of forty squadrons and more than half the aircraft were now fitted with ASV radar. Joubert's overriding task was to increase the effectiveness of his ASV aircraft and create airborne U-boat killers. He

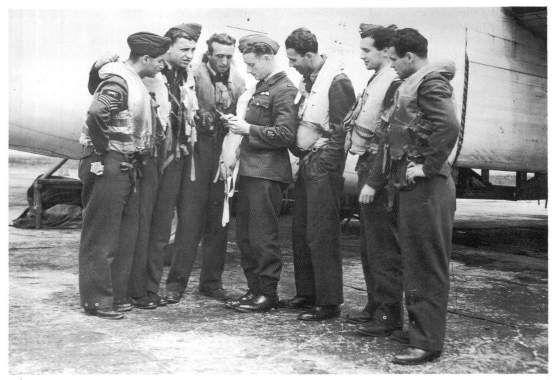

311 (Czech) Squadron crews gather beside their Wellington of Coastal Command. *(IWM)*

pressed for heavier types of anti-submarine bombs, bomb sights for low level attack, and depth charge pistols which would detonate at less than fifty feet below the surface. He encouraged tests, first started by Bowhill, with various forms of camouflage, in order to render the attacker invisible for as long as possible. As a result all anti-U-boat aircraft were painted white on their sides and under-surfaces.

By September 1941 increased shipping losses again prompted the Admiralty to explore the possibility of employing bombers in the war at sea. Air Marshal Harris had steadfastly refused to allocate any of his four-engined bombers to Coastal Command but had turned over large numbers of Welling-tons and other twin-engined types. In Sep-tember No 221 Squadron moved to Iceland, returning in December for transfer overseas. Three crews flew their Wellington Mk VIIIs to Malta while the remainder of the squad-ron flew to Egypt in January 1942 to begin anti-shipping patrols from bases in the Canal Zone.

Meanwhile, the shipping losses in October

and November 1941 showed a reduction over those of September. During early 1942 Coastal Command was helped by the transfer of further aircraft from Bomber Command. In April a squadron of Whitleys, eight Liberators and a Wellington squadron (No 311 Czech), were transferred to Coastal Command. On 7 May Bomber Command relinquished control of No 304 (Polish) Squadron, which flew to its new base at Tiree in the Inner Hebrides. Both squadrons were needed urgently and they took up their new role almost immedi-ately. No 304 commenced operations on 18 May and No 311 Squadron took off from its new base at Aldergrove in Northern Ireland on 22 May 1942 for its first operation.

The Poles had a very eventful career in Coastal Command, moving on 13 June 1942 to Dale in South Wales where they joined No 19 Group Coastal Command. They flew some 2,451 sorties up until 30 May 1945 and attacked 34 U-boats out of 43 sighted. The Czechs also gave sterling service in Coastal Command. No 311 operated the Wellington until June 1943 when it converted to the Liberator.

Meanwhile, advances had been made in the technical field. Very early in the war Coastal Command had realised that its anti-submarine aircraft would need something more reliable than the quickly consumed flares they were using at night to illuminate U-boats. As a result, in 1940 Squadron Leader H. de B. Leigh was encouraged by the then Chief of Coastal Command, Air Chief Marshal Bowhill, to develop the idea of an airborne searchlight. In October 1940 Leigh experimented with a 24 inch searchlight in the dustbin turret of a DWI (Directional Wireless Installation) Wellington, complete with generator. Despite early difficulties, Leigh had his prototype installation ready by January 1941. By May, the first successful trials were carried out and any weight problems were overcome by substituting batteries for the generator.

However, the Leigh Light had a rival; that of Group Captain Helmore's Turbinlight. In mid-June 1941 Bowhill was succeeded by Joubert and the latter asked for Helmore's invention to be fitted to two ASV Wellingtons. The Leigh Light eventually won acceptance over the heavier Helmore Turbinlight which was developed originally for night fighting and which proved totally unsuitable for anti-submarine work.

On 7 August 1941 Joubert called for six Wellingtons and six Catalinas to be fitted with the Leigh Light. Three months later he called for another thirty Wellingtons to be so equipped. However, the Air Ministry had misgivings and needed the guarantee of successful trials by the first six Wellingtons before it would sanction more suitably equipped aircraft. Under pressure from Joubert they finally agreed, in February 1942, to the formation of a full squadron of Leigh Light Wellingtons. On April 1942, No 1417 Flight at Chivenor was expanded to become No 172 Squadron but suitably equipped aircraft were slow to arrive. By May the squadron could only call upon five Wellingtons.

Joubert, knowing that only a successful operational demonstration of the capabilities of Leigh Light Wellingtons would carry the day, threw caution to the wind and despatched four of the five aircraft into the Bay of Biscay on the night of 3/4 June. One of the Wellingtons illuminated an Italian submarine and badly damaged it with depth charges. It was finished off by No 10 Squadron, RAAF,

Wellington GR XIV of 304 (Polish) Squadron. *(IWM)*

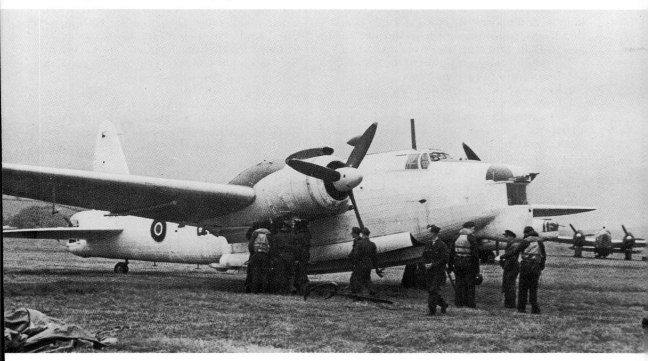

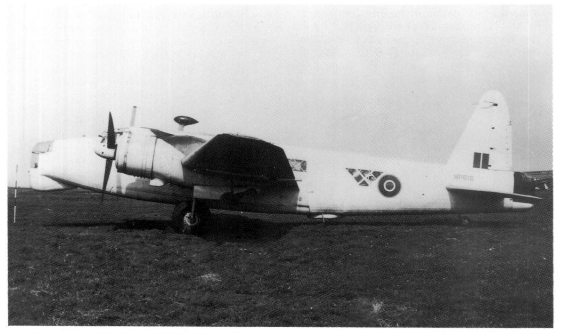

Coastal Command Wellington XII MP512 in January 1943. *(RAF Museum)*

three days later. The same Wellington also strafed another submarine with machine-gun fire, having used all its depth charges on the first attack. The three other Wellingtons sighted no U-boats but the ease with which they illuminated fishing vessels proved the merits of the Leigh Light.

The Leigh Light operator had to switch on the light at the last possible moment just as the ASV reading was disappearing from the radar screen because the blip, which grows clearer up to about three quarters of a mile from the target, then becomes merged in the general returns from the sea's surface. The detached object was then trapped and held in the beam allowing the crew to release its bombs.

During the remainder of June 1942 the five Leigh Light Wellingtons sighted no fewer than seven U-boats in the Bay of Biscay. Whitleys using conventional methods failed to find any enemy vessels during the same period. The Leigh Wellingtons proved so successful that on 24 June Dönitz ordered all U-boats to proceed submerged at all times except when it was necessary to recharge batteries. The morale of U-boat crews slumped with the knowledge that darkness no longer afforded them protection.

On the night of 5/6 July 1942 the Leigh Light Wellingtons chalked up their first U-boat kill and the following month the Air Ministry approved the formation of a second squadron. On September 1942 a detachment from No 172 Squadron, operating from Skitten, Caithness, was expanded and became No 179 Squadron. Early in November 1942 the Squadron was stood down from anti-shipping operations and by the end of the month had moved to Gibraltar.

Meanwhile, No 544 Squadron had formed at Benson on 19 October 1942 with two flights. 'A' Flight operated Ansons and Wellingtons from Benson while 'B' Flight operated Spitfires in the PR role from Gibraltar. 'A' Flight Wellingtons began flying experimental night photographic operations over France in January 1943. (In February the squadron handed its Wellingtons over to Nos 172 and 179 Squadrons and reverted to the Whitley, which it flew until April 1943 when it was re-equipped with Wellingtons again.)

By January 1943 Coastal Command aircraft had almost ceased to locate U-boats by night. The only solution was to replace the ASV Mark II, which only had a 1½ metre wave-length, with the long overdue ASV Mark III of ten centimetre wavelength. This apparatus was already in operation having originated from an adaptation of centimetric A1. An American version, developed with the help of British scientists, had been successfully tested in May 1942 although British models would not be available until spring 1943.

In 1943 Coastal Command underwent many changes to its Wellington squadrons. A summary of which follows:

Wellington movements Coastal Command October 1942–October 1943		
Date	Squadron	Remarks
1942:		
October 21	547	Established at Holmsley South as maritime recce unit with Wellington XVIII
December 5	612 (RAFA)	Replaces Whitley with Leigh Light Wellington
December 13	612	Begins CC operations
December 17	547	Begins CC ops at Chivenor
1943:		
January 29	407 (Demon) RCAF	Equipped with Leigh Light Wellingtons at Docking, Nfk
April 1	407 (Demon) RCAF	Begins anti-shipping ops
June	311 (Czech)	Converted to the Liberator
June	407 (Demon) RCAF	Receives Wellington XIV
August	172	Receives Wellington XIV
September	415 (Swordfish) RCAF	Receives Wellington VIII fitted with Leigh Light

Blackpool-built Wellington XIII JA144 torpedo bomber fitted with 'Stickleback' ASV radar. *(IWM)*

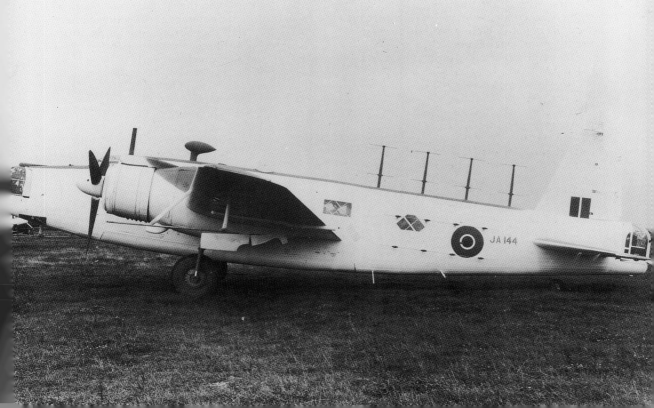

In November No 547 Squadron converted to the Liberator. On the 15th No 415 (Swordfish) RCAF, moved to Bircham Newton, Norfolk, for operations using Leigh Lights to illuminate targets for its Albacores to attack E-boats. The Royal Navy was also involved, as Fred Dorken, a WOP-AG in the squadron, recalls: 'The Navy would stay a few miles beyond the convoy route in their MTB and MGBs and when the E-boats were within range, working singly we would drop flares and illuminate them for the Navy. The E-boats had impressive armament and we longed for bombs instead of flares. Our CO, Wing Commander Rutton, got a DSO for sinking a sub in a two-minute action.

'We also flew eight-hour patrols against enemy convoys and several ships were destroyed. (We carried 500 lb bombs on these trips.) All told, it was hours of boredom and every once in a while, wild excitement. The North Sea in wartime is a cruel place and a goodly number of crews just disappeared.'

1944 ushered in fresh hopes of improving the U-boat kill ratio, although the early success of Leigh Light operations was now very much reduced due to U-boats being fitted with Schnorkel equipment enabling

them to re-charge their batteries at periscope height. By June 1944 Coastal Command operations had reached a peak, with the priority task of keeping the English Channel free of German shipping in preparation for the imminent invasion of Europe. Included in Coastal Command's Order of Battle were seven Wellington squadrons: Nos 172, 304, 407 RCAF and 612 AAF at Chivenor while No 179, returned from Gibraltar, was at Predannack. The remaining two squadrons, Nos 415 RCAF and 524, were located at Bircham Newton and Davidstow Moor respectively.

Early in September 1944 Arthur Rawlings joined No 179 Squadron at Predannack. He recalls: 'My position was that of wireless operator-air gunner in Squadron Leader E. E. M. Angell's crew. Most of our operations in the Wellington Mk XIV were night sorties, using radar search and homing procedures, descending to fifty feet (using radio altimeter) to inspect suspect contacts. The Leigh Light was switched on at about a quarter mile range.'

Squadron Leader Angell himself recalls: 'With overload tanks and carrying six depth charges, we used to patrol at about 1,500 feet

Coastal Command Wellington XIV MP818 in April 1944. *(RAF Museum)*

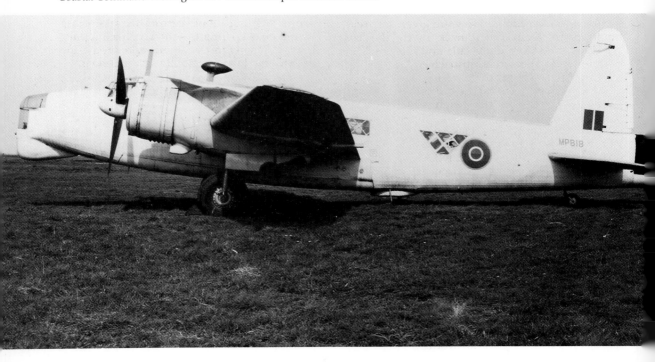

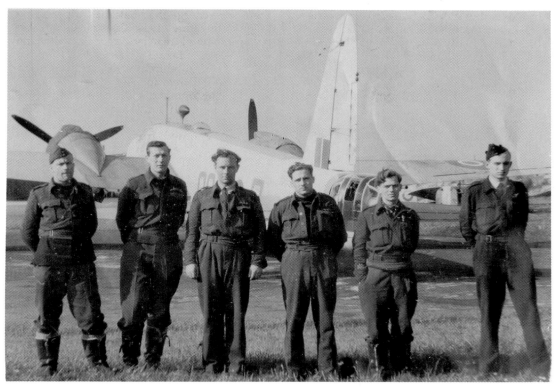

A very tired looking Flt Lt Chambers and crew pictured after an all-night sortie: left to right, F/O Rawlings; F/O Taughey RCAF; Flt Lt Chambers; W/O Pettigree and F/O Burgman RAAF. *(Rawlings)*

for up to ten hours. We were given set areas to patrol from Predannack in the Bay of Biscay and from Benbecula and Limavady in the North Western Approaches. On making a radar contact the drill was to home in going down to sixty feet on the radio altimeter and illuminating with the Leigh Light at three quarters of a mile.

'In preparing to attack, the bomb doors would be opened and the depth charges armed. The Leigh Light would be lowered and lined up with the target in accordance with radar reports by the second pilot who had remote controls in the nose. He would switch on and search for the target on the instruction, "Leigh Lights on!" from the captain. The front guns would be manned by the navigator sitting astride the second pilot and he would open fire if the submarine was surfaced. The pilot would release the DCs by eye, spacing them 60 to 100 feet apart. The rear gunner would be ready to fire at the submarine after the aircraft had passed over it.

'The wireless operator would already have sent a sighting report before the attack and would be preparing to send an attack report. Like so many aircrew on anti-submarine operations, I never actually saw a U-boat.'

Gord Biddle's crew were also involved in anti-submarine operations in September 1944. Biddle's crew were part of No 407 'Demon' Squadron, one of the few all-Canadian squadrons serving with Coastal Command, stationed at Wick. Harvey Firestone, one of the Wireless Air Gunners, recalls. 'Shortly after midnight on Tuesday 26 September we were briefed for a routine patrol off the coast of Norway. We feared that the trip would be cancelled because of persistent bad weather. A few days earlier we had missed an operation when Biddle had come down with a very high fever. We did not want to miss two trips in a row, so we hurried to board "S-Sugar", a Leigh Light-equipped Wellington.

'Despite the wild and stormy weather we were given the green light to take off. With visibility down to about a quarter of a mile and with a fifty-knot wind from the west, we

Wellington movements Coastal Command April 1944–November 1944		
Date	Squadron	Remarks
April 30	524	Begins anti-shipping role equipped with Wellington XIIIs off French coast
July	415 RCAF	Posted to Bomber Command
September 26	36	Joins CC (Chivenor)
October 24	14	Joins CC (Chivenor) using the Wellington GR XIV fitted with the Leigh Light
November	179	Converted to the Warwick

managed to become airborne at 00:50 hours. We headed out over the North Sea and proceeded to our patrol area.

'We were about thirty miles out from the Norwegian coast on a course roughly parallel to it, when suddenly, at 04:52 hours, our starboard engine coughed and spluttered but commenced running smoothly again. Biddle climbed hurriedly to 3,000 feet. A short time later it coughed once and a large fireball gushed out of the exhaust. Biddle throttled back immediately. George Deeth, the Second Pilot, feathered the propeller and pushed the automatic fire extinguisher on. He switched the engine off and closed the fuel cocks and gills.

'George Grandy, at the wireless set, sent out a QDM-5 (SOS) signal to Group. Fortunately, radio reception was good but Group informed us that the headwind we faced was not expected to abate but rather increase. They suggested we should try to reach the Shetlands and told us to continue sending signals so they could plot our course and attempt to monitor our position.

'Everything that we could do without was

Crew of 'S-Sugar', 407 'Demon' Squadron: standing left to right, George Grandy, Gord Biddle, Ken Graham; seated, Maurice Neil and Harvey Firestone. George Deeth, the second pilot, remained in England and is missing from this photo. *(Firestone)*

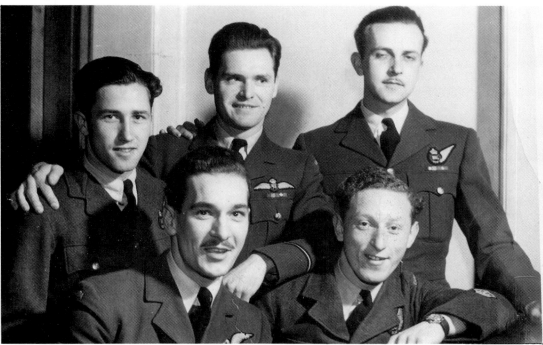

thrown out of the aircraft to maintain height and reduce strain on the one engine. Deeth and Neil threw the batteries that powered the Leigh Light out of the forward hatch. Graham threw out the radar equipment. Even the Leigh Light went, after quite a struggle for Graham and myself. We rid ourselves of the ammunition through the opening where the Leigh Light had been. The parachutes went too. Meanwhile, Neil and Deeth got rid of the ammunition for the single nose gun. Biddle, who had turned for home, had jettisoned the depth charges but we were still losing altitude.

'At 1,000 feet Biddle decided, after consulting with Neil and Deeth, that as we had about 5,000 lb of petrol still in the wing tanks, we could jettison about three quarters of it and still reach the Shetlands. The jettison valve was open for about twenty seconds, then closed but Graham, watching from the astrodome, reported that petrol was gushing from the wing outlet even after the jettison valve had been closed. Biddle and Deeth tried several times to stem the flow but the meter finally showed no petrol in the wing tanks.

'We could no longer hope to reach the Shetlands against the fifty-knot head-wind. We had only 92 gallons of petrol in our reserve tanks. We were over 100 miles from Sumburgh, the nearest British base and less than that from the Norwegian coast. Group ruled out an ASR operation for many hours and that to attempt to ditch in the raging sea would be suicidal.

'We all agreed, very reluctantly, that our only hope would be to turn round and head for Norway. Group were advised. They acknowledged and wished us luck. Our ground speed picked up considerably with the wind at our back and at the break of dawn we sighted the mountainous coastline of Norway. We heard Ken Graham softly praying over the intercom as we neared land.

'We could see nothing but mountains with low hanging clouds obscuring the tops. Biddle spotted an entrance to a fjord and headed towards it. We could see some ships ·escorting a submarine. We had little choice but to fly over the small convoy as our petrol at this time was just about all gone.

'As we neared the ships we were met by heavy machine-gun fire. Biddle took what little evasive action he could. I fired off a Very cartridge in the hope that we would confuse the gunners into thinking that we were a friendly plane. They stopped firing momentarily but started to fire again when they realised our deception. I fired off another but fooled no-one. Tracers entered just beside Graham in the astrodome. Our good engine had also been hit. Biddle and Deeth searched for a place to put the plane down as we had lost all power. They told me to tell Grandy and Graham to take crash positions.

'Grandy sent a final message and tied down the key. He strapped himself in at the wireless set. Neil was on the navigator's table. Biddle was in the pilot's position. Deeth, after first pumping down the flaps and opening the top hatch, took up his place behind the door. Graham and I braced ourselves on the floor behind the main spar. Silently, we turned to each other, shook hands and waited, wondering if we were going to make it.

'Biddle swung the plane around into the wind and without power, at over 100 knots per hour, attempted a wheels up landing on what appeared to be the only spot possible. We hit some trees with our port wing, shearing some branches about four feet from the ground. Biddle brought the tail down first to slow us up and then jammed the nose in. We slewed around and came to a very sudden stop, having landed in just about 65 feet. Grandy and the radio fell on top of Deeth, Neil was thrown from his table and had a gash in his head and a cut on his hand. Biddle was jolted but not hurt physically. The astro hatch, which had been removed in order for us to leave the plane, and which had been thrown to the rear of the aircraft, came plummeting forward toward Graham and me. I instinctively ducked and when we hit the second time, I hit my head on the main spar, dazing myself momentarily.

'Graham and I fully expected to see water come pouring into the aircraft but we had made it safely to land. As we jumped to the ground I saw that we had attracted a small crowd of people.'

Biddle's crew had crash-landed at Haughland on the outskirts of Os, three kilometres south of Bergen. They destroyed their maps and detonated the IFF equipment before burning their aircraft and headed in a south-easterly direction. Fortunately, they fell into the hands of the 2nd Company of the Milorg Resistance in Os and were later aided by the

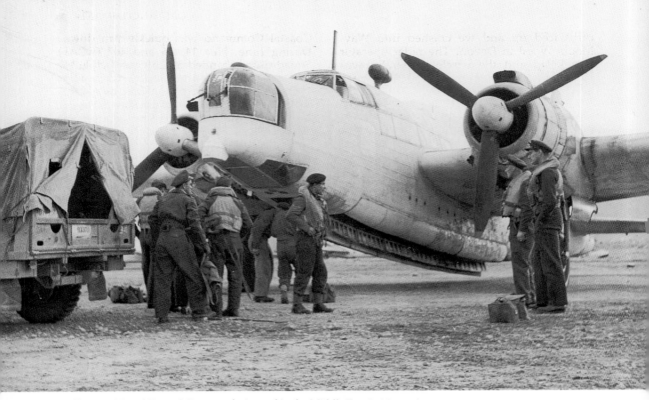

Wellington VIII of Coastal Command pictured in the Middle East in November 1944. *(IWM)*

Norwegian SOE. On 6 October the Canadians witnessed at first hand the first all-Canadian daylight bomber raid, on U-boat bases at Bergen and Hattvik. After many adventures, eventually the crew made its way back to England on 12 October via Leif Larson's 'Shetland Bus'; a service run by Norwegians in exile. Next day the BBC broadcast 'Cocohuts on holiday', to tell their Norwegian friends that the Canadians had reached England safely.

The war continued for other crews in Coastal Command. On 21 October Squadron Leader E. E. M. Angell's crew were posted to No 172 Squadron at Limavady, Northern Ireland and on 14 November 1944 Angell was posted to command a Halifax squadron. Flying Officer Chambers took over as pilot. Arthur Rawlings recalls: 'We only had one sighting of a U-boat just before the end of the war. We saw a periscope which was immediately submerged when we turned to attack. This was in the area of the Mull of Kintyre and the coast of Northern Ireland. At this time the enemy were increasingly entering the vicinity of the Clyde and North Channel in a last ditch effort against our shipping.

'Although Liberators and Sunderlands did most of the convoy escort duties' we once did an escort for the *Queen Elizabeth* on one of her troop carrying trips. She was too fast for the convoy system and both she and the *Queen Mary* were always independently routed. Of course, we had to keep a respectful distance but we could see the decks covered with thousands of GIs.'

Apart from enemy action, changing weather was a constant source of anxiety to Wellington crews on long, over water patrols. Icing could cause severe problems, as Gordon Haddock, a WOP-AG in No 36 Squadron recalls: 'With radar being somewhat primitive it was deemed one man should not have to gawk at the screen for more than 1½ hours at a time. So, by having three people in the same category, one could play musical chairs every hour or so from being radar operator, to the wireless operator, to the rear gunner. Invariably, we would toss a coin as to who would choose the position for take-off. While on a anti-U-boat course at RNAS Maydown, Northern Ireland, on 26 December, I was lucky in winning the toss and choosing to start the trip as rear gunner. In flight the carbs iced up and we crashed into Way-Moors Wood in Devon. The radar operator was killed and the wireless operator was facially burned. Neither he nor the captain ever flew again.'

Arthur Rawlings concludes, 'We had the pleasure of escorting in a surrendering U-boat off the west of Ireland a few days after hostilities ended on 4 May.' Then Coastal Command was quickly run down. During June, Nos 14, 36 and 407 (RCAF) Squadrons disbanded at Chivenor while No 172 disbanded at Limavady in Northern Ireland. On 14 June No 304 (Polish) Squadron was posted to Transport Command. By 7 July Nos 524 and 612 AAF Squadrons had disbanded at Langham, Norfolk.

Chapter 5
Night offensive

Early operations against German shipping had proved, at the cost of many valuable crews, that unescorted daylight bombing was out of the question. The losses seemed to have shaken the War Cabinet out of its chivalrous attitude towards the German civilian population, but it would not be until March 1940 that the so called 'niceties' of war were dispensed with and Bomber Command was allowed to bomb land targets for the first time. The RAF night offensive had opened in February 1940 with 'Nickel' raids with propaganda leaflets or 'Bumphlets' being dropped on Germany. They at least provided an opportunity for crews to gain some valuable experience of flying at night.

Unfortunately, the darkness was to prove no greater ally than daylight had been. On 2 March a Wellington of No 149 Squadron intending to drop leaflets over Bremen crashed shortly after take-off when one engine developed trouble and the other cut out altogether. All the crew perished in the crash. The following night a Wellington 1A of No 99 Squadron crashed at Barton Mills, killing all six crew, after being recalled from a 'Nickel' sortie to Hamburg.

In March significant changes occurred at RAF Mildenhall. The headquarters of No 3 (Bomber) Group moved from Mildenhall to Harraton House at Exning, near Newmarket. On 3 March the first Wellington 1Cs were issued to No 149 Squadron, quickly followed by No 99 Squadron. The Mk 1C had re-designed hydraulics and a 24-volt electrical system which permitted the use of the new directional radio compass. Crews, ever mindful of the the beam attacks made by the Luftwaffe, soon installed hand-held machine-guns in the long narrow side windows. Mark

Formation of Wellington IAs of 75 (NZ) Squadron during a training flight from Feltwell on 1 August 1940. AA-L is P9206. *(Robert Shepherd)*

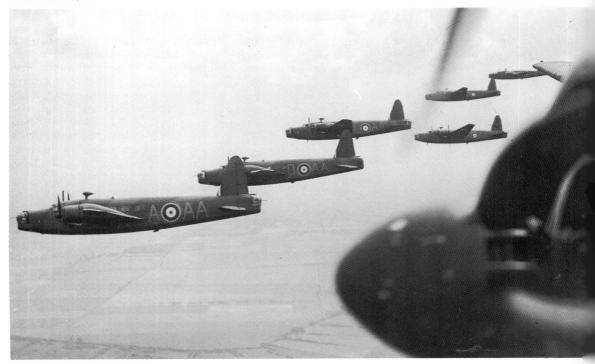

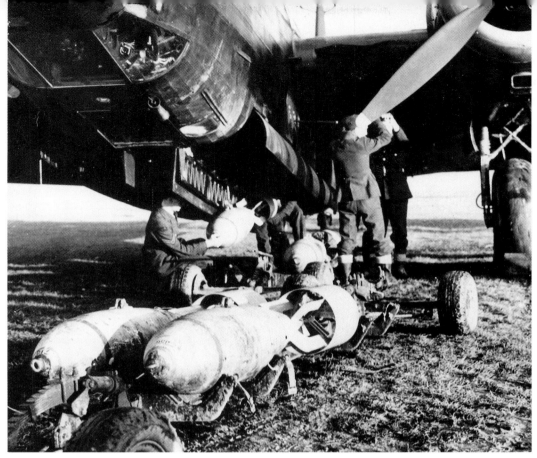

Bombs are loaded into the bomb bay of a Wellington IA of 75 Squadron at Feltwell. *(via Bob Collis)*

1Cs were first used on 20 March during a sweep over the North Sea.

Next day Wellington 1Cs of No 149 Squadron made a night reconnaissance over Germany. Then, on 23 March, Wellingtons reconnoitred the River Elbe and the port of Hamburg. One crew, which lost its way, was shot down by anti-aircraft fire near Dunkirk. All the crew managed to abandon their aircraft and reach the safety of Allied lines.

On 7 April Wellington crews were brought to a state of readiness when it was realised that German ships sighted heading for Norway and Denmark the day before were part of an invasion force. During the afternoon Blenheims attacked but their bombs missed and another attempt by two squadrons of Wellingtons was thwarted by bad visibility.

On 12 April six Wellingtons of No 149 Squadron took off from Mildenhall and followed in trail behind six Wellingtons of No 38 Squadron from Marham. They were ordered to head for the Norwegian coast near Stavanger and search for German warships. No warships had been sighted when the Wellingtons were intercepted by a group of Me 110s. The enemy pilots, again employing beam attacks to excellent advantage, shot down two bombers of No 149 Squadron. Twelve Wellingtons of Nos 9 and 115 Squadrons, which were ordered to make a bombing attack on two cruisers, the *Köln* and the *Königsberg* in Bergen harbour, fared little better. None of their bombs did any lasting damage.

The next bombing operations against German forces were made at night on the airfield at Ålborg in Denmark where the Luftwaffe had established a large supply base for their Norwegian campaign. On the night of 17/18 April No 75 Squadron despatched three Wellingtons to Stavanger for its maiden bombing operation. (Three Wellingtons had been despatched from Feltwell on 4 April but had been recalled.) On the Stavanger operation two aircraft managed to bomb the target. Then, on 25

April, six Wellingtons of No 149 Squadron took off late at night in another attempt to bomb Stavanger. It proved abortive. Thereafter, the Wellingtons were again employed on North Sea sweeps and night reconnaissance operations over the island of Sylt to prevent mine-laying seaplanes from operating.

On 9 May a Wellington of No 38 Squadron at RAF Marham was brought to readiness for a security patrol to Borkum in the German Frisian Islands. The front gunner, LAC G. Dick, recalls: 'The object was to maintain a standing patrol of three hours over the seaplane base to prevent their flarepath lighting up and thus inhibit their mine-laying sea-planes from taking off. We carried a load of 250 lb bombs in case a discernible target presented itself.

'We took off at 21:30 hours. Holland was still at peace and their lights, though restricted, were clearly visible, the Terscheling lightship in particular, obliging by giving a fixed navigational fix. After three hours monotonous circling and seeing next to nothing, I heard Flying Officer Burnell, our Canadian pilot, call for course home. The words always sounded like music to a gunner in an isolated turret with no positive tasks to take up his mind, other than endless turret manipulation and endless peering into blackness.

'I heard the Navigator remark that the lightship had gone out and the pilot's reply, "Well give us a bloody course anyway". One only had to go west to hit Britain somewhere, or return on the reciprocal of the outward course — drift notwithstanding. After an hour's flying with the magic IFF box switched on for the past thirty minutes, I gave the welcome call, "Coast ahead!" Much discussion occurred as to where our landfall really was. I told them I thought north of the Humber, which was 150 miles north of our proper landfall at the Orfordness corridor. I was told to "Belt up"; as a gunner, what did I know about it? (I had flown pre-war with 214 Squadron for two years up and down the East Coast night and day and was reasonably familiar with it.)

'Probably pride would not let them admit that they were 150 miles off course, in an hour's flying. Eventually, a chance light showed up and we landed on a strange

'Bashful', Bill Williams' Wellington IA of 75 (NZ) Squadron, at Feltwell. A number of the Squadron's aircraft were similarly painted with Disney characters. *(via Bob Collis)*

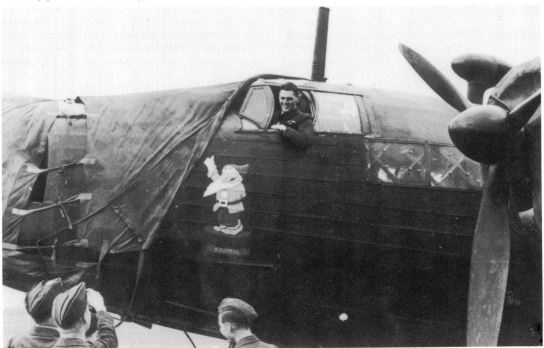

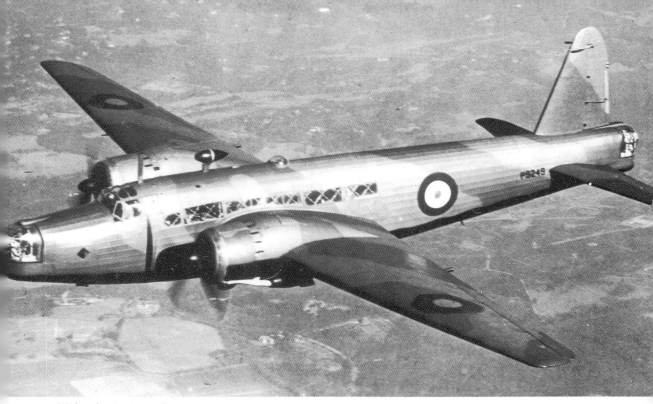

With only 62½ hours flying time logged, Wellington IC P9249 HD-T of 38 Squadron suffered an engine failure and crashed on approach to RAF Marham on 16 June 1940 killing its pilot P/O E. W. Plumb and seriously injuring two other crew. It is pictured here on a pre-service test flight. *(Vickers)*

aerodrome which turned out to be Leconfield. Overnight billets were arranged at 04:00 hours for the visiting crew. However, others were on an early start. They switched on the radio at 06:00 hours and gave us the "gen" that at around midnight Germany had invaded Holland, Belgium and France — hence the extinguished lightship. The odd thing was, we had returned with our bombs as it wasn't the done thing to drop them indiscriminately. We returned to base later on the tenth to be greeted with "We thought you'd gone for a Burton" — good news was slow in circulating in those days.'

At Honington Wing Commander Andrew McKee, the New Zealander CO of No 9 Squadron, could tell his crews little more than they had gleaned from their wireless sets. Rupert 'Tiny' Cooling, second-pilot in Sergeant Douglas' crew, one of two new crews who had arrived on the base barely three days before, recalls: 'The mess was quiet at lunchtime. Serious groups gathered round the radiogram, listening silently to the news. A lot was said but little was learned: things did not seem to be going well.

'The murmur of voices stilled as McKee walked briskly into the crew room, followed by his flight commanders. The target was the aerodrome at Waalhaven. It had been seized by German troops. Junkers Ju 52s were flying in men, munitions and supplies. Dutch troops were to attack at last light. The Wellingtons would crater the airfield, destroy the transports and soften up the defences. Each was to carry sixteen 250 lb bombs, nose and tail fuzed for maximum fragmentation. Weather was forecast to be fine. Flak, said the intelligence officer, would be light stuff, mainly 20 mm. The Germans had had no time to bring in heavy anti-aircraft weapons. Single-engined fighters were unlikely but there were reports of Bf 110 activity. He did not mention that five out of six Blenheims had been shot down by '110s earlier in the day and over the same target.'

In all, 36 Wellingtons would be despatched by Bomber Command. At Honington, No 9 Squadron began taking off for Holland at 17:30 hours. Sergeant Douglas piloted 'U for Uncle', a Wellington 1A. Second Pilot 'Tiny' Cooling continues, 'Away to starboard,

England was reduced to a dark shadow, separating sea from sky. With it strangely, went those last niggling doubts; those faint tremors of fear were swamped by a rising tide of excitement.

'"Wireless operator to front turret. Second pilot to the astrodome." Sergeant Douglas made his dispositions. We were 6,000 feet above the polders. In the distance I saw that the flickering curtain of flak was hemmed with orange flame and rolling curls of dense black smoke. "Bomb doors open. Target in sight. Right a little, right." The last word was drawn out, then chopped as the nose came

Sgt Jock Gilmour, Observer on 'Y-Yorker', lights up seated near bombs and fuel for Haddock Force at Salon-sur-Mer, near Marseilles. On 31 May Rupert Cooling flew the CO of 9 Squadron, Wing Commander Andrew McKee, to the airfield to make arrangements for operations against Italy. The bombs were never used. *(Rupert Cooling)*

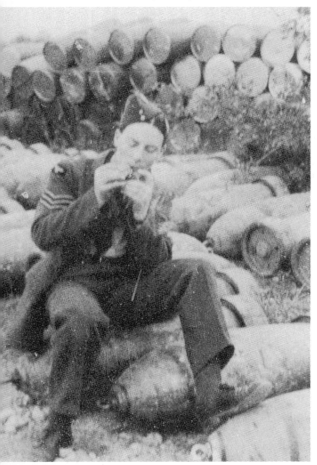

round to the required heading. Now the lights were directly ahead. "Left, left. Steady. Bombs gone." The Wellington jerked perceptively, as 4,000 lb of metal and high explosive plunged from the gaping belly. There was a sharp "twack" like some large and floppy fly swat striking the upper surface of the starboard wing. A triangle of the camouflage covering leapt up to dance upon the upper surface of the starboard wing.'

Surprised at his own calm and composure, Cooling said, 'Pilot, we've been hit. Starboard mainplane. There's a patch of fabric flapping just outboard of the engine.'

'U-Uncle' flew on past the Dutch coast. Out over the North Sea Sergeant Douglas handed over control to 'Tiny' Cooling before going aft to see the damage for himself. 'It was dark when "U for Uncle" crossed the Suffolk coast. Electric blue flashes from Honington beckoned us to within sight of the flickering gooseneck flare path. With a gentle bump the wheels touched, the tail settled. Then the Wellington tugged determinedly to starboard. In the light of the downward recognition lamp the flattened starboard tyre was clearly visible. Still hot, the engine exhaust rings ticked and cracked above our heads in the cool night air as we examined the wing, the wheel and the undercarriage doors by the light of our torches. A ragged piece of torn fabric as big as a dinner plate dripped intermittently, exuding the sweet smell of high octane petrol. One undercarriage door, perforated like the surface of a cheese grater, reflected a scatter of silver streaks on the matt black paint.'

The following night six Wellingtons of No 149 Squadron again bombed Waalhaven. The German violation of Dutch and Belgian neutrality had opened up a path for British bombers to fly directly from England to the Ruhr where sixty per cent of Germany's industrial strength was concentrated. However, political infighting between the French and British commands delayed matters. The French, with their hands full trying to repel an enemy force from its borders, were alarmed at the repercussions of such an action and Bomber Command, with its sixteen squadrons of Wellingtons, Whitleys and Hampdens, was prevented from carrying out the action.

For the time being RAF Bomber Command had to content itself with inland targets in Germany. On the night of 14/15 May Wellingtons of No 149 Squadron bombed Aachen and the following day the War Cabinet authorised Bomber Command to attack east of the Rhine. On the night of 15/16 May Bomber Command began its strategic air offensive against Germany when 99 bombers, 39 of them Wellingtons, bombed oil and steel plants and railway centres in the Ruhr.

Throughout May 1940 the Wellingtons attacked tactical targets with limited success. By early morning of 2 June the remaining troops of the BEF had been evacuated from the shores around Dunkirk. Thousands of French troops had still to be evacuated and during the daylight hours of 3 June Wellingtons stood ready, bombed up, to attack German positions near Dunkirk. 'Tiny' Cooling at Honington recalls: '9 Squadron were to wait by the Wellingtons, prepared to take off at 15:30 hours. The target had yet to be decided. We lay on the grass by our allotted aircraft in the warm sunshine. A daylight operation was a daunting thought. Take-off was delayed by two hours; hopes rose. Take-off would be 20:00 hours, the target Bergues, German positions on the southern edge of the Dunkirk perimeter.

' "For God's sake," said McKee with uncharacteristic emotion, "make sure you drop your bombs over enemy occupied territory. Our troops have enough to cope with without the added burden of someone's misdirected aim. And keep well away from the Channel. The Navy will fire at anything overhead. In present circumstances, who can blame them?"

Sergeant Douglas decided 'Tiny' Cooling would carry out the take-off and approach to the target. 'It was still daylight when I took off. As the coast appeared at Orfordness, I looked to port. A few hundred feet ahead was another Wellington, beyond it a third.' The moment of pride to be in such company made Cooling recall Shakespeare's Henry V before another famous battle in France. 'We few, we happy few, we band of brothers', he thought. The navigator's voice sounded over the intercom. 'Set course one-seven-one from Orfordness. ETA target 42 minutes.'

'The starboard wing dipped; the other aircraft were lost to sight. The turreted nose travelled round the horizon until, within the cockpit, the compass grid wires were aligned with the north-seeking needle. Level out, on course, the light is draining and darkness, like sediment, deepens in the eastern hemisphere. The sun has set and yet, due south beyond the bulbous nose, there is another sunset, a golden glowing arc resting upon the distant skyline. It is puzzling for a moment until we realise the glow is above Dunkirk; the light is from fires blazing ninety miles away.

'Douglas took over the controls; it was the second pilot's job to drop the bombs, whilst the Navigator kept track of our wanderings as we sought out "targets of opportunity." From the bomb aimer's position the sight was awesome. Six thousand feet below, Dunkirk was a sea of flame glinting like a brightly spotlit plaque of beaten copper. We turned and flew south, avoiding the coast; skirting the column of smoke like a deep grey stake into the heart of the town. A flare ignited and drifted above a pale grey sea of smoke. We might have been flying over a lake of milky water. Spot a gun flash in that sea of featureless mist; line up its imagined position to track down the aiming wires of the bombsight and then let go a stick of three or four. Did we deceive ourselves? Scatter enough bombs about and chance will ensure that something is hit. It was time we were buying, fragments of time to load another boat; to allow another ship to sail. We left the burning beacon behind and headed home.'

Italy's decision, at midnight on 10 June, to declare war on Britain and France caused Bomber Command to re-direct its bombing strategy. Mussolini's intentions had already been anticipated and it was agreed that as soon as Italy joined the war her heavy industry in the north of the country would be bombed by Wellingtons and longer-range Whitleys. Accordingly, on 3 June, preparations were begun to transform Salon in the Marseilles area into a refuelling and operational base.

At 15:30 hours on 11 June Wellingtons of No 99 Squadron flew in from England and landed at the forward base. Behind the scenes chaos reigned as first one order to bomb Italy was given, then countermanded by the French. Finally, an exasperated Group Captain R. M. Field, the CO of 'Haddock' force at Salon, ordered the Wellingtons off (a force of Whitleys, having refuelled in the Channel Islands, was already en-route to Turin and Genoa). The Wellingtons were prevented from taking off when at the last moment a procession of French lorries were driven directly into their path and left there!

When the political shenanigans had been sorted out, more Wellingtons made the seven-hour flight from England to Salon. On 15 June, two Wellingtons of No 99 Squadron and six of No 149 Squadron, took off from Salon for a raid on Genoa. Violent thunderstorms en route prevented all but one of the Wellington crews from finding their targets and seven bombers were forced to return to Salon with their bomb loads intact.

On the night of 16/17 June, nine Wellingtons made another attempt to bomb Italy but only five crews were able to find and attack the Caproni works at Milan. Crews returned to Salon to discover that the French had sued for an armistice and effectively, all future operations were brought to an end.

Meanwhile, on the night of 14/15 June, No 214 Squadron at Stradishall flew its maiden Wellington operation when it was despatched to the Black Forest. June was also a month when Wellington crews in Norfolk and Suffolk 'got their feet wet'. On the night of 20 June Wellingtons of No 99 Squadron were engaged in operations over the Rhine Valley south of Kalsruhe. Acting Flight Lieutenant Percy Pickard's Wellington IC was hit over Munster and he was forced to ditch about thirty miles off Great Yarmouth. Pickard and his crew were picked up by a high speed launch thirteen hours later and landed at Gorleston. (Group Captain Percy Pickard, DSO, DFC, and Wellington, 'F for Freddie', were later featured in a propaganda film, *Target for Tonight*. Pickard would lose his life leading the now legendary attack on Amiens prison in 1944).

During July 1940 the Wellingtons of No 3 Group carried out attacks on west and northwest Germany, with the occasional raid on targets in Denmark. During the mid-morning of 8 July New Zealand and Commonwealth crews stationed at Feltwell, home of No 75 (NZ) Squadron, knew there was a 'flap' on when they were commanded to air test their Wellingtons. Sergeant Robert Shepherd, a nineteen year-old WOP-AG and front gunner in Flying Officer 'Joe' Larney's crew, recalls: 'We went out to dispersal to carry out our checks. In my case, I checked the radio and the front turret guns and changed the accumulators. Later on in the war radio and R/T checks were limited because the Germans were listening out on all frequencies. It

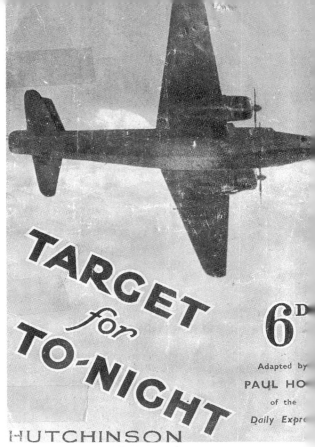

TARGET for TO-NIGHT

6D

Adapted by
PAUL HO
of the
Daily Expre

HUTCHINSON

Programme for 'Target for Tonight' which featured 'F for Freddie' flown by Flt Lt Percy Pickard (later Group Captain, DSO, DFC). 'F for Freddie' had never actually taken part in an operational mission against the enemy — the original had been wrecked when it ran into the earth bank of the bomb dump at Mildenhall when returning from a raid. *(via Bob Collis)*

would indicate to them what preparations for a raid were in the offing.

'Having completed the DI we flew a forty-minute NFT (Night Flying Test) for checks on engine and flaps, etc. After lunch we went back to the squadron for lectures on aircraft recognition and radio and gunnery. At 17:00 hours in the station HQ we were briefed that our target would be Mors in Denmark. Our station commander, Group Captain Modin, was respected by all ranks. He was posted to the Far East in 1941 and was unfortunately taken as a PoW in Singapore. Wing Commander Buckley, our squadron CO, and Flight Commander, Squadron Leader Cyrus Kay, both of whom were Kiwis, were great commanders, highly respected and loved for the way they led the squadron on operations.

'After briefing we went back to the mess to pass the time away until after take-off, which in our case was scheduled for 21:45 hours. Security was fairly lax. After briefing was over one could leave the station and quite unintentionally divulge the "target for tonight". Later, from the time briefing commenced, the main gate was closed and nobody allowed out until aircraft were over the target.

'Up to take-off one felt tense. We went out to our kite, P9206 L ("for Larney"), and Joe, our Kiwi skipper, and Pilot Officer Harry Goodwin, the Navigator, inspected the bomb bays and flaps. Then it was all aboard. Larney ran up the engines. All OK. We got the green light from the control tower and soon were airborne. After take-off we were more relaxed; our minds occupied with our jobs. I put the "J" switch over to intercom and radio to enable me to listen out on base frequency for any messages like "BBA" (return to base) or change of target.

'There was none. We crossed the coast and

Sergeant Robert Shepherd while an air gunner with 75 (NZ) Squadron. *(Robert Shepherd)*

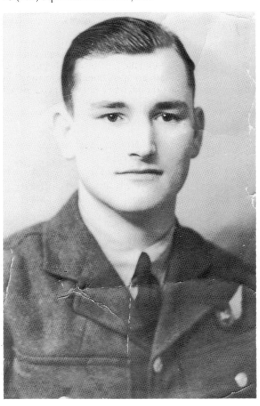

our IFF was switched off. I test fired my guns with a short burst and reported to Larney by intercom that all was OK. I remained in my turret right up to the bombing, assisting the Navigator by getting him fixes. The target loomed and I saw flak and searchlights for the first time. I thought, "We won't get through that", but as we got nearer it seemed to disperse. We dropped six eighteen-hour delay bombs, together with incendiaries and 500 lb bombs from about 10,000 feet.

'Crossing the enemy coast I got on the radio and checked in with base. The skipper was limited as regards communication by R/T. The equipment then was the TR9 with a range of only fifteen miles. Pilot Officer "Hank" Hankins, our Second Dickie, took a brief spell at the controls. Nearing the base we were given permission to land. Joe turned and landed without incident. Malfunctions were reported to the ground crews. One cannot praise them highly enough. How could we operate without them? They were highly skilled in all trades. Our lives were indeed in their hands every time we took off. We headed for debriefing, anxious to get it over so we could go to the mess for egg, bacon and milk before bed.'

Unrestricted warfare now threatened from both sides of the Channel. On the night of 23/24 August the Luftwaffe rained bombs on London, the first to fall on the capital since 1918. Bomber Command was quick to retaliate, for on the following night, 24/25 August, it despatched 81 Wellingtons, Hampdens and Whitleys to Berlin as a reprisal. The flight involved a round trip of eight hours and 1,200 miles. Seven aircraft aborted and of the remaining force, 29 bombers claimed to have bombed Berlin and a further 27 overflew the capital but were unable to pinpoint their targets because of thick cloud. Five aircraft were lost to enemy action, including three which ditched in the North Sea.

Bombing results had been unimpressive but the RAF had scored a great victory for morale. Berlin was again bombed on the night of 30/31 August while in September Wellingtons of No 3 Group made repeated night attacks on invasion barges massed in the Channel ports ready for Operation 'Sealion' the proposed German invasion of England.

Other desperate measures were called for by Bomber Command. Unrestricted warfare manifested itself again on 4 September when the Intelligence Officers told crews they would be despatched to the Black Forest, where the Germans were massing heavy armament. They were to carry a new incendiary device called 'Razzle'. This consisted of a wad of wet phosphorous placed between two pieces of celluloid which ignited to produce an eight-inch flame when the phosphorous dried

An experiment had first been tried on the night of 11/12 August by Wellingtons of No 149 Squadron, carrying fifty biscuit tins each filled with up to 500 examples, but Churchill, fearing that such tactics could lead to German reprisal raids, had ordered the scheme to be postponed. Bob Shepherd of No 75 (NZ) Squadron, recalls: 'I took the lids off the tins and there were wads swimming about in a solution. I opened the flare chute and, one by one, tossed out the contents of three tin loads from about 10,000 feet. We also dropped a full load of incendiaries and six 250 pounders. There was hardly any flak at all.'

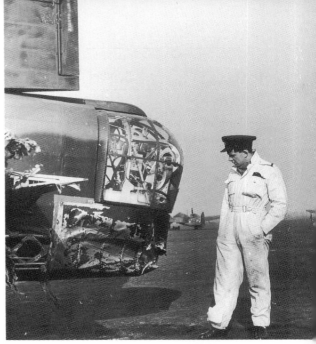

Bill Williams, pilot of 'Bashful' in 75 Squadron, makes a close inspection of damage to the rear tail section of a Wellington at Feltwell. *(via Bob Collis)*

A wide range of flying gear is evident in this picture of 149 Squadron crews as they prepare for a night raid at Mildenhall in 1940. *(via Dr Colin Dring)*

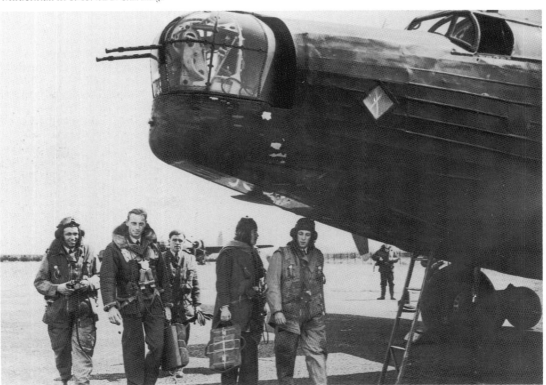

Date	Squadron	Remarks
Wellington movements **Bomber Command September 1940–January 1941**		
1940: Sept 10/11	311 (Czechoslovakian)	Flew inaugural Wellington operations when three a/c bombed the airfield at Antwerp/Deurne, Belgium
Oct-Nov	300 (Masovian) 301 (Pomeranian) 304 (Silesian) 305 (Ziemia Wielkopolska)	All four of these Polish Fairey Battle squadrons converted to the Wellington IC; none was operational until 1941
November	38	Deployed to Middle East
December 20	218	Started ops from Marham
Dec 21/22	15	Flew inaugural Wellington op, to the docks at Bremen
1941: January	57	Flew inaugural Wellington op, having converted from the Blenheim

Mk IAs OJ-W P9245 (which failed to return from a raid on Ostend on 8/9 September 1940), OJ-M R3206 (which later served with 311 Squadron) and OJ-N P9273 (lost on 9/10 October 1940) of 149 Squadron over Thetford Forest early in 1940. *(Rupert Cooling)*

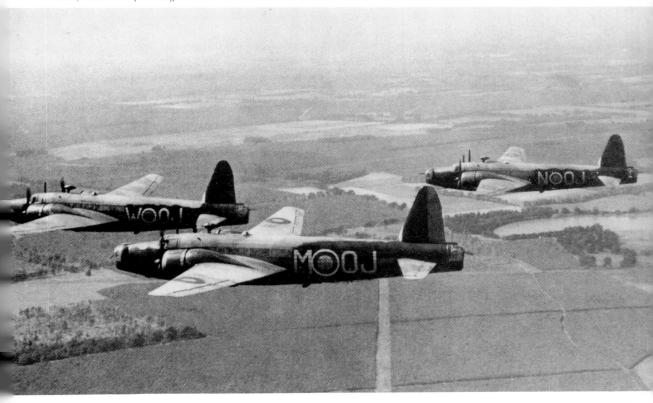

The RAF bombing directive of 21 September gave support to priority attacks on oil refineries, aircraft factories, railways, canals and U-boat construction yards while electric power stations and gas works in Berlin should also be bombed. On the night of 23/24 September Berlin was selected for a special retaliatory attack and was bombed by 119 Whitleys, Hampdens and Wellingtons. However, most of the objectives were missed and many bombs failed to explode.

In September 1940 the Luftwaffe had been forced to abandon massed daylight bombing and the invasion fleet was dispersed. Bomber Command could again turn its attention to city targets. On the night of 16/17 November, 127 bombers, the largest number yet despatched, raided Hamburg. By the end of 1940 Berlin would have been bombed on ten occasions. A trip to the German capital on 26 November proved to be Bob Shepherd's 30th and final op of his first tour. 'I flew with Pilot Officer Saxelby; "Joe" Larney (later Squadron Leader Larney) having completed his tour on 29 September on our trip to the oil refineries at Magdeburg. We got through and I left for a long rest before returning, in 1942, to fly a second tour, on 57 Squadron Lancasters at Scampton. Saxelby did not make it. He was shot down in 1942 and was made a PoW.'

Bob Shepherd had certainly led a charmed life in No 75 Squadron. He was one of the last of the original pre-war air gunners stationed at RAF Feltwell to survive a first tour. Others were not so lucky and many of his pre-war contempories, like nineteen-year-old Bill Hitchmough, had been killed. Hitchmough was a gunner in Pilot Officer W. J. Finlayson's crew which failed to return on the night of 23/24 October 1940 when Bomber Command had despatched some 79 Wellingtons to many targets including Berlin and Emden. Next morning Shepherd was airborne with Pilot Officer 'Spanky' McFarlane with orders to mount a search off the Dutch coast. A dinghy was found but there was no trace of the crew.

These continual high losses of crews could only be made good by young men passing out of the OTUs, even if they were not fully trained or as familiar with their aircraft as they would have liked.

Chapter 6
Bombers' Moon

The RAF was so desperate that training courses were nortoriously short, as Sergeant Alfred Jenner, a WOP-AG, who in mid-November 1941 joined No 99 Squadron at Newmarket Heath from No 15 OTU at Harwell recalls: 'The gunnery course should have been one month: it was in fact two and a half weeks. I did at least make one flight over enemy territory — a "very scary" trip to Paris on a leaflet dropping sortie.

'At Newmarket we were quartered in the Rowley Mile grandstand near the aircraft. The stand was always dirty and we could never keep our clothes clean. We ate below the seating enclosure and boiled our guns clean in the saddlery, which served as an armoury. Crews were very keen and the ground crews knew their job. Although bomb loads were small and we did not always hit our targets, we firmly believed we were very good for morale. It did people good to see and hear us going out.'

Alf Jenner made his first operational trip on the night of 16/17 December 1940 when he flew as front gunner in Sergeant Fletcher's crew. Jenner recalls: 'We were to scatter-bomb Mannheim in a "town blitz".' Operation "Abigail", as it was code-named, would be in retaliation for the German bombing of Coventry and Southampton. In all, some 134 bombers, including 61 Wellingtons, were despatched; the first "area" bombing raid on a German industrial target.

'Aircraft were despatched to the target singly. At this time we could not afford crew losses from collision or bombs falling on each other's aircraft so this was the only practical way. It was cold and lonely in the front turret but my Brownings never froze up on any of the operations I would fly. However, if one

A grim-faced crew from 99 Squadron prepare to board their Wellington IA at a desolate and snow covered corner of Newmarket Heath during the winter of 1940-41. *(via Eric Masters)*

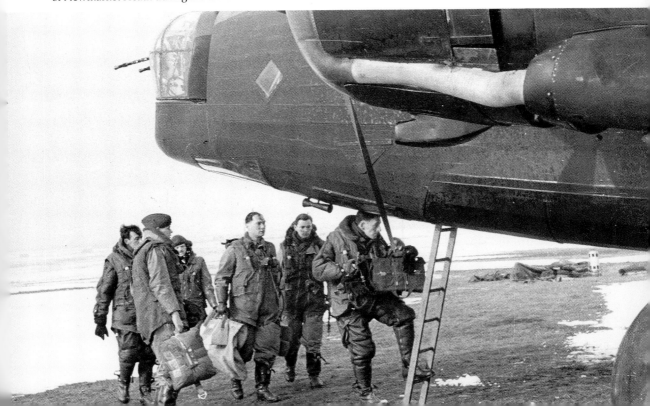

carried an apple, we were warned not to eat it; it would break your teeth!

'From a safety point of view, the front turret was preferable to the rear, which could be an exhausting trek to reach in our flight gear. The rear gunner was protected by two slabs of armour plate which could be joined together to protect his chest. However, in the front turret I could only rely on armour plate behind the pilots to stop bullets hitting me from the rear. The primary function of an air gunner at this time was to be a heavy flak spotter for the captain. He told us to keep our eyes peeled and report enemy aircraft and flak gun flashes immediately.

'We dropped our bombs on Mannheim from about 12,000 feet and although it was my first experience of flak, we came through all right. We landed back at Newmarket after being in the air for six hours and ten minutes.' Unfortunately, incendiaries carried as markers by eight leading Wellingtons were dropped in the wrong place and the subsequent bombing had been widely spread.

In the New Year Jenner was on ops again. 'On 29 January 1941 we were told to bomb the *Tirpitz* at Wilhelmshaven. My pilot was Pilot Officer Coote, an ex-Public school type who would stand no nonsense. All he wanted was to do a good job. He taught us that each man was reliant on the others. He was also a great "jinker" [taking avoiding action against flak and fighters]. Coote stayed over the target for three quarters of an hour with German guns popping off at us. Our Observer, who was in something of a panic, shouted, "Why don't we drop the bloody bombs and get out?" Coote said in no uncertain terms, "I'm the skipper of this ship and you'll drop the bombs when I tell you!" In fact we never did see the ship and we brought our bombs home.

'On 11 February we brought our bombs home again. Our target was Bremen but there was 10/10ths cloud and we got hopelessly lost. We flew back and saw a strip of coastline but we were not sure whether it was France, Germany, Wales or England. We flew up and down. I suddenly spotted two towers and realised it was the entrance to Lowestoft harbour (the town where I was born and had spent my childhood). We flew back to Newmarket and landed through a gap in the cloud with the bombs still aboard. We had not noticed they hadn't been dropped! We lost a lot of aircraft that night.'

(Of a total force of 79 bombers, 22, including eleven Wellingtons, crash-landed in England.)

On 14 March Alf Jenner flew with Sergeant Kitely, a Canadian, on a trip to Gelsenkirchen. 'No-one could ever find Gelsenkirchen because of the industrial haze. Kitely decided to bomb and shoot up an airfield in Holland on the homeward trip. It was very exciting and we dropped our bombs. He dived the Wimpy down to 300 feet and I fired about 1,000 rounds at chance lights and searchlights and the rear gunner had a go as well.

'Ten days later, on 24 March, 99 Squadron were briefed to attack the *Von Hipper* in Brest Harbour. Brest was very clear. From about two miles away I could see two ships when the Sergeant Pilot ordered, "Bomb bay doors open". The bomb aimer, surprised, said, "But we're too far away". We dropped them anyway. Our pilot, who was only one short of his tour, was determined to survive. It was the only case of "sugaring" I recall during my operations.'

Meanwhile, Eric Masters, a Sergeant Pilot who had recently arrived at Newmarket from an OTU, waited impatiently to fly his first op with No 99 Squadron. Squadron Leader Stanley Black, the CO, explained that Masters would captain a crew whose previous captain had been grounded. Black added that he would fly as an observer on the first two operations. In the first three weeks five operations were cancelled because of the weather. Masters recalls: 'I was becoming desperate to get the first op under my belt, to discover for myself whether I would make it — to find out just how scared one would be. Whilst I knew I had a super crew, I also knew they would be watching me very closely to see if I had any of the faults of their previous skipper.

'Finally, the day arrived and we set off to bomb Cologne. I was very nervous, not at the prospect of enemy action, but having the CO along as my second pilot! It was in fact quite enjoyable and the ack-ack fire was nothing more than a nuisance. At times the Germans seemed keen on playing possum rather than give away the locality of a town by defending it too vigorously. One felt sorry for the crew of the other aircraft, coned in ten searchlights, weaving this way and that, trying to get away, but we were glad they were taking the attention of the enemy.

'My landing back at Newmarket was my one "black". I dropped the Wimpy on the deck from about 25 feet instead of the normal five-ten feet and she bounced quite violently. I had to give her a quick burst on the throttles to keep her flying and let down again more gently. Squadron Leader Black suggested that it was because I had been used to concrete runways which reflected what little light there was and enabled one to judge "hold-off" more accurately. Grass was comparatively non-reflective and one had to judge height entirely by the flares. I was feeling rather miserable about it myself. However, no harm was done. I did my second trip a night later, with the CO coming along, to Cologne again.'

Over at Mildenhall 27-year-old Flying Officer Trevor A. 'Happy' Hampton, who had joined No 149 Squadron in February, also found himself flying to Cologne, accompanied by his Flight Commander. 'We had been assigned a brand new Wellington IC [*R1474*], which should have made me a little suspicious and my ground crew painted on it

our squadron letters "OJ" and our identification letter "M-Mother". Secretly, I was delighted. I had a good mother and she would look after me — it was an omen.

'After a few days in the Officers' Mess I seemed to detect a subtle sort of deference being bestowed upon me by other junior officers. Nothing was said, but everyone was so "very nice". At first I thought it might be that I had arrived as a fully fledged Flying Officer, with 600 flying hours in my logbook, rather than the more usual humble Pilot Officer straight from training school. For a day or two I basked in my fool's paradise.

'I began to notice that my crew, also, were being treated with a touching courtesy quite alien to the wartime RAF. I mentioned the phenomenon to my rear gunner, Sergeant George "Junior" Gray, who had previously been a commissioned pilot but was accident prone. Junior looked at me incredulously. "Don't you know Skipper? There have been eleven 'M-Mothers' since Christmas!"'

An early infra-red camera captures an air crew of 149 Squadron being driven to dispersal for a raid on Kiel docks on 11 March 1941. Left to right, Wng Cdr (later Grp Capt) Powell OBE, DSO, Squadron CO; Sgt Petter, WOP of Wellington 'M-Mother'; P/O Coryat; Squadron Navigation Officer. Standing, F/O T. A. Hampton. Sitting, Sgt George Gray. *(T. A. Hampton)*

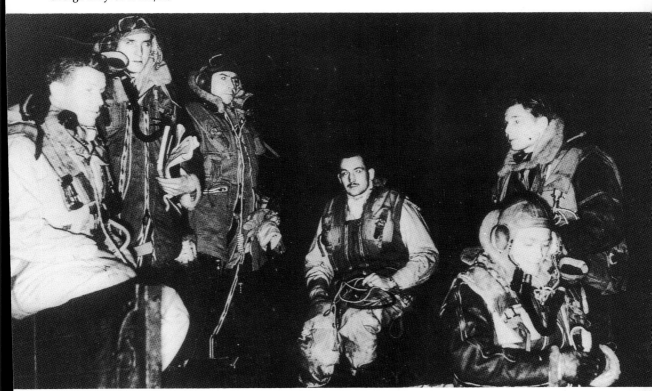

'I was a bit shaken but I soon consoled myself — I still had faith in mother. Out of our squadron of eighteen aircraft, they must have been losing one 'M-Mother' every week.

'The first trip was, more or less, a "blitz" on Cologne. The Germans had had a go at Coventry in November 1940, which I had seen burning from my own aircraft, so I didn't feel too badly about it. My Flight Commander, Squadron Leader Sawry Cookson, accompanied us just to show us the ropes and let me see how "easy" (his words) it was. He naturally assumed command and we left my second pilot behind.

'With an inferno below we steamed over the city at 140 knots, at 8,000 feet, the ceiling for a Wellington with a bomb load. Having done two runs over the target area, we were chased off by ground fire and searchlights, diving into the protective cloak of darkness clear of the city and levelling out at 2,000 feet. Cooky let me take over and he went aft for a word with the crew. When he returned to the cockpit I was climbing but he stopped me — 2,000 feet would be OK.

'We cruised along quietly and eventually came across an enemy airfield, all lit up for night flying. "Go down and stir them up a bit," said Cooky, so down we went. Once round the circuit and they realised there was a cat among the pigeons and let us have some flak and light tracer fire. I looked at Cooky and he nodded towards home. I set course and started to climb but again he told me to stay at 2,000 feet. It didn't seem right to me — but he should know.

'We stooged along for some time and I was beginning to feel confident. I noticed intermittent flickering lights immediately beneath the aircraft. So much for black-out precautions — I was looking straight down the chimneys of a large city, probably Rotterdam, but I didn't get the chance to confirm with the Navigator, Sergeant Cymbalist.

'At that moment there was a blinding flash and "M-Mother" was on the instant the focal point of countless searchlights and we seemed to be trapped in a cage of golden rods. I was petrified into immobility but it did slowly dawn on me that the air was composed of vicious tracer shells and bullets. The crack of exploding shells could be heard above the noise of our engines — that meant they were close, and then a much louder one rocked the aircraft. The starboard wing went down, followed by the nose.

'I had the stick right back and the wheel hard over to port but "M-Mother" was diving out of the sky and I was quite helpless. The altimeter was unwinding like a mad thing, I watched it go past five hundred feet in numb despair and I knew we were "going in" — this was it and on our first trip — Oh, Mother!

'Under such circumstances imminent death brings with it no acute agony of mind as one would expect, but a hopeless numb realisation of the end. I knew it was no good struggling anymore and I was just about to let go of the controls and cover my face for the final blinding crash when Cooky's voice came over the intercom, "Come on, hold it!" We might have been on a training exercise. I hung on, with Cooky leaning across me, helping to take some of the weight and we eventually levelled off at 200 feet, the searchlights and flak losing us as we dived earthwards.

'Our speed was down to 85 knots and we were flying in a semi-stalled condition, tail down and nose up. Our engines were at full boost but we couldn't gain speed or height and I dared not let our nose or wing go down the slightest degree. We staggered home across the North Sea, every moment expecting the aircraft to drop a wing and spin in but as we burnt up our fuel, inch by inch we made a little height and crossed the English coast at 500 feet. Cooky could see that I was exhausted and he managed to slide underneath me into the pilot's seat.

'Cooky saved "M-Mother" that night. He was a remarkable person who just did not acknowledge danger and was quite fearless. I felt I had the edge on him as a "safe" pilot, but who wanted "safe" pilots in 1941? I expected Cooky to make a full power approach and do a wheel landing but too late I realised he was holding off to do a "three pointer". The starboard wing naturally stalled first, a great chunk of it was missing and down we came into Mildenhall, a shaken crew.

'At dawn the ground crew pushed off for breakfast, having written us off as one more "M-Mother". However, they were soon out on "M site" again, and seemed genuinely pleased to see us back, although it meant the fitting of a new wing.

'I was rather looking forward to the

interrogation by our Intelligence Officer, one John Cobb, of water and land speed record fame. "Everything OK?", asks John. "Yes, bombs on target", says Cooky. "Come on, let's get some breakfast." I was learning fast

'After some sleep, to my surprise, I found that the night's experience had improved my morale and my faith in "M-Mother" had been justified. My crew were not convinced and Junior privately expressed the hope that he would be re-commissioned before he got the "chop".

'A new wing was fitted and I carried out an air test. On reporting the aircraft serviceable again Cooky informed me that he was lending my "M-Mother" to "A" Flight for the coming night's operation. I could stand down with all my crew except for my second pilot, Sergeant E. R. Cook, who they wanted to borrow.

'During the afternoon of 17 March a Sergeant Pilot, the captain of the unserviceable "A" Flight aircraft, sought me out in the "B" Flight crewroom. He was in a dreadful state and made little effort to hide it. "I'm told I have to take your aircraft tonight, Sir — and it's "M-Mother"." I said "Yes, look after her; she's flying nicely with the new wing".

'The poor boy was nearly speechless but in a rambling disjointed manner he told me he had done some 28 operations without incident, had only two more to do of his present tour and now fate had dealt him "M-Mother". In 149 Squadron she really was the "end". I felt a little piqued. I didn't like to think of my aircraft as a leper. In truth, there was little expressed sympathy wasted in the wartime RAF and none was expected. This expression of fear to an officer he hadn't even spoken to before, was unprecedented in my experience. It was more than just a premonition to the boy. He had made up his mind they were for the "chop". Instead of trying to laugh him out of it, I found myself comforting him and my last words were, "I guarantee "M-Mother" will bring you right back."

'I lived off the camp and the following morning, 18 March, driving along the road from Barton Mills to the airfield, I saw the tail end of a Wellington bomber sticking up out of the roof of a house. Just clear of the slates I read "M-OJ".'

"M-Mother" had returned safely from the raid on Bremen, but had been jumped by a Ju 88C night intruder flown by Leutnant Rolf Pfeiffer of 1 Staffel, NJG 2, as it was coming into land near Beck Row. Sergeant R. Warren, the pilot, and the other five crew were killed in the attack. The occupants of the house, an insurance agent named Titchmarsh and his wife, escaped unhurt as they had taken refuge under their bed when they had heard machine-gun fire.

'A new Wellington [R1587] was towed out to "M" site and yet another "M-Mother" was prepared for operations. In this one we completed a few operations and to everyone's surprise, returned intact. One night, intent on blasting Hitler's three pocket battleships lying in Brest harbour, we were being shaken up by the combined defensive fire of the three battleships and all the Brest Peninsular flak. The Navigator was chanting over his bombsight for my benefit "Left. Left. Steady. Right. Steady", when I heard Junior shout something about a fighter.

'Without any conscious intention on my part I had "M-Mother" in a vertical diving turn to starboard. The Navigator shouted, "Bombs gone" but added that he didn't know where, and from the rear turret Junior howled, "Hell, Skipper. What are you doing? You frightened the daylights out of the Jerry fighter. You turned right across his bows." It wasn't only the Jerry who was shaken.

'Back at base Junior got me on one side; he had been delegated by the others. "Skip, you really must see Doc about your ears." I did, and was grounded for further examination. To my surprise the news caused consternation in the crew. Squadron Leader Anthony W. J. Clark, just posted to the squadron, took over "B" Flight from Cooky, who was promoted to Squadron Commander. Clark also took over "M-Mother" and my crew for the time being and decided on a daylight training flight to get to know the aircraft and the boys. He had only been on the camp a few hours and could not have known "M-Mother's" reputation. Being a senior officer and on such short acquaintance, my crew wouldn't have presumed to mention such a subject and I didn't say anything; what good could it have done?

'I watched "M-Mother" climb away with mixed feelings on 17 May. It is not nice being grounded, even temporarily, and I had a guilty sense of having let my crew down. I wandered into the crewroom, wondering what I should do until their return but hearing the commotion of the fire engine and

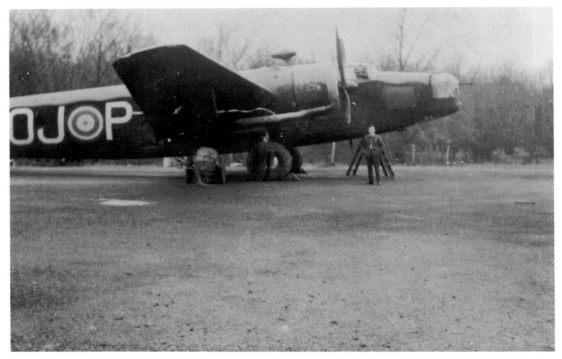

The last 'unlucky' 'M-Mother' had its letter changed to 'P'. *(T. A. Hampton)*

the ambulance getting underway, I went outside to see what was up. Someone shouted across to me, "Your aircraft has gone in. A Hurricane flew smack through her." I jumped into my car and headed for the distant column of black oily smoke that marked the end of one more "M-Mother".'

Clark had been leading a box of four Wellingtons, and a Hurricane I of the Meteorological Flight (also based at Mildenhall) flown by Flying Officer I. R. MacDiarmid, DFC, had been carrying out fighter affiliation tactics when the incident occurred. MacDiarmid 'attacked' the leading Wellington, and severed the tail. The Hurricane lost its port wingtip and both aircraft fell near Soham. Although some parachutes were seen to leave the Wellington late, all seven men in the two aircraft were killed.

'Happy' Hampton arrived on the scene: 'In the middle of the potato field I stumbled amongst the still smouldering remains of my aeroplane and friends until the station doctor walked me away. "You shouldn't be here. You can't do any good." It was, of course, bad for morale; my morale.

'One of the fire crew came up and told me that the tail and rear gun turret were in the next field, unburnt. My unspoken question was answered before I dare ask it. "The rear gunner didn't have time to get out. They were only at 2,000 feet." I walked over to a stretcher on which was the only body they had recovered. From beneath army blankets protruded two beautifully polished boots. It was the last I was to see of Junior, the "tail end captain" of "M-Mother". To the others around it might have seemed that I was staring morbidly at my dead friend but they didn't know I was trying to get a final message through to him and the intercom was worse than usual. "You very nearly made it Junior — your commission has been approved."

'I had a talk with Cooky, who laughed at me at first but once he realised I was dead serious he agreed to drop "M-Mother" from the squadron aircraft board and replace it with "P-Peter". I was posted away for training as a test pilot and lost touch with Bomber Command friends but I hope the trick worked. However, "M-Mother" had looked after me. I felt she would — I had a good mother.'

Other squadrons had their unlucky aircraft too. Officers and crews of No 99 Squadron considered they had two. In 'A' Flight it was 'B-Bertie', while 'R-Robert' was considered the 'jinx kite' in 'B' Flight. 'B-Bertie' (*R1333*) was possibly so named because it was dubbed the 'Broughton Bomber', having been bought by aircraft workers at the Broughton factory. On the night of 18 December 1940 'B-Bertie' crashed on take-off into Devils Dyke with Pilot Officer G. S. Ogilvie at the controls during its maiden operation to Ludwigshaven. 'B-Bertie' caught fire and exploded. Four crew were killed and two more, including one who was pulled clear by Sergeant Hansen, a Dane serving in the RAF, were seriously injured.

By mid-March 1941 No 99 Squadron had moved ten miles distant to the newly completed base at Waterbeach and on 30 March the Wellingtons began their campaign against the German battle cruisers *Scharnhorst* and *Gneisenau*, or 'Salmon and Gluckstein' as they were known, while the Halifaxes went after the cruiser *Prinz Eugen* at Brest. The campaign was to last for more than ten months.

On the night of 31 March/1 April, 4,000 lb bombs were used operationally for the first

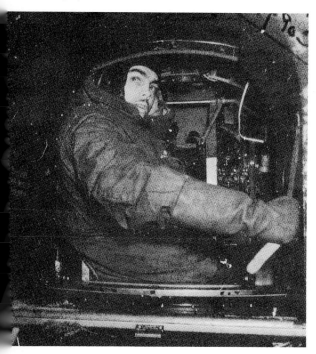

Sgt Alfred Jenner in the front turret of his 99 Squadron Wellington at Newmarket Heath, 1940. *(Alfred Jenner)*

time when two were dropped on Emden by modified Wellington IIs of Nos 9 and 149 Squadrons. Four aircraft were detailed for this operation, two acting as cover for the two Wellingtons carrying the bombs. No 149 Squadron's 'X-X-Ray', piloted by Pilot Officer Franks, successfully completed its mission but the second squadron Wellington failed to get airborne and slid to a halt in a barley field near the runway. The 'Wizard of Oz' painted on the aircraft had failed to work its magic.

On the night of 9 April Alf Jenner flew his first operation from Waterbeach, with a new crew captained by Squadron Leader David Torrens, an ex-Battle of Britain pilot. 'Torrens was our new Flight Commander. As he was new to Bomber Command it was decided to give him the most experienced crew. I was by now something of a veteran with twelve ops and I became Torrens' front gunner. First WOP was Arthur Smith; a splendid wireless operator who had served in the pre-war RAF in Iraq. The second pilot was Eric Berry, who came from a well-off Yorkshire family and who had flown private aircraft before the war. His wartime training had been short; converting straight from a Tiger Moth to a Wellington. Although he had only flown two or three ops he was well thought of and was about to skipper his own crew. Our rear gunner was Pilot Officer Palmer and our Observer, Flying Officer Goodwin, was from Ipswich.

'At Waterbeach we played a guessing game. If there was a "breeze" that an op was on that night we would watch the petrol bowsers refuelling the Wimpys and note the number of gallons. If it was about 400 gallons that meant a trip to the Ruhr; if it was over 650, it must mean Berlin! Everyone was worried but did not show it. We had things to do to pass the rest of the afternoon. The wireless had to be checked and guns cleaned.

'At 5 o'clock on the afternoon of 9 April we entered the briefing room and sat down. At the end of the room was a large map, covered with a curtain. The Briefing Officer dramatically pulled the curtain aside and we were startled to see a red ribbon that seemed to go on for ever! It meant a four and a half hour trip to Berlin. The RAF hadn't been to the big city since the previous September. We all thought, "Jesus Christ! Why me?"

'After briefing finished we ate our Flying Supper in the mess. It was rather poor fare;

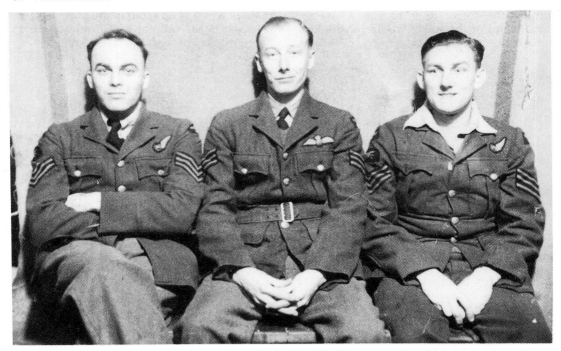

99 Squadron 'kriegie' triumvirate at Stalag Luft III shortly after Alfred Jenner was shot down on the night of 9 April 1941. Left to right, Jenner, Eric Berry, Albert Smith. *(Alfred Jenner)*

usually corned beef and chips, bread pudding and tea. Everyone was in a high state of nervousness and excited hysteria, although no-one showed any sign of despondency. We were quite well trained and highly motivated.'

This was Jenner's 13th op and although he was not superstitious, he felt prompted to write to his wife. At 19:00 hours the crew truck nicknamed 'Tumbril', took the crew to the infamous 'R-Robert' waiting at dispersal. Jenner recalls: 'It was was really dark, cold and clear. A bomber's moon shone overhead. I climbed into the astrodome area and stowed my parachute. Our pilots wore theirs in flight. As we taxied out and lined up on the new tarmac runway I gripped the astrodome hatch clips, in case I needed to get out quickly, as I always did. We were away first. Torrens thundered down the runway (our bomb load was small because of the need for extra fuel). With flaps full on we climbed slowly into the sky above Waterbeach. I climbed into the front turret immediately (enemy fighters might already be about).

'Grinding away slowly we headed for Southwold, our point of departure. Nearing the coast of Holland I exclaimed, "Enemy coast ahead!". There were a few shots then all was quiet again. The captain talked quietly to us, telling us to keep our eyes peeled. Then the fun began. A succession of searchlights picked us up and passed us on from one to another until we could see the multitude of coloured flak bursts over Berlin. We had been told that there were 1,000 guns at Berlin. They couldn't all fire at us but it felt like it. Down below, Lake Wannsee shone in the moonlight. Buildings, or imagined buildings, appeared in the Berlin suburbs below.

'We could actually smell flak. The Germans were very good gunners. A shell knocked out one of the engines. Fortunately, it did not catch fire. Torrens feathered the prop. We dropped our bombs and droned away. Nearing Brunswick Torrens came on the intercom. "Sorry to tell you chaps but we will not make it back. You will each have to decide if you want to bale out or stay in the aircraft for a crashlanding."

'I had previously decided that should such an occasion occur, then I would jump. I looked at the altimeter. It read 1,100 feet (300 feet less than recommended). The ruddy bulkhead at the front prevented me from turning the turret door handle. (To bale straight out of the turret would have taken me into the turning props.) To my relief, Eric Berry opened it from the other side. Flying Officer Goodwin, the Observer, and I baled out. The remaining four crew, including Pilot Officer Palmer, the rear gunner, and Sergeant Albert Smith, the WOP/AG, stayed with the aircraft and crash-landed at Wolfenbuttle, near Hannover. They set fire to the aircraft before being captured and made PoWs. Goodwin and I joined them.'

The following night, 10/11 April, No 12 Squadron made its operational debut when the squadron despatched Wellingtons to Emden. In April-May No 15 Squadron flew its Wellingtons for the last time before converting to the Short Stirling.

At 23:50 hours on the night of 16 April a Wellington of No 3 PRU, piloted by Flight Leiutenant R. P. Elliott, took off from RAF Oakington in Cambridgeshire for a photo-reconnaissance operation. The Wellington carried eight personnel, including Wing Commander Bennett, who was flying as an observer to watch some night photography with a new colour camera which was being carried.

At first all went well. The Wellington crossed the enemy coast at 10,000 feet and arrived in the vicinity of the target area where there was a considerable ground haze. Elliott found a clear patch about twelve miles south west of Bremen and a parachute flare was launched. Almost immediately it was extinguished by anti-aircraft fire. Undaunted, the Wellington crew made a run-up on a dummy aerodrome and photographs were taken.

About five miles from the enemy coast the port engine burst into flames. Although the crew managed to extinguish the flames all was not well, as Sergeant R. F. 'Chan' Chandler, the rear gunner, explains: 'Eventually the airscrew fell away. I drew Flight Lieutenant Elliott's attention to this fact and after throwing everything we could, out of the Wimp' and finding that we could not maintain the height required, we ditched!

'We ditched approximately nine miles from the enemy coast. It was 5 am and the water was cold. The first thing we saw was an He 111 flying east at about 5,000 feet. We hoped it would "go away". Sergeant Evans, the cameraman, and myself, spent the whole time in the sea, hanging on to dinghy lines,

as there was just no room in the dinghy. The side had been badly holed on release from the Wimp' and despite chewing gum and the multi-pressure of flat hands on top of the tear, the dinghy was going down very quickly.

'It was a most welcome PRU blue Spitfire, piloted by Squadron Leader Ogilvie, that found and circled us. On the horizon came smoke and very soon, HM Transport *River Spey* came alongside our rapidly deflating dinghy and took us aboard. They were painting an emblem on the funnel as they had just had a successful engagement with an E-boat. We were given a warm change of clothing and large quantities of hot drink and rum. At Lowestoft Evans and I were rushed off to the local hospital. Eventually we arrived at Oakington to be given a royal reception in the Sergeants' Mess.'

At Waterbeach, one day late in April, No 99 Squadron crews were awaiting the call to briefing when they were surprised to hear Merlin engines, as if two Spitfires were landing together. Sergeant Eric Masters recalls: 'We all rushed to the windows to see a very unusual Wellington landing. It had Merlin engines instead of Pegasus radials. I was told to report to Wing Commander Black, who told me it would be my aircraft and that I had better have a chat with the ferry-pilot who had brought her in to learn of any different handling features. He told me it handled very well except for being extremely nose heavy due to the in-line Merlins moving the c-of-g forward. He said the trimming wheel was right back with very little more adjustment and he hated to think how she would handle with "the" bomb on board. He then told me this Mk II Wellington was made to carry one 4,000 lb bomb — the first of the blockbusters!

'Next day I took the new aircraft up for a test flight and found that the increased power from the Merlin engines was most noticeable, especially on take-off and climb. The usual bomb bay, with its opening and closing doors, was not big enough, so the doors had been dispensed with, leaving a large indentation along the bottom of the fuselage. It was not rigged for any other selection of bombs and had just the one release gear. This harming of the aerodynamics of the airframe made the aircraft somewhat "lumpy" to handle but the smoothness of the in-line engine power with the

Wreckage of T2963 of 115 Squadron which crashed into council houses at Debach in the early hours of 24 June 1941. *(via Bob Collis)*

increase in airspeed, outweighed every possible criticism.

'I still had my standard Wellington Mk 1A assigned to me and in fact did five more missions in the aircraft before my first in the modified Wellington. It was on 5 May that I first took a 4,000 lb bomb on ops, to Mannheim. By then the squadron had received another Mk II Wellington and there were twelve others distributed amongst squadrons in the Group. There were plenty of spectators, including myself, at the bombing up to see the massive bomb being winched into the bomb-bay. It appeared to be a number of metal barrels welded together with a slightly pointed nose cap stuck on one end — merely, I thought, to tell which was the forward end. It was quite a shock to see that quite a proportion of it was protruding and I wondered what effect this would have on the handling of the aircraft. I thought, too, that the bomb would not fall in the way a normal bomb would, but would most likely tumble over and over. However, our flash photo later showed the bomb bursting; a real fluke.

'Following this we had a very busy period. We went to Brest on 7 May and to Hamburg (with the second 4,000 lb bomb) on the night of 8/9 May 1941. [360 aircraft (plus another three on mining operations), the largest number of aircraft so far despatched, were sent to mainly Hamburg and Bremen.] On the 10th we went to Berlin (with another), then one to Mannheim on 12 May and another, to Cologne on 17 May, before receiving my commission to Pilot Officer.'

There was no let up. On the night of 12/13 June 1941 No 405 (Vancouver) Squadron at Driffield, Yorks, made its operational debut when the Canadian squadron despatched four Wellington IIs to Schwerte. On the night of 23/24 June 1941, 44 Wellingtons and eighteen Whitleys made a heavy raid on Cologne. One of the Wellingtons, despatched by No 115 Squadron, was flown by Pilot Officer Douglas Sharpe. His rear gunner, Sergeant R. F. 'Chan' Chandler, who had been involved in a No 3 PRU Wellington 'prang' the previous month, recalls: 'After bombing Cologne things seemed to go wrong. There was a lot of chatter on the intercom between the pilot and the navigator. There was no doubt whatsoever that we were lost.

The crew were repeatedly instructed to keep constant watch for any sign of land through the cloud.

'Shortly we saw the coastline. There were repeated comments about "fuel state". The aircraft was throttled back and a gradual descent was made. I was invited by Pilot Officer Sharpe to bale out over land. I declined, thinking it was best to stay with the aircraft and crew.'

Sharpe nursed the ailing bomber back to Suffolk, where almost out of fuel, he decided on a crash landing. Chandler recalls: 'It so happens that the area around Bredfield, Burgh and Pettistree is very flat and a suitable length of pasture land was selected. Sharpe made a gradual descent and approach. I jettisoned my turret doors and my back was to the starboard side as we dropped to a height of about fifty feet. I lowered my goggles and eased myself out on the edge of the turret. Looking out and down with the ground rushing past at an alarming 100 knots, I thought of rolling out of the turret. Looking along the fuselage I could see tall trees ahead and slid back into the turret. The next second there was the most tremendous crash and I lost consciousness.'

The Wellington had hit the trees and crashed into some council houses at Debach. Incredibly, a man with a child in his arms jumped to safety from the bedroom window of the smashed house. 'Chan' Chandler suffered serious leg, head and arm injuries but would recover. Fred Tingley, the second pilot, died later as a result of his injuries. He was the only fatality. Sharpe was unhurt but was killed on his next trip.

The night of 7 July was full of incidents. One crew member was killed in a Wellington of No 75 Squadron when it hit a tree during a night flying exercise while trying to land on one engine at Methwold. A Wellington of No 115 Squadron crash-landed at Marham

F/O B. G. Cook of 101 Squadron flew this IC home on one engine after an attack by a night fighter near Hamm on 7 August 1941. P/O Milton Pelmore, 2nd Pilot and Cook were wounded and Sgt Lackie, the rear gunner, who was hit badly by a cannon shell, could not bale out because two parachutes were badly burned. With hydraulics out, Cook skilfully bellied in at Oakington and the crew were evacuated before the Wimpy caught fire. It was only then that a 500 lb bomb was discovered still in the bomb bay! *(B. G. Cook via Dave Brighton)*

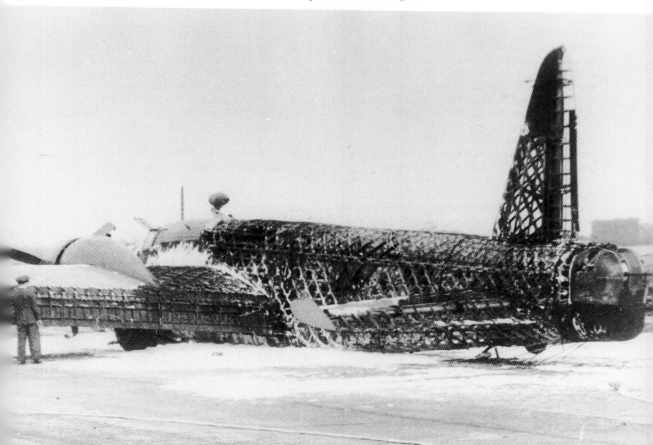

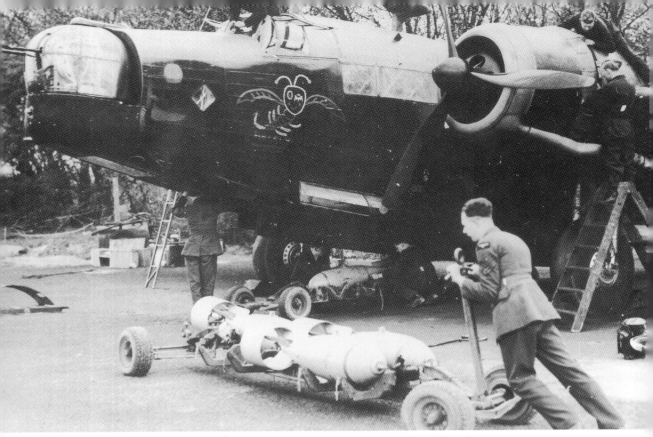

R1593 'N-Nuts' of 149 Squadron, which on 14 July 1941, following a raid on Bremen, was taken away in pieces, later repaired and served throughout the rest of the war with various OTUs. The insignia is of a drunken firefly representing, variously, WOP (antennae), pilot (wings), tail-gunner (Scorpion sting) and the eyes of the half-blind navigator. The whole portrayed a crew that flew by night and was supposedly drunk by day. *(Lord Sandhurst)*

after being damaged in combat with a Ju 88C intruder of NJG 2 and another squadron Wellington, piloted by Sergeant O. A. Mathews, RNZAF, crashed in the North Sea with the loss of all the crew.

That night, Eric Masters of No 99 Squadron, was flying the 30th and final operation of his tour, a sortie to Cologne. Masters was philosophical about it: 'Our losses were running at approximately five per cent so one believed one was living on luck after the 20th trip. One was just as likely to "buy it" on the first as on the thirtieth.' All went well until Masters' crew approached the Rhine. 'Pilot Officer Don Elliott, my Canadian navigator, came to stand beside me. There were two areas of AA activity ahead and I decided to head between them so that Elliott could pick out the river reflecting the moonlight from the south, and from his map would be able to place us exactly. We discovered we were just south of Cologne. I wanted to get a really good run at the target and needed to get north of the city.

'There was no need for navigation now and having passed over the river I turned north and flew past Cologne on its eastern side watching the flak exploding, flares dropping, flash bombs illuminating huge areas and bombs bursting. I felt remote from it all. North of Cologne I turned over the river and headed south. Elliott was now in the prone bomb aiming position, just below and in front of me, getting a very clear view of the river and giving me course corrections to keep us in line with the target.

'The activity over the target had practically ceased and it became very peaceful. One of the gunners remarked, "Everyone else seems to have gone home, skipper". In these last minutes I had kept straight and level and at the same speed for much too long. The Germans must have wondered about this crazy lone raider. We were caught in the bluish-white beam of a master searchlight. Six more standard searchlights coned us. Now the whole fury of the Cologne defences concentrated on us. I increased speed, still heading for the target. The flak followed us expertly, throwing the aircraft about. Johnny Agrell, the Second Pilot, who was watching it all at the astrodome ready to deal with the flash-bomb, called out that we had been hit.

'I had felt a judder in the control column and then found it rigid in the fore and aft direction (elevator control). As I had been holding it in the dive I was now unable to bring the nose up.' In vain Masters tried to correct. 'The flak was still after us. I told Don to jettison the bombs (live) in a last hope to get the nose up but when this failed, I realised we were virtually out of control at 10,000 feet and losing height rapidly. I had no alternative but to give the order, "Bale out!" I was thankful my chest parachute pack was in its storage position. At times I had been known to forget to take it on a trip and I had delegated Don Elliott to make sure it was always on the "tumbril". I was glad that on this occasion he had not let me down.' Eric Masters baled out and was captured. He spent the remainder of the war as a 'guest of the German government'.

The following night, 8 July, Wellingtons of No 75 Squadron raided Münster. On the return flight at 13,000 feet over Ijsselmeer, Squadron Leader R. P. Widdowson's aircraft was attacked by a Bf 110 night-fighter. The rear gunner was wounded in the foot but managed to drive off the enemy aircraft. Incendiary shells from the fighter started a fire near the starboard engine, and fed by a fractured fuel pipe, soon threatened to engulf the whole wing.

Sergeant James Ward, RNZAF, the Second Pilot, climbed out of the astrodome into a 100 mph slipstream in pitch darkness a mile above the North Sea, and by kicking holes in the fabric covering of the geodetics, inched his way to the starboard engine and smothered the fire which threatened to engulf the aircraft. Ward's actions earned him the Victoria Cross. (Sadly, he was killed two months later, shot down in a Wellington over Hamburg.)

Other Wellingtons came home on a wing and a prayer. On the night of 14 July Sergeant Tony Gee of No 149 Squadron brought 'N-Nuts' home to Mildenhall after being coned in searchlights at 8,000 feet over Bremen and fired on by accurate flak. Gee finally escaped but he was down to 2,000 feet. His Navigator/Bomb Aimer, The Right Honorable Terence Mansfield, who was flying

Wellington II W5360 PH-C of 12 Squadron, Binbrook which failed to return from a raid on Brest on 7 July 1941. *(RAF Museum)*

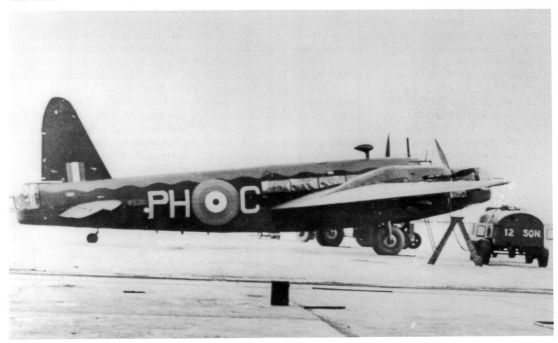

his 11th operation recalls: 'No-one was wounded but, as daylight came we found lots of it coming in everywhere. Our wireless was not working so we could not tell base that, although we were a long way behind schedule, we were still coming. By the time we got back to Mildenhall we were classed as overdue. Someone classified the damage to *R1593* as not repairable and "N-Nuts" was taken away in pieces.

In the half light of dawn on 15 July Sergeant J. C. Saich and the crew of a Wellington 1C of No 9 Squadron was returning to Honington with six 500 lb bombs still in her bomb bay after a raid on Bremen. Three hours and forty minutes earlier, 'T-Tommy' had been caught in the glare of searchlights over Bremen at 11,000 feet, hit four times by flak and set on fire. Sergeant English, the rear gunner and Sergeant Telling, the Second Pilot, were wounded by shell splinters. Flares stored in the port wing ignited and two large holes were blown in the starboard wing and rear fuselage. Much of the fabric covering the tail fin was burned away before the fires were finally extinguished. The bombs could not be jettisoned because of damage to the hydraulic and electrical systems. One main wheel refused to lower, the flaps were inoperative and the fuel gauges had read 'zero' for the last two hours of the flight.

The area picked out for an emergency landing was a large field near Somerton, Norfolk. However, telegraph poles had been erected in all fields in the vicinity as an anti-invasion measure in 1940 and these could not easily be seen in the dim light. 'T-Tommy' touched down, went into a swing and slammed into one of the wooden poles, finishing with its fuselage broken in two. Incredibly, all six crew emerged from the wreckage with little more than a few bruises.

Saich and Telling were each awarded the DFM for their exploits. Saich and five other crew, including Sergeant Trott, who had been aboard 'T-Tommy, were killed when their Wellington was shot down in flames by a German night fighter near Terwispel in Holland during the costly raid on Berlin on 7/8 September 1941. Sergeant Telling was killed six months later when his Wellington broke up during a training flight near Thetford, Norfolk.

Meanwhile, on 24 July 1941, Wellingtons, Hampdens and Fortresses made daylight attacks on the *Gneisenau* and *Prinz Eugen* at Brest while Halifaxes attacked the *Scharnhorst* at La Pallice. Sixteen bombers failed to return and two other aircraft were lost when they ditched on the way home. On the night of 11/12 August the first service trial over enemy territory of the Gee navigational and identification device was carried out successfully by two Wellingtons of No 115 Squadron during a raid on Mönchen Gladbach. On 28 August, three of the squadron's Wellingtons were lost landing back at Marham after runway lighting had been damaged by enemy bombers.

No 458 Squadron, the second Australian bomber squadron to be formed, arrived at Holme-on-Spalding Moor, Yorkshire, where they joined No 1 Group, Bomber Command. On 1 September 1941 Wing Commander N. G. Mulholland, DFC, assumed command of the squadron and led its first raid, on the night of 20/21 October, when ten Wellington IVs attacked targets at Emden, Antwerp and Rotterdam. On 15 November No 460 Squadron, the second Australian Wellington unit to form, was established from 'C' Flight of No 458 Squadron, RAF Molesworth, Huntingdonshire. (Initially, No 460 Squadron joined No 8 Group, Bomber Command, but it flew no operations as part of this command. In January 1942 it was transferred to Breighton, Yorkshire to join No 1 Group and the first bombing operation followed in March of that year.)

Meanwhile, in September 1941, the Wellingtons were flying further afield, as Terence Mansfield, of No 149 Squadron, recalls: 'On 26 September, while en route to Genoa, we had been recalled over France due to forecast bad weather at base.' Three days later the Wellingtons went all the way. Mansfield continues: 'We had a lovely view of the Alps but Genoa was mostly covered by cloud so bombing was on estimated position using the coast. After leaving Genoa our wireless blew up and cloud developed solidly below 10,000 feet so navigation was solely on astro fixes. Fortunately, we hit the Mildenhall Lorenz beam almost on ETA. Duggie Fox, my pilot, turned on to it and descended in the low cloud. Honington had been alerted and they fired a massive assortment of pyrotechnics as we approached and we crawled in under a cloud base of, at most, 200 feet.

On 30 September the Wellingtons carried a

new weapon, as Terence Mansfield recalls: 'We carried a new 65 lb incendiary for marking purposes. This horrid weapon was very light case, rather like a large oblong tin, the contents of which were spontaneously combustible on contact with air. The resulting fire was very visible but it was a menace, as a leak brought fire.

'On 12 October we again carried 65 lb incendiaries, to Nürnberg. We had orders to drop only on visual. It was totally dark and although we flew around the area for forty minutes, we could see no ground detail. Then bombing started but it was not Nürnberg. Anyhow, we went over to investigate at just over 4,000 feet and I was confident that I could make out a small town. Since the fires were well established, we added to them and sent a signal back that we had bombed a secondary target. Further astro fixes on the return trip confirmed my calculated positions. On landing, we were told that we were the only crew not to find the target but our photograph proved that we were right and that almost the entire attack had been against the wrong place. We got our haloes back!

'On 7 November, my last [trip] with Duggie Fox and 149, we carried the 65 lb incendiary again. All the outward route was appalling, with high cloud, very bad icing, turbulence and rattling hail. Using the occasional breaks in the tops, I managed to get a series of astro fixes, so that at least we thought we were almost on track. Total cloud cover at the target meant that we could not drop our bombs and we brought them all the way back! That we crossed the Suffolk coast almost on track and only five minutes late on ETA proved the value of my sextant. We saw no signs of any defensive action and felt sure that the high losses, 21 of 170, were due solely to the weather.'

In the closing days of 1941, No 149 Squadron at Mildenhall began exchanging its Wellington IIs for the Short Stirling. No 3 Group, since it operated Bristol-engined bombers, had, in August 1941, been selected for re-equipment with the Short Stirling. On 24 December there was a taste of things to come when the Avro Lancaster entered service with No 44 Squadron at Waddington. It seemed that the Wellington's days in Bomber Command were numbered. But were they?

Wellington II W5461 EP-R of 104 Squadron failed to return from a raid on Berlin on 12 August 1941. *(via Mike Bailey)*

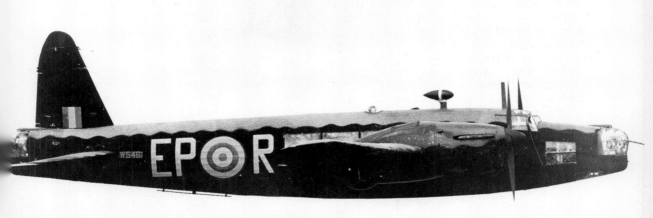

Chapter 7
Millennium

The year 1942 began badly for Britain and her allies. January could hardly have been less auspicious with extremely bad weather conditions and operations being curtailed by heavy falls of snow. At Holme-on-Spalding Moor, for instance, Wellingtons of No 458 Squadron had to have their wing surfaces brushed clear of snow before they could take off. The operation, to Brest, then went ahead as planned shortly before midnight, but one aircraft, suffering from severe icing, crashed on take-off, killing two crew members.

In warmer climes overseas British and Commonwealth forces received bad reverses in both the Middle East and the Far East. On 11 January the forces of Japan invaded Java and paratroop attacks on Sumatra soon followed. On 19 January Burma was invaded. By 31 January all British units in Malaya had been forced to withdraw across the straits to Singapore and it was only days before the island fell. Meanwhile, on 21 January Erwin Rommell had begun his second counter-offensive in the Western Desert and British forces were falling back everywhere.

Urgent steps were at once taken by the British Chiefs of Staff to bolster their flagging forces in both theatres of war. Although bomber squadrons were too valuable to be spared in January 1942, No 99 Squadron at Waterbeach received the news that its Wellingtons and crews were to be transferred to India. Meanwhile, on the night of 28/29 January 1942, two Wellington IVs of No 458 (RAAF) Squadron returned to their base at Holme-on-Spalding Moor from Boulogne amid rumours of their imminent move abroad. Any doubts were quickly removed with the arrival on the station of Wellington 1Cs fitted with tropicalised Bristol Pegasus

Wellington IC of 99 Squadron at Gibraltar while en-route to India in mid-1942. *(Grp Captain Jones)*

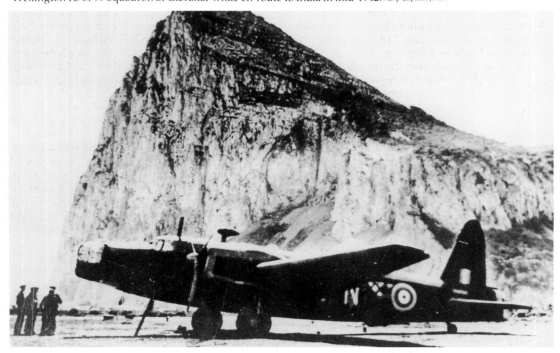

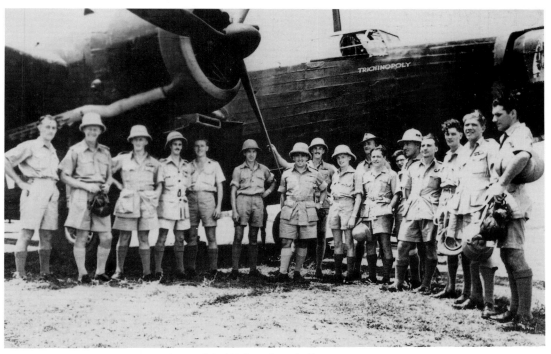

Officers and men pose before 'Trichinopoly' of 99 Squadron, India. *(via Grp Captain Jones)*

engines which the squadron was to swap for their Pratt and Whitney twin-row Wasp-engined Wellington IVs, for operations under desert conditions. Another change in January-February 1942 saw No 218 Squadron re-equip with the Short Stirling.

It was not all one-way traffic though. On 11 January 1942 No 419 Squadron at RAF Mildenhall made its operational debut in Bomber Command when the Canadian squadron despatched two Wellingtons to Brest where the German battlecruisers *Scharnhorst* and *Gneisenau* were bottled up by the Royal Navy. Amid general speculation that the two German capital ships must soon leave the port, the bombers stood by. When, on 12 February, they finally made their dash for their home ports the RAF and Royal Navy were found wanting. In the late afternoon, when all else had failed, three Wellingtons and two Stirlings from RAF Mildenhall were despatched to attack the German ships. However, they failed to find them in poor weather and two of the Wellingtons failed to return. Almost immediately, the squadron was declared non-operational again when its Wellington 1Cs were replaced with the Hercules-engined Wellington III.

On 21 February the Canadians were stood down while conversion took place.

The following day, having been recalled from the USA where he was head of the RAF Delegation, Air Marshal Arthur T. Harris arrived at High Wycombe, Buckinghamshire, to take charge of RAF Bomber Command from Sir Richard Peirse, who had been posted to India on 8 January. Harris's concept was to break the German spirit by the use of area rather than precision bombing and the targets would be civilian, not just military. Such a concept two years before would have been unthinkable but Harris saw the need to deprive the German factories of its workers and therefore its ability to manufacture weapons for war. Mass raids would be the order of the day, or rather the night, with little attention paid to precision raids on military targets.

However, Bomber Command did not possess the numbers of aircraft necessary for immediate mass raids. On taking up his position Harris found that only 380 aircraft were serviceable. More importantly, only 68 of these were heavy bombers while 257 were medium bombers. Undaunted, Harris selected the Renault factory at Billancourt

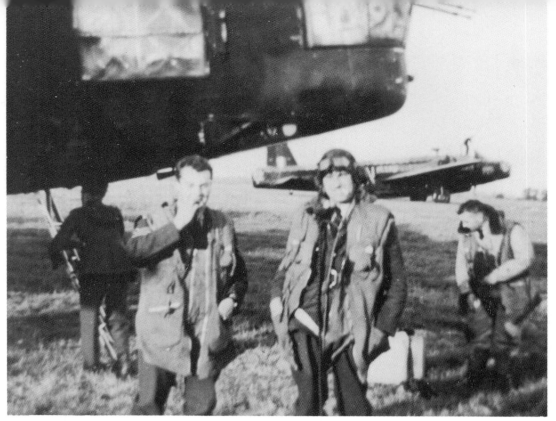

Reg Singerton (centre) in front of 9 Squadron Wellingtons at Honington in March 1942. *(via Bob Collis)*

near Paris, which had been earmarked for attack for some time, as his first target.

A full moon was predicted for the night of 3/4 March so Harris decided to send a mixed force of some 235 aircraft, led by the most experienced crews in Bomber Command, to bomb the French factory. It was calculated that approximately 121 aircraft an hour had been concentrated over the factory, which was devastated, and all except twelve aircraft claimed to have bombed.

While the experienced crews formed the spearhead of Harris's new policy, fledgling squadrons continued to swell the ranks of Bomber Command. On the night of 17/18 February, No 156 Squadron, RAF Alconbury, had flown its inaugural Wellington operation when three aircraft joined the Bomber Command stream attacking Essen.

During March the first Gee navigational and target identification sets were installed in operational bombers and these greatly assisted bombers in finding their targets on the nights of 8/9 and 9/10 March in attacks on Essen. On the latter, 187 bombers, including 136 Wellingtons, set out for the target. One of the Wellingtons, a Mk III of No 9 Squad-

ron, which took off from Honington, was piloted by Sergeant James Cartwright.

Shortly after taking off from Honington a radio message was received stating that the Wellington was returning to base with engine trouble. It was not the first time Cartwright, and his air gunner, Sergeant David Nicholas, had encountered trouble with a Wellington. Both were veterans in the squadron and on their sixth operation, on the night of 9 November 1941, they were involved in a dice with death while returning from a raid on Hamburg. Cartwright was flying as Second Pilot to Sergeant Pendleton when their Wellington developed engine failure in the vicinity of the target. They returned to East Anglia on one engine but stalled and crashed in a wood near RAF East Wretham. The aircraft was totally burnt out but none of the crew suffered any lasting injuries. Cartwright was later given his own crew and Nicholas went with him.

On the occasion of the Essen operation Cartwright and Nicholas were not so fortunate. Near Harleston, Suffolk, an eye witness saw the bomber circle once with the engines spluttering then saw an engine on fire and flames streaming behind it. Cartwright went around for a second time. The note of the engines then rose to a high-pitched whine as the aircraft dived to earth. None of the six crew baled out before the Wellington crashed in a ball of flame in a meadow, scattering a number of propaganda leaflets about the area. Among those who died was the WOP-AG, Sergeant Albert Singerton whose brother Reg was a radio technician at RAF Honington. The two brothers often conversed on the radio on the Wellington's return flight to base and Reg had been best man at Albert's wedding in May 1941.

On the night of 12/13 March, No 460 RAAF Squadron, RAF Molesworth, made its operational debut when five Wellington IVs joined the bomber stream, again attacking Emden. Meanwhile, Harris had decided that the incendiary bomb was his best weapon in the war against German civilian centres and he had chosen Lübeck, an historic German town on the Baltic, with thousands of half timbered houses, as an ideal target for a mass raid by RAF bombers carrying incendiary bombs.

On 28/29 March 234 bombers, mostly carrying incendiaries, set out for Lübeck. Eight bombers were lost but 191 aircraft claimed to have hit the target. A photo-reconnaissance a few days later revealed that about half the city, some 200 acres, had been obliterated. For four consecutive nights, beginning on the night of 23/24 April, it was the turn of Rostock to feel the weight of incendiary bombs. By the end only forty per cent of the city was left standing. The raids on Lübeck and Rostock prompted the Luftwaffe into reprisal, or 'Baedeker' raids (named after the German guide book to English cities) on Canterbury, Exeter, Norwich and York.

On 23 April Air Vice Marshal Edwards, Chief of the Air Staff of the RCAF, visited Mildenhall to inspect No 419 Squadron, commanded by Wing Commander John 'Moose' Fulton, DSO, DFC, AFC. This squadron was one of several which had perfected the technique of dropping bomb loads of 4 lb incendiaries over Lübeck and Rostock.

On the night of 25/26 April 1942 No 311 (Czechoslovakian) Squadron flew its last operation of the war before it was posted to Coastal Command, when five aircraft were despatched to Dunkirk. Also in April No 214 Squadron began converting to the Stirling and No 405 (Vancouver) Squadron, RCAF, at Driffield, Yorks, began converting to the Halifax.

Meanwhile, top level consultations between Harris and his subordinate commanders had revealed that the raids on Rostock had achieved total disruption. Whole areas of the city had been wiped out and 100,000 people had been forced to evacuate. The capacity of its workers to produce war materials had therefore been severely diminished. Harris had for some time nurtured the desire to send 1,000 bombers to a German city and reproduce the same results with incendiaries. Although RAF losses would be on a large scale, Churchill approved the plan. Harris (now Sir Arthur), gave the order 'Operation

Wing Commander 'Moose' Fulton, DSO, DFC, AFC, and Flt Sgt Alexander stand beside the splintered port prop blade following a 'scuffle' with a Bf 110 on 28/29 April 1942 after bombing Kiel. Flt Lt Bob O'Callaghan, Gunnery Leader, was wounded. The hydraulic system was damaged and the undercarriage and bomb doors stuck in the down position. Fulton failed to return from a raid on Hamburg on 28/29 July 1942 and 419 adopted his nickname in his memory. (via Dr Colin Dring)

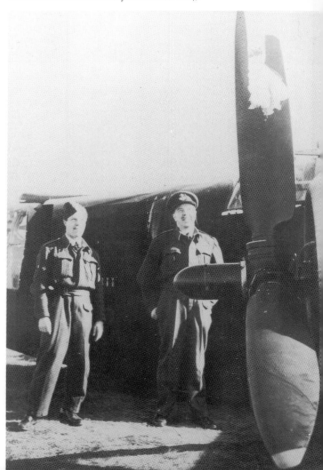

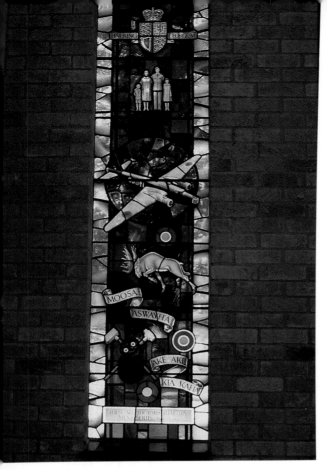

Memorial window at Mildenhall chapel showing (from top) the Royal arms of HM King George VI, the Commonwealth family, Wellington and elements from the crest of 75 New Zealand and 419 Squadron. Quotation was written by Thomas Paine. *(Author)*

Plan Cologne' to his Group Commanders just after midday on 30 May so that 1,000 bombers would be unleashed on the 770,000 inhabitants.

All bomber bases throughout England were at a high state of readiness to get all available aircraft airborne for the momentous raid. No 12 Squadron at Binbrook, for instance, managed to put a record 28 Wellington IIs into the air. To accomplish this task, however, all aircraft had to fly without second pilots and this placed added strain on the crews. Many aircraft came from OTUs and were flown by instructors.

At Mildenhall, No 419 Squadron had eighteen first-line Wellingtons ready. Flight Lieutenant The Honorable Terence Mansfield, the squadron Bombing Leader, who would be flying with his CO, Wing Commander 'Moose' Fulton, recalls: '419 was wholly

equipped with Wellington Mk IIIs and there were crews for every aircraft. "Moose" was not one to take over someone else's aircraft, so he borrowed an elderly 1C from the Blind Approach Training Flight. This normally spent its time flying along our Lorenz beam, training pilots to use it.

'We took off at 23:25 hours. Although 419 was in the first wave, we were not. At approximately 50 mph slower than the Mk IIIs, our 1C was also handicapped by trying to get to the briefed height of 18,000 feet, some 4,000 feet higher than I had ever been before in a Wellington.'

A quarter of the 1,046 aircraft despatched came from No 3 Group which operated in a fire-raising capacity, carrying loads of 4 lb incendiary canisters. In all, some 599 Wellingtons, including four belonging to Flying Training Command, and 338 Stirlings, Halifaxes, Manchesters, Halifaxes and Lancasters made up the attacking force.

Not all of the aircraft reached the target. At 23:28 hours, only 41 minutes after becoming airborne, disaster struck a Wellington II of No 12 Squadron, piloted by Sergeant G. H. Everatt. As the bomber approached the village of Lexham near Dereham in Norfolk, it lost height rapidly and ploughed into woodland at the rear of Lexham Hall.

One of the chief hazards for each crew was the risk of mid-air collision in the highly congested target area. For 98 minutes a procession of bombers passed over Cologne. Stick after stick of incendiaries rained down from the bomb bays of the Wellingtons, adding to the conflagration. Almost all aircraft bombed their aiming point as briefed. Flight Lieutenant Pattison, who piloted a No 419 Squadron Wellington wrote: 'When I bombed there was a huge fire on the east bank of the Rhine and another just starting on the west bank. When I left the target area both sides were getting it thick and fast and eventually, large concentrations of fires were spread practically across the length and breadth of the entire built-up area.'

Terence Mansfield adds: 'We made visual identification on arrival at Cologne and made one circuit of the city before our attack. We then flew round the target again as Moose had a pair of night binoculars which were remarkably effective, but I made no notes of what I could see. I think I must have been more interested in looking down from what seemed such a great height, this being the first occasion on which I had dropped bombs from over 10,000 feet. Our attack was made as ordered; height 17,500 feet; night photograph taken and later plotted within 800 yards of the aiming point. The weather over the target was remarkably clear and not as we had come to expect from the Ruhr area.'

The defenses, because of the attacking force's size, were relatively ineffective and flak was described variously as 'sporadic' and 'spasmodic'. Some enemy fighters were encountered and forty bombers failed to return. In all, 898 crews claimed to have hit their targets. Post-bombing reconnaissance photos certainly showed that more than 600 acres of Cologne had been razed to the ground. The fires burned for days and almost 60,000 people had been made homeless.

Squadrons repaired and patched their damaged Wellingtons and within 48 hours they were preparing for a second 'Thousand Bomber Raid' — this time against Essen. On the night of 1/2 June a force of some 956 aircraft was ready. Again, some bombers returned early with mechanical and engine problems. Although seemingly lacking the concentration of the earlier raid on Cologne, the bombing was nevertheless effective enough to saturate the defences. One skipper went as far as to say that the fires were more impressive than those of Cologne. A belt of fires extended across the city's entire length from the western edge to the eastern suburbs. Many fires were also spread over other parts of the Ruhr.

Losses occurred after the raid. A Wellington II of No 305 (Polish) Squadron, piloted by Flight Lieutenant Hirszbandt, developed engine failure on the homeward leg. The pilot turned into the dead engine while attempting to make an emergency landing and the bomber stalled and crashed in a field at Billingford, Norfolk. All six crew perished in the resulting inferno.

The third 'Thousand Bomber Raid' took place on the night of 25/26 June when 1,006 aircraft, including 102 Wellingtons of Coastal Command, attacked Bremen. Included in the number were at least two crews from No 425

149 Squadron Wellington ICs and their crews at Mildenhall. *(via Dr Colin Dring)*

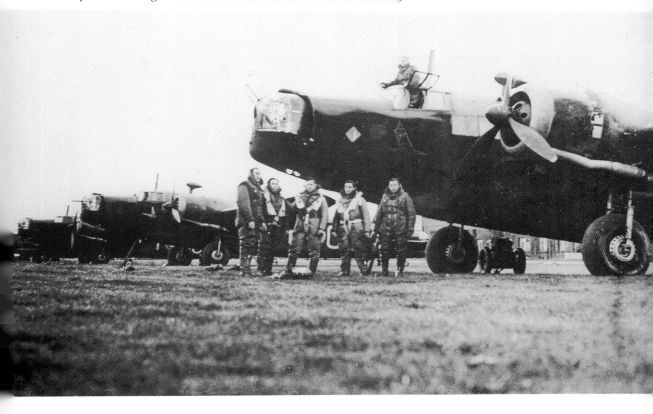

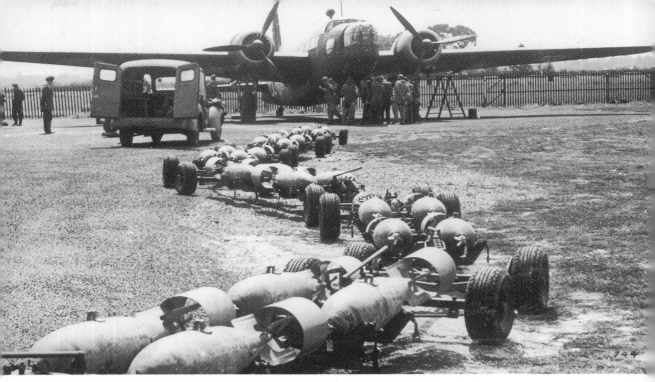

Bombing up a Wellington of 149 Squadron at Mildenhall. *(via Wally Gaul)*

Wellington IC R1230 NZ-E of 304 Squadron was one of seven Wellingtons which failed to return from a raid on Essen on 11 April 1942. *(RAF Museum)*

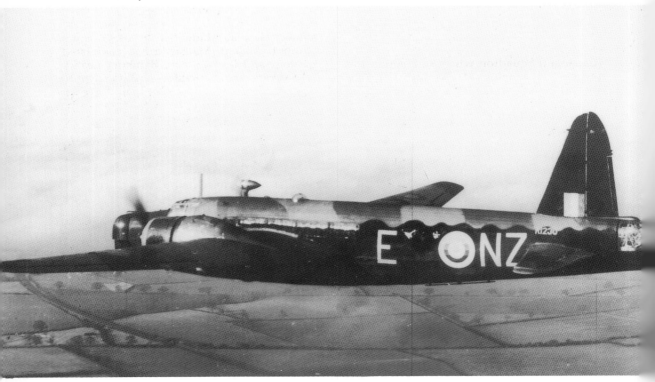

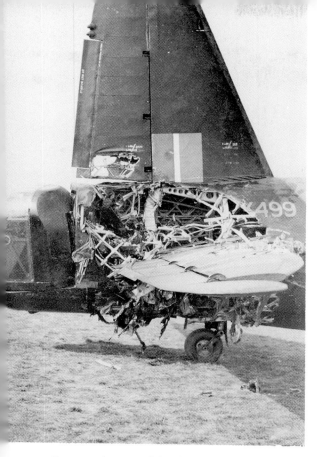

Enemy action caused this damage to Wellington III BK499 of 429 'Bison' Squadron. *(Dr Colin Dring)*

(Canadian) Squadron which was still in the process of forming at Dishforth on the Wellington III. The CO, Squadron Leader 'Joe' St Pierre and his flight commander, Flight Lieutenant Logan Savard, captained their own crews and flew in No 419 Squadron's formation led by Wing Commander 'Moose' Fulton, this time in a Wellington III.

Terence Mansfield, Fulton's Navigator/Bomb Aimer, who was on the 30th and final operation of his tour, recalls: 'We took off at 23:25 hours. Although briefed for a greater height, we found the target area completely covered by cloud and came down to 12,000 feet in the hope of getting some visual identification from which we could start a timed run. We ended up doing what others did, namely bombing what we thought was the most likely place. Not very satisfactory and nor were the results.'

Crews were given the opportunity of either bombing the red glow of the fires, using Gee as a check, or proceeding to a secondary target in the vicinity of Bremen. The cloud conditions prevailed at many of the targets of opportunity and many crews, unable to bomb, brought their lethal cargoes home.

The risk of collision and enemy fighter activity proved a constant threat and crews had to be ever watchful. Squadron Leader Wolfe's No 419 Squadron Wellington was involved in an engagement with an Me 110 night fighter north of Borkum at 4,200 feet over the North Sea. Sergeant D. R. Morrison opened fire and the enemy fighter's port engine was seen to burst into flames, which almost at once engulfed the entire wing. It dived into the sea, leaving a large circle of fire around the point of impact.

'Moose' Fulton and Terence Mansfield landed back at Mildenhall at 04:45 hours without incident. Mansfield had completed his tour and later became Bombing Leader on a squadron of Lancasters. Fulton failed to return from a raid on Hamburg on the night of 28/29 July 1942 and his nickname was incorporated in the official title of the unit.

Bremen was the third and final 1,000 bomber raid in the series of five major saturation attacks on German cities. The German High Command was shaken — while on the home front, morale soared.

Chapter 8
One of our aircraft is missing

As the RAF night bombing offensive gained momentum during the summer of 1942 the stark obituaries began to fill the newspaper columns. More often they read, 'Dead, MIA — believed killed.' One crew, fresh from an OTU, arrived at Marham, Norfolk, to join 'A' Flight, No 115 Squadron, which had managed thus far to keep out of the despairing columns, and was skippered by a Canadian, Flight Sergeant Del Mooney. The front gunner and bomb aimer was Sergeant Joe Richardson; the tail-gunner, Sergeant Bill Margerison. At 21, Sergeant Eddie Killelea, the WOP-AG, was quite a ladies' man and could sing and dance well. His easy rhythm on the dance floor had helped him during Morse training and he had finished top of his course. Sergeant Don Bruce, a 21-year-old Londoner, was the observer. He had already escaped serious injury in an Anson crash at Air Navigation School.

It was the practice for 'green' crews to fly with other operational crews for experience. Thus, Sergeant W. C. 'Norrie' Norrington took the new crew under his wing. On the morning of 6 June they went aloft in *KO-A*, a new Wellington, for an hour of air firing, 'George' (automatic pilot) tests and homing practice using Gee. When they landed the crew passed through the flights and saw the instructions for the ground crews chalked on the boards. It read: '600 gallons of petrol and a standard high explosive bomb load (six 500 pounders and a 1,000 pounder to drop the middle of the stick) for *KO-A*.'

Bruce recalls: 'We knew then we would be on "stand-to" that night. Had the petrol load been 450 gallons it could have meant "Happy Valley" (the Ruhr) or perhaps a "cushy" trip to Paris and the Renault factory. After lunch we spent the time sunbathing and relaxing as far as possible and then around tea time we were briefed and told that the target was Emden.'

Bombing up a Wellington. *(via Wally Gaul)*

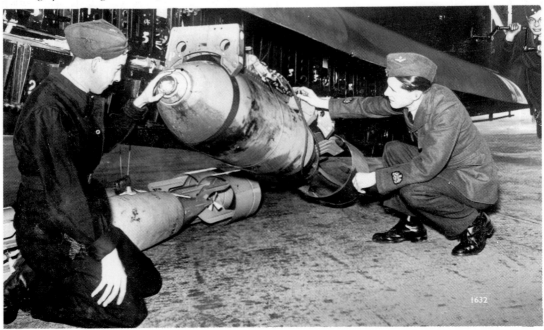

Norrington took off at 23:35 hours. During the trip out he had difficulty getting the 'S' Blower (supercharger) in. Bruce recalls: 'If he had failed we would have stayed at 10,000 feet. He was also worried that the oil temperature on the port engine was too high so he throttled back. Bill Margerison experienced difficulty with his rear turret and it could only be operated manually. Should we turn back? Norrington decided to carry on.

'At 12,000 feet we could see the glow from the target. Apart from the odd flak gun popping off miles out of range we experienced very little hostility. The gunners now began shouting over the intercom warning the pilot of pockets of flak. We started weaving violently.'

Joe Richardson moved forward to the bomb aimer's position, setting the course on the pilot's compass as he passed. He lay prone along the bombing hatch and for the first time got a good view of the target. It was well alight, like a running red sore in the blackness of the night. For a brief moment a bomb aimer could feel sick with horror and the thought, 'My God, there are human beings down there' could enter his mind. Then, too busy to care, the bomb aimer

would return to the task in hand. Richardson set the rotor arm that spaced the stick of bombs. He removed the bomb release from its holder (this automatically fuzed the bombs) and lined up the target in the wires of the bombsight.

The flak was heavy and Norrington weaved desperately as red balls of light flak rose lazily from the ground. They gained impetus, heading straight for the bomb aimer's stomach. Bruce sucked in his breath but the tracer passed like lightning to one side of the aircraft and arced above them. The light flak at Emden did reach to 14,000 feet.

The gunners yelled for the bombs to be dropped so they could be away. The intercom crackled. 'Get over to port, man. Hold it! Bombs gone!' The plane rose, unburdened and free. The Wimpy swung on course and Richardson scrambled back to his cabin. Norrington left the target behind in a shallow dive to increase speed.

The crew relaxed as the Wimpy re-crossed the comparative safety of the open sea. The English coastline came into view and IFF was switched on. Crossing the coast and moving inland everyone had his eyes peeled for Norwich and its balloon barrage. Nearing

Wellington III X3662 KO-P of 115 Squadron, Marham. *(via Mike Bailey)*

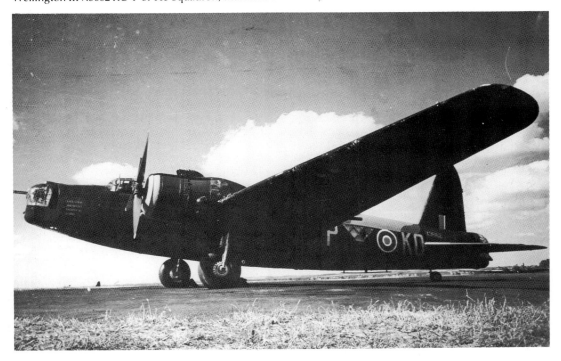

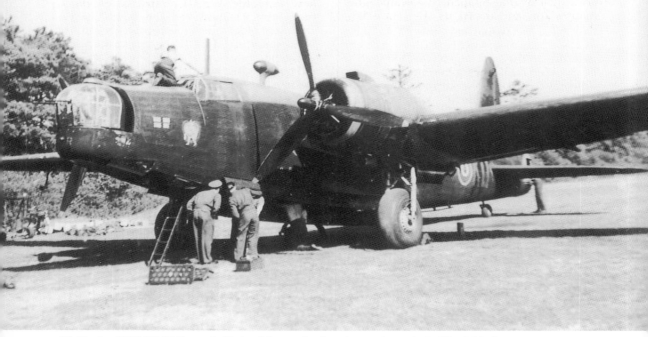

Wellington III Z1657 'R' (formerly 'A-Apple' as retained on the nose) near Lady Wood, Marham, in August/September 1942. *(Jack Goad)*

the aerodrome Norrington started to circle. The undercarriage red light remained on, indicating that the wheels would not lock.

Killelea called up the ground 'Hello Waggon Control, this is "Reveille A-Apple".' There was no reply. After trying several times it was realised that the transmitter had packed up. The receiver was working but the voice was not 'Waggon Control'. They were over the wrong airfield! There was momentary panic until they arrived over Marham. The Wellington crossed the flare path at right angles and fired the double green distress signal. Then Norrington flew over again and 'A' was flashed on the downward identity light.

'Waggon Control' radioed other aircraft to get out of the circuit and Norrington tried a landing. He overshot and the crew braced for a crash landing. Second time round they made it; a beautiful landing. The undercart light was not working. Bruce concludes: 'We climbed out and suddenly my parachute harness weighed a ton. We had returned to base at 04:30 hours on 7 June. A quick de-briefing and then smooth white sheets and a wonderful sleep.'

In between 'ops' air crews 'let their hair down' when they could. On 12 June Bruce, Killelea and Margerison visited nearby King's Lynn. Killelea, attracted by a blonde in the doorway of the 'Eagle' hotel, suggested they paid it a visit. Bruce and Margerison were hungry so they decided to go their own way to a cafe. A short time later, a Dornier, exploiting a hole in the clouds to excellent advantage, made a hit and run attack on the town. Bruce and Margerison finished up under their table. Further down the road the 'Eagle' was flattened. Killelea was among the 42 bodies pulled from the wreckage.

Jack Goad replaced Killelea and Flight Sergeant Del Mooney took over again as captain. On 17 June the crew of *KO-A* flew an operation to the French port of Saint Nazaire. However, the target could not be identified so they could not drop their fourteen 250 lb bombs (RAF crews were not allowed to release bombs over France if the target could not be determined). Returning, Bruce had trouble with his compass, and the ETA for landfall in France came and went. When Bruce finally got his pinpoint worked out he 'nearly had a baby on the spot! I shouted over the intercom. ''Christ, we're right over Brest! Just at that moment the searchlights snapped on and coned us. Del started to weave the Wellington like Hell but flak was already bursting closer. He climbed 500 feet and then dived 500 feet. It was rather sickening for us and as we dived the gravity sucked the fuel from the engines and they cut out. We did not know if we had been hit — only Del knew that. I was absolutely paralysed with fear and what with the table going up and down I couldn't plot a thing.'

Suddenly, Del Mooney snarled over the intercom, 'Give them a stick.' Eight 250-pounders whistled down into the night and as they exploded the searchlights went out. However, the port engine, which ran the hydraulics and the radio, had been put out of action. Mooney turned and limped away from Brest in a northerly direction. Over the sea the remaining eight 250-pounders were jettisoned. The WOP-AG managed to get his transmitter working off batteries and sent out a Mayday distress call which was acknowledged. Bruce was so dejected that he swore that if they got back, he would never fly again.

They did get back. Mooney suggested they

crash-land but the Englishmen aboard warned how hilly the West Country is. Mooney thought they should crash-land on the beach but the crew were worried about mines. Bruce, now standing in the Second Pilot's position, saw runways passing below the bombing panel. 'Hey! We're over an aerodrome!' he exclaimed. It was Exeter. Mooney banked carefully and the aerodrome put its light on. As they made their approach a searchlight was swung onto the Wimpy, almost blinding the swearing Canadian.

Exeter was a fighter airfield and had a different system of lights which no-one understood. Mooney ended up going downwind at 110 mph! Bruce looked back at the undercarriage and could see the wheel banging down. Grimly, he gripped Mooney's seat and as they touched the concrete runway, the wheels folded and the Wimpy collapsed on its belly. Great streaks of sparks shot back from the fuselage. Fortunately, the starboard engine was still operating and it slewed the bomber around in a 180° arc as 'blood wagons' chased them along the runway. They finished up facing the opposite direction.

Everyone got out safely but *KO-A* was

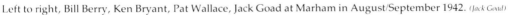

Left to right, Bill Berry, Ken Bryant, Pat Wallace, Jack Goad at Marham in August/September 1942. *(Jack Goad)*

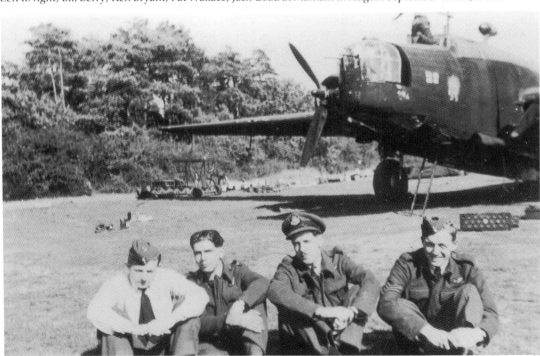

finished for the time being. No-one was sad to see the end of it for the gun turrets had never worked properly. In the afternoon Squadron Leader Cousens flew down from RAF Marham to take the crew home. Next day, 19 June, Bruce had got over the Brest episode and on 20 June the crew returned to operations with an uneventful trip to Emden. Two days later they returned to the German city, this time with a 4,000-pounder in the bomb bay. On 25 June the RAF mounted a thousand bomber raid on Bremen. Mooney's crew visited the city again two days later.

This run of operational bombing sorties was interrupted towards the end of the month. On 30 June Mooney's crew made two search operations over the North Sea for a missing aircrew. Bill Margerison moved from the rear turret to the front and a new rear gunner, Sergeant Ron Esling, joined the crew. Pilot Officer Bill Hancock became the new WOP-AG and flew on the 2 July operation when No 115 Squadron again bombed Bremen.

On 13 July Mooney's crew were alerted for an operation to Duisburg, Germany. They were given a new Wellington, *KO-K*, to replace *KO-A*. By now Mooney's crew were old hands on the squadron, with six weeks' operational experience. This operation would be Don Bruce's eleventh trip; unlucky thirteenth if he counted the two search sweeps over the North Sea.

All through briefing Bruce's mind was on the bomb load they would be carrying deep into Germany. It was a lightly-cased 4,000 lb dustbin-shaped bomb studded with detonators. For maximum blast effect it had a protruding rim to prevent it penetrating too far into the ground. The Wellington had to be stripped of its bomb bay doors and flotation bags to accommodate the sinister weapon and this meant that the bomber would not be able to fly on one engine, or float for long if they had to ditch.

Mooney's crew were to follow in the wake of the main bomber stream. There would be a lull after the main force had finished bombing and the Germans would assume that the raid was over. The rescue services

Wellington IC R1448 'Akyem-Abuakwa' of 218 (Gold Coast) Squadron at Marham in the summer of 1941. *(via Mike Bailey)*

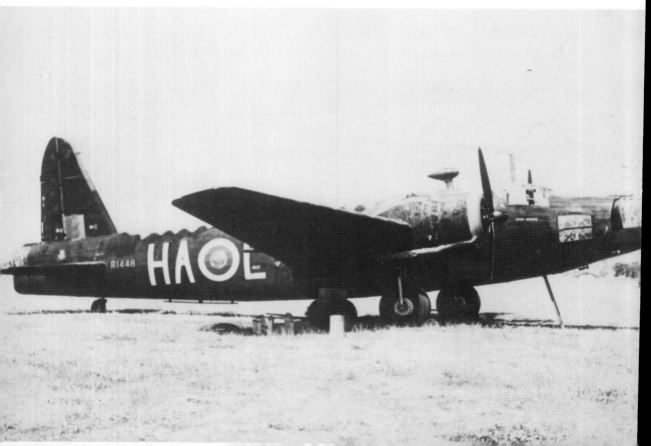

WIRELESS OPERATOR PILOT AND CAPTAIN FRONT GUNNER

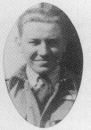

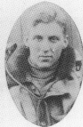

P/O BILL HANCOCK   F/SGT DEL MOONEY   SGT BILL MARGERISO

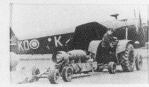

BASE – 115 SQUADRON MARHAM

SGT DON BRUCE   SGT RON ESLING

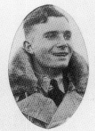

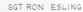

DUISBURG

NIGHT 13/14ᵀᴴ JULY 1942
BAILED OUT NIJNSEL/SON

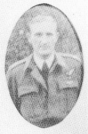

OBSERVER   REAR GUNNER

Photo montage of the crew of KO-K July 1942.
(Don Bruce)

would be in full swing and then *KO-K* would arrive over Duisburg to drop its 'maximum blast' bomb, effectively wiping out any rescue services.

The briefing room was crowded and hot. Wing Commander Dixon-Wright, who was to die a fortnight later bombing Hamburg, addressed the Wellington crews. 'Go for the centre of the town, boys. Plenty of dry timber there. It will burn well. . . after all, they do it to our towns so we do it to theirs.'

In the early hours of 14 July Mooney's crew prepared to take off for Duisburg. Bruce recalls: 'Prior to take-off I was busy preparing the Flight Plan. I collected my bag of navigational instruments, a Met report and operational rations for the crew — usually chocolate, oranges or raisins, chewing gum and six thermos flasks. Finally, we were seated outside the Flights, complete with flying kit and parachutes, ready for transportation to the dispersal points. As each

crew dropped off at their dispersal point we wished them luck. We sat on the grass by *KO-K*. It was still sunlight and we had a long wait. Twenty-eight aircraft from two squadrons [No 218 Squadron's Stirlings shared Marham] got airborne at approximately two minute intervals.

'Tense and nervous, we urinated against the wheels of the aircraft for good luck. As take-off time approached I climbed into the aircraft and set the detonators and diffusers on Gee and its map containers. It was warm inside the aircraft and strangely quiet compared to the noise of the engines outside. Alone for a moment, I looked around the Observer's compartment and wondered what it would be like with a hail of cannon shells from a night fighter ripping through the cabin. Then the rest of the crew began climbing aboard. Del started the engines and we taxied along the perimeter track, maintaining strict W/T silence. The aircraft ahead of us got the "green" from the Aldis lamp and then we were swinging round to face the take-off strip.

'No-one spoke to the pilot, Del must not be distracted. The bomber was heavy and it took all his concentration to get it off the ground. The heavy tail turret, complete with gunner, was raised off the ground as Del jammed on the brakes and pushed the throttles up the gates. The plane shuddered and roared as he pushed the stick forward until it touched the control panel. Slowly, the tail lifted and when the nose pointed slightly downwards he released the brake and we trundled off. We gathered momentum and at 100 mph Del held her down. At 120 mph we lifted off and as I took my hands off the log to note the time, I saw that the place where they had been resting was damp with sweat. Take-off with fuel and bomb load was extremely dangerous.

'We climbed on course, passing out to sea without incident. Still climbing, the gunners asked permission to test fire their guns. The whole structure shuddered as their .30 calibre guns opened up and the reek of cordite filtered through into the cabin. We hoped that no patrolling night fighter had spotted the one in five tracer shells.

'Approaching the Dutch coast we unfolded and locked into position the armour plate doors. These were ostensibly to protect the cabin and pilot's position from rear attack. Still climbing on course, the WOP-AG in the astrodome assisted Ron Esling in his search for night fighters. This was their area. Del started to weave the Wimpy gently from side to side to uncover the blind spot below us for the gunners. 10,000 feet; cold but not unpleasant, we started to use oxygen.'

Approaching Duisburg and running in at 13,000 feet, Mooney became cautious, steering the bomber around the town. Suddenly, he spotted what he had been seeking, another Wellington about 500 feet below and making its run across the target. It was attracting the flak and the searchlights. KO-K followed unmolested. When things became too hot for its crew, the other Wimpy banked away in a dive. KO-K maintained its position, right in the centre of the target.

The Wellington bucked as the 4,000 lb bomb was released. The defences tried to bring them down. All Hell was let loose and the blue 'radar' searchlight on them was joined immediately by other searchlights which formed a cone around them. Mooney had forgotten to put his goggles on and was blinded by the glare. Esling, who had been wounded by flak once before, was shouting over the intercom for Mooney to get out of the beams. Bruce thought, 'We have very little time before our height and course are predicted. Can't shake them off. They are hitting us. A sound like a stick rattling on corrugated iron. The port engine is hit. The pilot in desperation pulls the nose up and up.'

There was an inert sensation before a stall then Mooney swung the bomber over in a stall turn. The Wimpy was now diving in the opposite direction. The searchlights lost the bomber in its exacting gyrations but would the Wellington stand up to the great stress and strain Mooney was imposing upon it?

The bomber plunged to 9,000 feet. Inside, the crew were floating in space. Only the navigation table held Bruce down where it pinned his knees. Accumulators, maps, nuts and bolts and pencils floated past his face. All the time his eyes remained glued to the Observer's airspeed indicator. The needle had started on the inner circle: 320, 330, 340, 350 mph! He read the ever-increasing airspeed indicator with alarm, thinking of the red warning plate mounted on the pilot's control panel which read: 'THIS AIRCRAFT MUST NOT BE DIVED AT SPEEDS IN EXCESS OF 300 MPH'!

Down and down the Wellington dived.

Gravitational force pressed on the hands and arms of the crew, making them feel as heavy as lead and forcing Bruce down into his seat and onto the navigational table. His eyelids began to close involuntarily. Before the 'final squashing process' Mooney somehow managed to pull the Wimpy out of its near fatal dive. The crew could hear him, panting with exertion through his microphone. The crew were as one with the terrible strain that was wrenching at every rivet in the aircraft.

As suddenly as it had begun it was over and, incredibly, the bomber was back on the straight and level. Nuts and bolts and other debris littered the table and floor. The case containing the 'ops' rations had burst open, showering the Observer's table with raisins. In the dim cabin light Don Bruce watched an earwig emerge from the sticky heap.

Bruce gathered his maps from the floor near the bed while Mooney was still fully employed with the joystick and rudder, desperately trying to keep the port wing, with its dead engine, on an even keel. He climbed 500 feet but the starboard engine could not do the work of two and began overheating. As the aircraft levelled out it dropped back again 500 feet. It lost height so rapidly that the crew realised that they would not make the coast. A hurried consultation between Mooney and Bruce resulted in the immediate order of 'Jump, reargunner!' There was no reply from Esling. Bruce was about to investigate when Mooney cried out, 'Don't bother — he's gone.' The Canadian could tell from the trim of the aircraft, which was now flying light in the tail, that he had baled out. If Bruce had been required to turn the turret using the 'dead man's handle' it is doubtful whether he and Mooney would have got out in time.

The forward escape hatch in the Wellington was for use by the Pilot, Wireless Operator, Front Gunner and the Observer. Bill Margerison went through the forward escape hatch first after taking some time to find his parachute, which had been dislodged during the stall turn. Bill Hancock started but almost at once returned to his position to retrieve his gloves! Bruce removed his intercom to prevent strangulation during the parachute descent, loosened his tie (the RAF dressed for war!) and fastened his parachute to his harness. Mooney grinned and gave Bruce the thumbs up. 'Good old Delmer, he's a great guy', thought Bruce.

The Wellington had a diamond-shaped escape hatch on the starboard side, near the bed. It was cut away in the geodetics and either covered with fabric or a trapdoor. This was to be used only in extreme emergency but Don Bruce doubted whether anyone could exit through it with a parachute pack. He was not about to try. He removed his intercom, loosened his tie, fastened his parachute to his harness and moved to the forward escape hatch. Gingerly, he lowered his legs through the hatch. The slipstream caught them like chaff in the wind and he was swept along the underside of the fuselage, his parachute pack jamming against the hatch in the process. Finally, Bruce was wrenched away into the night.

'THE RIPCORD! Pull the ripcord, you fool!' Bruce said to himself. There was a sharp slither of fabric as the pilot 'chute tugged at the main fabric and then a crack like a pistol shot as the cords holding the harness across his chest broke free. There was a terrific jolt and the umbrella of silk opened. He felt sick and hung limply in his harness.

'Suddenly, there was the noise of an aircraft and a terrific whining roar as it dived. Stupidly, I thought it was a night fighter. Then, a flare illuminated me. I thought the fighter was going to fire. I collected my senses and realised it was *KO-K* making her last dive and the flare was *KO-K* erupting into a blossom of fire in the void. Her oxygen bottles burst in brilliant blue flashes. There was a rattle of exploding ammunition and rivers of fire spread with the gouts of petrol from the shattered tanks.'

Dim shapes began to form. Bruce got into a sitting position. The parachute trailing ahead in a light wind caught in a tree. He swung into soft earth and grazed his elbow. He had in fact landed near a farm at Nijnsel in Saint-Oedenrode owned by Mr Van Dijk.

Bruce shouted 'Hello!' A woman gave a piercing scream and both Van Dijk and his seventeen year-old son, William, who were outside thinking that a German aircraft had crashed, ran inside (there was a curfew and Dutch people were not allowed outside at this hour). They peered through a window and saw Bruce take off his Mae West and make off down the road. He was alone in a strange country.

The Wellington had been shot down at approximately 03:30 hours. Ron Esling, the first man to bale out, had landed in a farmyard. His first reaction was to go to sleep; a sure sign of shock. He did not sleep long. He decided to open his survival kit. Not wishing to be caught with what was essentially a 'spy kit', Esling proceeded to eat all the edible maps, water purification tablets, 'uppers and downers' pills and chocolate! Feeling drunk and after trying, unsuccessfully, one of the many farm labourer's houses around the farm, Esling tottered into the village of Son. Esling hammered happily on the door of a most imposing house which, as it turned out, belonged to the Burgomeister and his charming and pregnant wife. The Burgomeister was a pleasing fellow and he took the fallen flier in.

Esling was hardly the picture of sartorial elegance and so the mayor called for a barber. A shave and haircut improved the airman's morale. However, the mayor informed him that, much to his regret, he would have no option but to turn him over to the authorities because he had already attracted too much attention in the district. He asked Esling what branch of the military would he like to take him into custody. Esling replied, 'the Luftwaffe'. In his current state of mind he would not have been surprised to have said 'the Gestapo.'

The pills were having an effect and Esling dozed off to sleep again. He was awakened by a Luftwaffe field policeman standing before him and shouting at the top of his voice. Esling thought he looked like someone in a play. The German had just shaved because he still had talcum powder on his face. Around his neck hung an illuminated plaque and he wore the familiar 'piss pot' helmet on his head. There the comedy stopped. Amid a tearful farewell, Esling was marched into custody.

Meanwhile, Bill Hancock had also been captured. He had almost landed on top of the burning Wellington but had managed to pull the shrouds of his parachute and just missed a fiery death. He landed in a field full of cows, twisting his ankle in the process. While he struggled to his feet two very young German soldiers rushed him and arrested the fallen airman.

Meanwhile, Don Bruce had left the scene of the crash at the Van Dijk's farm. The farmer and his son, William, peered out through the window and saw the British airman make off down the road. Later, a

German patrol visited the Van Dijks. They asked, 'Where is the Tommy?' The Van Dijks gesticulated, using sign language, that he had 'gone away'. The Germans did not believe them and a soldier levelled a machine-gun at them while four others searched the farmyard and drove stakes into the hay loft.

Bruce met a man out of the darkness pushing a bicycle. He eyed the British airman suspiciously. Bruce discovered only much later that in this particular part of Holland the Dutch had not seen RAF personnel before and to them the RAF uniform was very similar to the German one. After an amusing tug of war over the bicycle the Dutchman realised that Bruce was not a German and he led him to a cottage. Bruce tried unsuccessfully to converse in English and then French.

Just at that moment footsteps could be heard along the road. They were Germans! The Dutchman panicked, shut the door and left Bruce standing alone on the porch. Luckily, the German patrol ignored him. Taking no further chances, Bruce ran down the road in the opposite direction. The following morning he had another close shave when a German staff car roared past but did not stop. It was just another example of what an RAF airman on the run could get away with at this stage of the war.

Bruce eventually arrived at Nijnsel. He remembered what he had been told at evasion briefings: 'Head for large houses where the inhabitants are thought to be better educated and therefore able to speak English.' Bruce chose a large building but it turned out to be the Presbytery of the village church. He knocked at the door and a grille opened to reveal the face of an elderly person (he could not determine who it was in the darkness). Bruce pointed to his RAF brevet and said, 'RAF'. The figure replied, 'Nein, nein'. Later, Bruce was to discover that it was a woman cleaner and that she was stone deaf!

It was the final straw. Soaking wet from a rainstorm and suffering from shock, Bruce wandered around the village in despair. He thought of giving himself up. No-one appeared to want to help. Although he did not know it, there was no resistance group in the area and there was little chance of getting back to England. In desperation he approached some of the congregation who were leaving the church. Van de Laar, a seventeen-year-

Wim Van Dijk's (2nd left in uniform) family in front of their farmhouse where Don Bruce landed (his 'chute hooked up in the tree on the right. *(Don Bruce)*

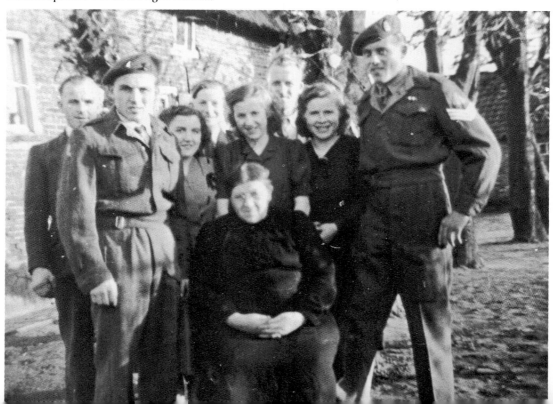

old Dutch boy, listened to the airman. He did not understand that Bruce wanted a telephone so that he could give himself up. The Dutch took Bruce to the house of Pieter Bekkers, the village baker who had a telephone. People from miles around came to see the British airman on whose country so many Dutch pinned their hopes. Many peered through the baker's windows and others came inside and shook Bruce's hand.

Anna Bekkers, the baker's wife, asked Bruce how old he was. By means of sign language he drew the figure '21'. Mrs Bekkers threw her arms in the air and began crying. Bruce thought, 'My God, does she think I'm too young to die?' He was physically and mentally exhausted by now and really believed he might be shot by a firing squad.

Meanwhile, Bill Margerison had had better luck. He had fallen in a wheat field about three miles from where Don Bruce had landed. He lay low until the following morning when a passing friendly Dutch civilian escorted him to a farmhouse between Son and Nijnsel. Van de Laar was despatched to find him. Margerison accompanied the young Dutchman on a bicycle and was reunited with Don Bruce at the Bekkers' house.

Pieter Bekkers wanted to hide both the British airmen but Bruce knew the situation was hopeless and told him he must hand them in; Bekkers reluctantly telephoned the Burgomeister. He agreed with Bruce. So many people had seen the two men that one might inform the Germans. The Burgomeister summoned Police Chief Eikenaar, head of the Dutch Police in the area, and aided by two Luftwaffe officers he arrested the two British airmen.

Bruce and Margerison were taken to the Burgomeister's house in Son where Ron Esling was under house arrest. All three men were taken to a Luftwaffe airfield at Eindhoven where they were joined by Del Mooney. The Canadian explained that he had baled out of the doomed Wellington with great difficulty. Hancock had clipped on Mooney's parachute but had only fastened it on one side. It was never easy to exit from a Wellington in distress because the pilot had to crawl underneath his seat and leave by the escape hatch in the floor.

As Mooney left his seat, the Wellington began rising on its one remaining engine and started circling. As if that was not enough,

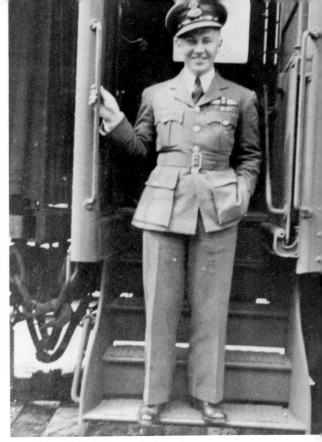

A smiling F/O Del Mooney in Canada after repatriation from Germany. *(via Don Bruce)*

Mooney had to get his parachute clipped on properly and fight his way down to the escape hatch. When he had finally got to the floor the 'Wimpy' had lurched into a dive, hurtling to earth at frightening speed. It had taken a frenzied surge of strength on the part of Mooney to extricate himself. He just managed to get clear at only five hundred feet. The time lapse between his baling out and the Wellington crashing was so slight that he had almost landed on top of the burning bomber.

The crew were re-united with Bill Hancock and after four days at Eindhoven were put on a train for Amsterdam. There they were put in cells below ground for two days. Hancock was retained for more questioning and then sent to Stalag Luft III but Mooney, Margerison, Bruce and Esling were sent to the Dulag Luft Interrogation Centre outside Frankfurt. (Stalag Luft III was for officers only.)

Their train steamed across the flat lands of Holland and through the German countryside to Cologne. The city had been devastated three weeks before by an RAF 1,000-bomber raid and feeling among the German civilians was running high. The station was extremely crowded with the evacuation still in progress. The sight of RAF uniforms aroused deep hatred and the prisoners had to be locked in a small room for their own protection.

Although the train was overcrowded the escort party and their prisoners had a reserved compartment. Bruce sat down and glanced casually through the window towards the platform. An elderly German rushed over, fixed his eyes on the British airman, swore profusely and then spat on the window. Apparently, he objected to the RAF having seats and, eventually, he succeeded in getting them moved out of the compartment. Bruce and his fellow crew members spent the journey to Frankfurt standing in the corridor.

At Dulag Luft, Mooney's crew signed the visitors' book, checking to see if there were any other crews that had been shot down on the Duisburg raid. It was not until after the war that Bruce discovered that they were one of five crews shot down on the raid and according to the visitors' book, the only survivors.

The four airmen were marched away to solitary confinement, interrogation and eventual processing for onward trans-mission to PoW camps. On 19 July they were despatched to Stalag Luft VIIIB at Lamsdorf to begin almost three years of tedious and sometimes painful internment behind barbed wire. Ironically, their route took them past Duisburg. Much to the amusement of the escorting German Officer, Bruce and his fellow crew members were surprised at the lack of bomb damage around the city.

Chapter 9
Bomber finale

'Hamburg lay behind us and we were on course, homeward bound, flying between Bremerhaven and Wilhelmshaven, when "Frizzo" Frizzell piped up from the rear turret, "What about a bloody drink? I'm gasping." Jack French, the WOP-AG, was just about to hand me a cup of coffee when, BANG! We were hit in the port engine.

'The smoke and havoc was appalling. I feathered the port engine and managed to bring her head round. Fortunately, no-one was hurt. Len Harcus came out of the front turret to hang on to the rudder bar to try to help counter the violent swing to port. I took stock of the situation and tried to increase boost and revs on the starboard engine, but to no avail. By this time we were losing height.'

It was the night of 26/27 July 1942; a week after *KO-K* had failed to return to Marham, its stablemate 'B-Bear', piloted by Jim Burtt-Smith on his ninth operation, was about to suffer the same fate. Burtt-Smith continues: 'I got Barney D'Ath-Weston, my Navigator, to give me a new course for home. Heavy ack-ack was still pounding away. We were heading for the open sea and try as I might, I could not gain any height. As we headed over the coast the searchlights pointed our way to the fighters. We were now down to 1,000 feet. I told Jack to let out the sixty-foot trailing aerial. We were having a terrible time trying to keep the aircraft straight and level. The drag of the dead engine was pulling us to port. I applied full rudder bias and Len hung onto the rudder for dear life. It was

Crew of KO-B, taken in the winter of 1941 at 11 OTU Bassingbourn, Cambs. Left to right, P/O E. H. D'Ath-Weston RNZAF, Observer; Sgt W. Frizzell RNZAF, Rear Gunner; Sgt Len Harcus, Bomb Aimer; Sgt Jim Burtt-Smith, Pilot; Sgt J. French, WOP. *(via Don Bruce)*

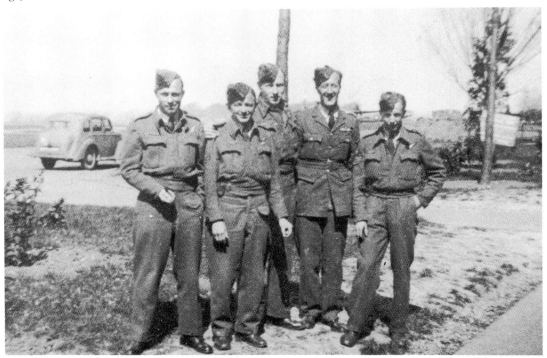

impossible to set a straight course. I gave instructions, ninety miles out over the North Sea, to take positions and prepare for ditching. It was as black as a November fog; no moon, no nothing.

'As Jack and Len left the cockpit I jettisoned the fuel, shut off the remaining engine and turned towards England. I had no idea of height because when the port engine failed, so did the lights and instruments. Jack clamped the morse key down so our people could get a fix on us. I told him to give me a shout when the aerial touched the water so I knew I had sixty feet of height left. I had to keep playing with the stick to keep her airborne, letting the nose go down then pulling her up a bit, just like a bloody glider. I prayed for a moon, knowing full well that if I couldn't see to judge which way to land we would plunge straight in and down. (One had to land towards the oncoming waves; any other way would be disastrous.)

'Jack shouted out, "Sixty feet!" and there we were, wallowing about like a sick cow. I shouted to the lads to hold tight, we were going in. "Frizzo" turned his turret to starboard so that he could get out when we crashed. This was it! Prepare to meet thy doom. Suddenly, the moon shone and, thank God, I could see the sea. The moon beams were like a gigantic flarepath. We actually flew down them. We were practically down in the drink when I saw we were flying the wrong way. I lugged "B-Bear" around, head on to the waves. I hauled back on the stick and there was one almighty crash. We were down!

'The water closed over my head and my Mae West brought me to the top. I got my head out of the escape hatch and there we were, wallowing in the sea. Then the moon went in! It was again as black as it could be. Len helped me out of the cockpit. Jack popped out of the astro hatch carrying the emergency kit, followed by D'Ath, who had stayed to destroy the Gee box and papers. "Frizzo" scuttled along the fuselage and we all scrambled into the dinghy which had popped out of the engine nacelle and was inflating in the water, still attached to the

New Zealand High Commissioner Mr Jordan shakes hands with W/O Bernet DFM during a visit to 75 (NZ) Squadron at Mildenhall on 8 October 1942. *(via Dr Colin Dring)*

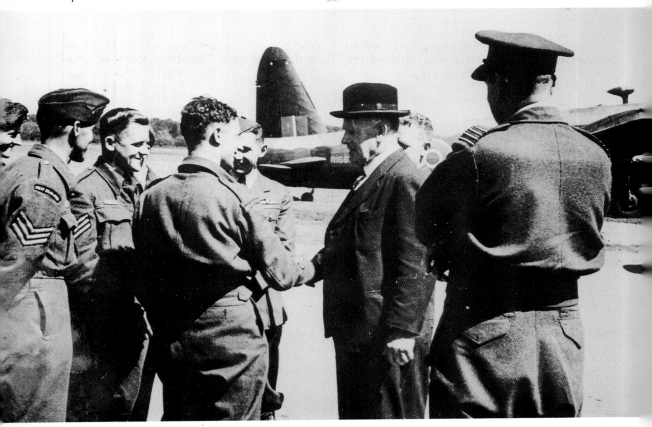

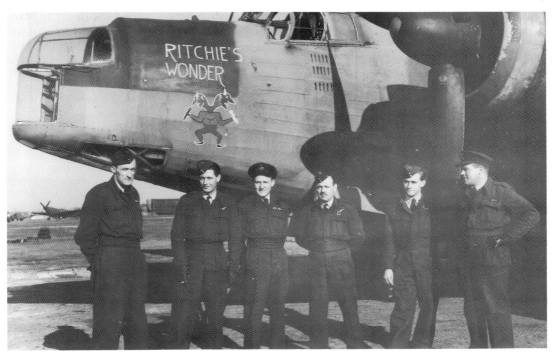

PR XIII 'Ritchie's Wonder' of 69 Squadron, 2nd TAF, at Melsbroek in October 1944. *(RAF Museum)*

Wimpy, which was sinking fast. D'Ath slashed the rope and we pulled away as best we could before we got sucked under.'

'B-Bear's' crew were picked up by a German seaplane from Nordeney and finished the war as PoWs. Three other crews, all from 'A' Flight, also failed to return to Marham.

In August it was decided to move Marham from No 3 Group to No 2 Group and when, on 24 September No 115 Squadron moved to Mildenhall, Marham's association with the Wellington came to an end. For the remainder of the war the station became the Main Operating Base for the Mosquito.

A few weeks previously, on 14 August 1942, No 419 'Moose' Squadron (re-named after its Commanding Officer, Wing Commander John 'Moose' Fulton who had been killed in a raid on Hamburg on the night of 28/29 July), had left Mildenhall for Leeming, to be replaced by No 75 (New Zealand) Squadron. The Canadians were renowned throughout the Mildenhall area for their high spirits and were greatly missed.

Meanwhile, on 27 August, at Waltham, Lincolnshire, No 142 Squadron prepared for a raid on a German army headquarters and garrison at Kassel. Norman Child, the Radio Operator in Pilot Officer Alan Gill's crew in 'B' Flight, recalls: 'At briefing we were told to expect the target to be heavily defended. We carried a mixed load of 500 lb bombs and incendiaries. The Met report was "good visibility" over the target. Wind, "light westerly". We were routed in ten miles south of Münster. Same route out.'

Gill's Wellington was airborne at 21:45 hours and they climbed to 9,000 feet. Child wrote: 'Flak ships were very active off the Dutch coast. No trouble so far. Visibility good. Lots of flak up ahead. Somebody must have wandered off course over Münster. Good pin-point. Approaching target and all hell let loose approximately ten miles ahead. Very heavy barrage — town ringed with guns and searchlights. Several kites have been hit and gone down.

'Running into target now — terrific smell of cordite — searchlights are blinding but drop bombs on schedule at 8,500 feet. Weave out of target area and for a few minutes everything is chaos. Set course for home. Same route as course in. Difficult to get a good pinpoint and aircraft ahead running into heavy flak . . . shouldn't be any flak on this course.

'Check the wind again. There has been a sudden terrific wind change round to the north and the whole force has been blown over the Ruhr Valley. Searchlights and flak are forcing us lower and lower and many aircraft are seen to go down. The flak is so bad and the searchlights so blinding, we decide to go right down full power to below a thousand feet. Front and rear turrets are firing at the searchlights and between them they account for five. We burst our way out of the Ruhr, knowing that we have been hit many times and climb up to 8,000 feet again. We make for "Over Flakkee" (an island off the Dutch coast just south of the Hook of Holland and an aiming point for a comparatively quiet exit from the Continent).'

Gill's Wellington was not the only No 142 Squadron aircraft to have trouble with the German searchlights. Flight Lieutenant Ron Brooks, DFC, and crew in 'A' Flight were returning from their target at Kassel when they saw several Wellingtons 'coned' by many searchlights. Arthur Johnson, the front gunner, recalls: 'Flight Sergeant Jim Oldham, our Navigator, told us later that several aircraft were shot down between Hamm and Münster. Our Skipper was unable to get out of the searchlights in spite of violent evasive action. He gave orders that we were to watch out for fighters; he was going down the lights. We managed to get five with our guns before the Skipper levelled out. All the lights went out and the flak stopped. Jim Oldham said we must be somewhere south of the Ruhr and gave us a rough course to the coast.'

Both Brooks' and Gill's Wellingtons succeeded in reaching England safely but both aircraft were forced to land at Harwell. Norman Child surveyed his Wellington and wrote later: 'Our aircraft looks a mess. Full of holes and big chunks off but, miraculously, except for cuts and abrasions, none of the crew is hurt.' Ron Brooks' crew found much the same scene at their dispersal. Arthur Johnson recalls: 'When we went out to the old Wimp later in the day the WAAF riggers had done a fine job patching the holes up and retrieving some of the shrapnel from the fuselage.'

Both Brooks' and Gill's crews had been lucky. The squadron had lost five aircraft. Norman Child wrote: 'The next day we were flown back to Waltham to discover, to our horror, that of the six aircraft from "B" Flight,

our crew were the only survivors. The Met report, or lack of one, could be held responsible for the debacle over the Ruhr Valley and the consequent loss of aircraft and crews force-landing all over south of England, out of fuel.'

On 8 September the Wellingtons of No 142 Squadron struck at Frankfurt-on-Main. Norman Child wrote: 'We carried one 4,000 lb "cookie". Our route out took us via Over Flakkee, south of Cologne, Koblenz and then due east to Frankfurt. The Met report said it would be probably hazy over the target but otherwise, good.

'Airborne at 20:20 hours. Set course for Over Flakkee and climbed to 10,000 feet. Cloud thicker than expected over Holland and we fly in cloud up to the German border. Break in the cloud and we get a good pinpoint on the Maas. Steered well clear of Cologne but plenty of flak to port suggests that a number of aircraft have wandered off course in cloud and are over the city. Cloud now clearing and only 3/10ths cover. North of Mainz we are attacked by a night fighter and he scores a hit on our tail fin. "Jock" Sloan, the rear gunner, gives him a burst and we weave and dive our way to safety.

'Approaching target we detect a Halifax just overhead with its bomb doors open. We take quick avoiding action and prepare for our own run in. Very heavy defences and well predicted flak. Enormous flash in the sky and flaming debris falling — looks as though two aircraft have collided.

'Dropped our "cookie" into the middle of a huge circle of explosions and fires and dived away into the night. Checked on the damage to tail but although it looked a ragged sight, it was still functioning satisfactorily. Steered course for home north of Koblenz and south of Cologne.

'Brief encounter with flak ship off Dutch coast and a few more holes punched into us. None of the crew hurt. Message from base: 'Weather closed in — visibility very poor. Divert to Waterbeach". Landed at Waterbeach. Duration of flight: 6 hours 55 minutes. Riggers inspected the tail unit and the damage was so severe they were amazed that the whole structure hadn't collapsed. The Wellington is a tough baby.'

At this stage of the war a number of Wellington ICs were still in use with OTUs and when a maximum effort was required, extra aircraft were used from OTUs to make up numbers. Noel 'Chris' Croppi, a Pilot Instructor with No 16 OTU at Upper Heyford and veteran of all three 1,000-bomber raids (on Lancasters), recalls: 'The Wellington IC was a shock after the Lancaster and I had a crew who had not completed OTU and had no operational experience! Our first op was to Düsseldorf on 10 September. There was the usual flak and searchlights but nothing particularly alarming.'

It was differerent two nights later, on 13 September, when Bomber Command struck at Bremen. Croppi recalls: 'This was a real horror. Our Wellington was a very old IC in poor condition. I could only obtain a maximum height of 10,000 feet and we ran out of oxygen before reaching the target. There was very heavy flak. I had been to Bremen many times before so I knew what to expect.

'After completing the bombing run I asked the Navigator for a course direct to base. He gave me 178° — almost due south. I told him

in very choice language that even if he wanted to finish up in China, I did not and I was going to fly 278 degrees! (Things were a bit desperate in 1942 — we were losing about nine out of ten aircrew before they finished their tour.)

'Long before we reached the coast of England, while over the North Sea, ALL petrol gauges were registering ZERO: more panic! The Wellington had two reserve fuel tanks, one in each engine nacelle, but the pilot could not turn them on and there were no gauges on them. We only knew that they held about fifty gallons each. Therefore, I sent the front gunner to sit on the main spar and hook his index fingers into each pull ring, which opened the valves and pull if we needed fuel. As it turned out we never used them. Duff gauges, but as I said, these aircraft were real old.

'We eventually hit the coast at least fifty miles north of track. The Navigator had by this time almost given up (he was grounded

An unscheduled visitor at Chipping Warden on 20 September 1944 was this Mk III HF754 OX-U of 22 OTU, Wellesbourne Mountford. On a cross country training flight the port engine failed; a forced landing was attempted at Chipping Warden but the approach was too fast and the aircraft over-shot. The damage caused when it hit an air raid shelter required works repair. *(Michael L. Gibson)*

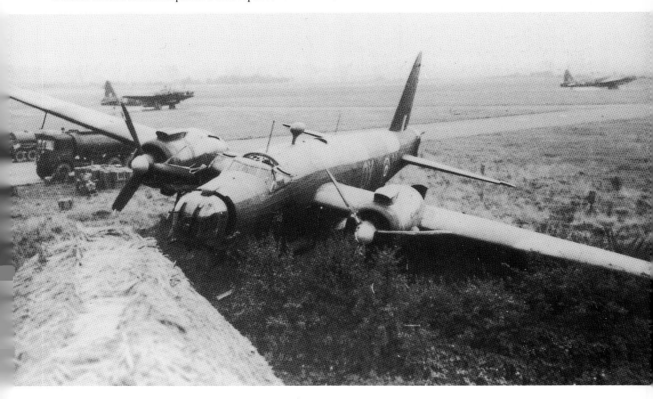

after this trip) but we spotted a beacon and eventually made it back to base.'

In October a directive was issued that crews stood down from night flying would be well employed on daylight intruder missions and so keep the enemy sirens wailing and the work benches empty. Norman Child recalls: 'Our black-painted Wellingtons were quite unsuitable for this type of work and, to the crews, plain suicidal, but orders were orders.

'On 23 October the order was to penetrate well into Germany, circle for a while and return. The Met report was two layers of cloud and 10/10ths at 6,000 feet with clear sky between the layers, "these conditions extending from the English coast to central Europe".

'Airborne at 12:40 hours. Climbed to 8,500 feet and flew in upper layer for approximately one hour. When over the Dutch coast, the cloud started to thin and we ran into clear sky. Immediately, we dived for the thick lower layer and continued on course at 6,500

feet. It was noticeable that the cloud was beginning to thin and after three quarters of an hour we suddenly ran out into clear sunshine, many miles short of the German border.

'We steep-turned back into cloud and headed home at full throttle, volubly cursing all the "duff gen merchants" and what they could do with their forecasts. We came unscathed through light flak at the Dutch coast and flew low in thick cloud to avoid fighters. Duration of flight: three hours thirty minutes.'

The following day Wellingtons of No 142 Squadron flew down to Manston in Kent to refill overload tanks for a bombing operation to Milan. Each Wellington carried a mixed bomb load of 500 lb bombs and canisters of incendiaries. The Met report indicated fine weather, good visibility and light, variable winds.

Child recorded: 'Airborne 16:30 hours. Landed Manston 17:30 hours. Took on fuel for overload tanks. Airborne again 19:15

German officers make a close inspection of Wellington III BJ780 of 12 Squadron, Wickenby, which was brought down near Lorient during a minelaying sortie on 9 October 1942. *(Rupert Cooling)*

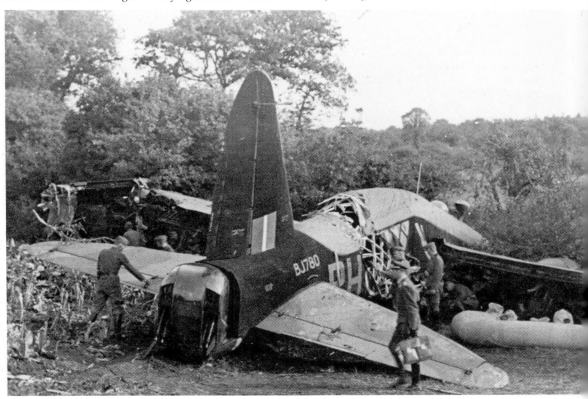

hours. Climbed to 9,000 feet over France. Clear starlit night. Fighter reported on starboard bow cruising at same speed so we throttle back and descend to 15,000 feet to clear Swiss Alps — extremely cold. Good pinpoint on Lake Geneva to port and mountain range looming ahead. Mont Blanc identified quite easily in clear night air and set new course for target.

'Box barrage over target which quietens down when bombing commences (unlike German targets) and we bomb through comparatively little opposition. Many fires started and large explosions seen. Bombed at 12,000 feet. Turned on course for base and climbed back to 15,500 feet. At course change at Haute Savoie we notice the port engine is leaking oil badly and beginning to overheat. The port engine is throttled right back and we start a very slow descent across France to keep up a reasonable airspeed. Everyone is keyed up and anxious.

'We reach the French coast at 3,000 feet and pinpoint St Valery. Everything is quiet and we steal out to sea untouched. The port engine temperature is now so high we decide on a forced landing at West Malling. They cleared us for emergency landing and when we taxied to a halt the port engine died. The fitters found an oil feed line had been damaged by a shell splinter and the engine was starved of oil. Across France we had the choice of feathering the prop and probably a forced landing there, or pressing on and risking the engine catching fire. We made the right choice — just. Duration of flight: seven hours fifty minutes.'

On 7 November No 142 Squadron ventured to the harbour approaches at Brest for a minelaying operation, three miles south of Point de St Mathieu. The Wellingtons were to drop the mines from a height of 700 feet at ten second intervals. The Met report indicated that visibility would be fair but deteriorating with an approaching front.

Pilot Officer Gill's Wellington was airborne at 21:10 hours. Norman Child recalls: 'We climbed to 6,000 feet and set course for Portland Bill. Cloud was thickening inland but clearer over the sea. We set course for Ushant Island from Portland Bill. Midway to Ushant our radio receiver reported U/S — but our transmitter was OK. We decided to continue to the target whilst the fault on the receiver was traced.

'Ushant Island was identified approx five miles to port. It was a dark night but visibility was reasonably good. No joy with the receiver. We made a wide turn out to sea and descended to dropping height. Engines throttled right back and mines dropped on time track in the harbour approach. Opened up engines and executed tight turn to port to avoid the town. Halfway on turn, and climbing, there was a terrific explosion aft and the aircraft was almost out of control. Ground fire continued for a few minutes but we were not hit again.

'We set course for base and climbed to 4,000 feet at reduced revs. The damage was inspected and we discovered an enormous hole blasted out of the underbelly and side. A freezing gale was raging through the aircraft and we brought the rear gunner forward of the damage. Over southern England the weather had worsened with thick cloud and light rain. We descended to 2,000 feet, still in cloud. We called base, reported the damage and the receiver U/S. We checked that the undercarriage would lock down and we landed. Cloud ceiling at base was 700 feet. Duration of flight: 7 hours 45 minutes.

'With our receiver U/S we did not know that there had been a general recall and, as a consequence, we were the only aircraft from No 1 Group flying that night! We should have aborted with a U/S receiver and earned ourselves a reprimand. However, a couple of days later we heard that an enemy freighter had struck a mine and blew up in Brest harbour approach which, to this day, we always claim as "ours".'

The decision to form a new Canadian command had been taken in 1942 and a headquarters was established at Allerton Park, Yorkshire, on 1 December 1942. Nos 420, 424 and 425 Squadrons of the RCAF were selected in January 1943, along with other Canadian bomber squadrons, to form No 6 Group RCAF, which officially became operational on 1 January 1943. At Leeming Nos 408 (equipped with the Halifax) and 424 Squadrons took up residence, and Nos 419 (also equipped with the Halifax) and 420 took up station at Middleton St George. Dishforth became home to Nos 425 and 426 Squadrons, while Croft accommodated No 427 Squadron. At Dalton, No 428 Squadron moved in. A sixth airfield at Skipton-on-Swale was still under construction.

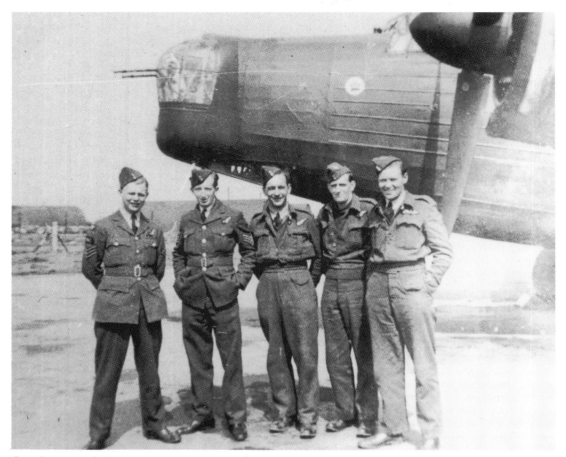

Canadian crew of 427 (Lion) Squadron at Croft on 12 April 1943. Left to right: Sgt Charles Lott, WOP; Sgt Jack Hamer RCAF, Rear Gunner; Sgt Stuart Brown RCAF, Navigator; Sgt Cletus Lunny RCAF, Bomb Aimer and Sgt Alex Mitchell, Pilot. *(G. Stuart Brown)*

On the night of 3/4 January 1943 No 6 Group flew its first operation when six Wellingtons of No 427 Squadron were despatched to lay mines off the Frisian Islands. By March some seven Canadian Wellington squadrons were operating within Nos 4 and 6 Groups of Bomber Command. On 10 March Sergeant Alex Mitchell (a Scot) and his crew, most of whom were Canadian, were posted to No 427 Squadron. At first the crew were given daily assignments to test the flight capabilities of their Mk X and to install new equipment. Stuart Brown, the crew's Navigator, from Brandon, Canada, recalls: 'On 16 April we flew our first op; an uneventful trip to Mannheim with 3,500 lb of bombs. On 28 April we flew a very dicey do, minelaying

near sea level on the Elbe estuary, from which only four out of ten aircraft from our squadron returned.

'Immediately following this trip 427 Squadron was reorganised to become 1664 Conversion Unit for the training of crews to fly the larger Halifax bombers. Senior crews were posted in from other Wellington squadrons and in May our crew was posted to 428 Squadron to continue operations from Dalton, Yorkshire. May 1943 saw the beginning of the Battle of the Ruhr and our crew flew five trips. Following the trip to Düsseldorf on 11 June we were posted back to 427 Squadron for conversion to the Halifax.'

Other movements of Canadian squadrons during January to November 1943 were:

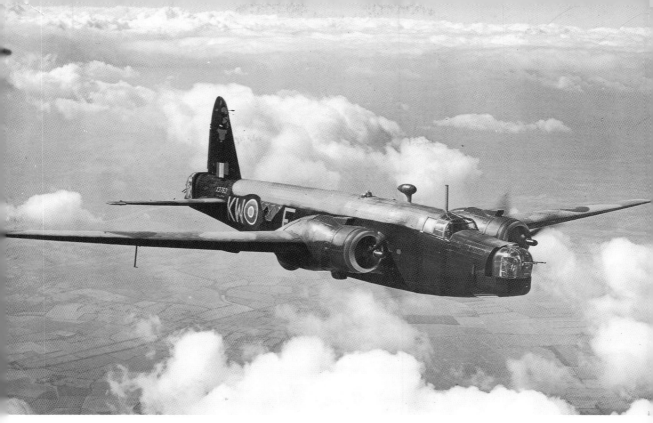

Wellington III X3763 KW-E of 425 (Alouette) Squadron RCAF which failed to return from a raid on Stuttgart on 15 April 1943. *(IWM)*

RCAF/RAAF Wellington Squadron Dispositions Bomber Command December 1942–November 1943				
1942:		**SQUADRON**	**GRP**	**STATION**	**REMARKS**
Dec	14	427 (Lion)	6	Croft, Co Durham	Debut, mine-laying off Frisian Islands
1943:					
Jan	13	466 (RAAF)	4	Leconfield, Yorks	Debut, mine-laying off Frisian Islands
Jan	14/15	426 (Thunderbird)	6	Linton-on-Ouse, Yorks	Debut, Lorient
Jan	15/16	424 (Tiger)	6	Topcliffe, Yorks	Bombing debut, Lorient
Jan	15/16	466 (RAAF)	6	Leconfield, Yorks	Bombing debut, Lorient
Jan	15/16	427 (Lion)	6	Croft, Co Durham	Bombing debut, Lorient
Jan	21	429 (Bison)	4	East Moor, Yorks	Debut, Mk III
Jan	26/27	428 (Ghost)	6	Dalton, Yorks	Debut, 5 a/c to Lorient
Mar	2/3	431 (Iroquois)	6	Burn, Yorks	Debut, 8 Mk X mines off Frisian Islands
Mar	5/6	431 (Iroquois)	6	Burn, Yorks	Bombing debut, Essen
May	23/24	432 (Leaside)	6	Skipton-on-Swale, Yorks	Bombing debut 14 Mk X to Dortmund
Oct	5/6	425 (Aloutte)	6	Dishforth, Yorks	Debut 4 a/c to Aachen
Nov	6	419 (Moose)	6	Croft, Co Durham	Last op, 3 a/c on 'moling' to Wilhelmshaven before conversion to Halifax II

Wellington movements Bomber Command May 1942–October 1944		
Date	Squadron	Remarks
1942:		
May	304	Posted to Coastal Command
June	158	Converted to the Halifax
July	103	Converted to the Halifax
August	9	Converted to the Lancaster
September	57	Converted to the Lancaster
September	460	Converted to the Halifax
October	101	Converted to the Lancaster
November	12	Converted to the Lancaster
November	75	Converted to the Stirling
November	419	Converted to the Halifax
December 6/7	199	Op debut, 5 bomb Mannheim
1943:		
January 27/28	166	Op debut, 7 Mk IIIs (mines)
January 29/30	166	Op bombing debut, Lorient
January	156	Converted to the Lancaster
February 4/5	196	Op bomb debut, Lorient
March	301	Trans to 38 (SD) Squadron
April	425	Posted to North Africa
May	424	Posted to Algeria
May	427	Converted to the Halifax
June	426	Converted to the Lancaster
June	428	Converted to the Halifax
June	199	Converted to the Stirling
July	196	Converted to the Stirling
July	431	Converted to the Halifax
August	429	Converted to the Lancaster
August	305	Converted to the Mitchell
September	466	Converted to the Halifax
September	166	Converted to the Lancaster
October	424	Converted to the Halifax
Oct/Nov	425	Return to UK to rejoin 6 Grp
1944:		
Feb 19/20	425	Resumes bombing ops
April	300	Converted to the Lancaster
October	425	Converted to the Halifax
October	150	Converted to the Lancaster
October	432	Converted to the Lancaster

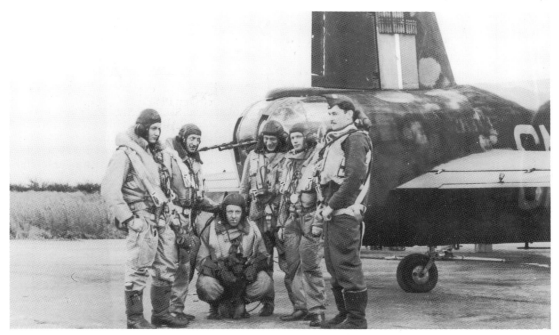

A Polish crew gather for a group photograph in front of Wellington II Z8343-SM of 305 Squadron. This aircraft first saw service with 142 Squadron and was struck off charge on 27 July 1944 when it was serving with 104 Squadron. Note the bomb log painted above the fin flash. *(RAF Museum)*

On the night of 8/9 October 1943 the last bombing operation by Wellingtons of Bomber Command was made by No 300 (Polish) Squadron, during a raid on Hannover. However, Wellingtons continued to serve with OTUs throughout 1944 and, on occasion, they were used directly against the enemy. Noel Croppi recalls: 'By 1944 we were trying everything possible to reduce losses and so many diversion raids were mounted when a few aircraft attacked one target while the main force went somewhere else.

'However, we then tried diversions with a difference. Firstly, I took off on 22 February but was recalled due to bad weather. Then, on 27 April we took off in a Wellington X to fly almost due east across the North Sea until we reached a position about seventy miles west of the Danish coast and about the same distance north of the Frisian Islands. We then changed course to fly south-east as if heading for Bremen or Hamburg. When we were just off the German coast we released masses of "Window" to confuse German radar. Apparently, this operation was a great success since Intelligence advised that we had drawn off about a third of the total German Night Fighter Force.'

Wellingtons also served until the end of the war with the 2nd Tactical Air Force in England and France. Len Aynsley, a bomb aimer in Pilot Officer Jack Haines' crew, recalls: 'We completed our course at OTU in May 1944 and after leave received orders to report to 69 Squadron, 2nd Tactical Air Force, at Northolt without delay. So much for indefinite leave! Worse was to come. On arrival at Northolt we discovered that the squadron did not have one plane to its name! A day or so later we had to parade before an Air Vice Marshal. He told us what our role would be — namely low level photographic reconnaissance. This sounded OK until he went on to say that we would be assigned Ansons, with no armament. His next remark was, "We want keen volunteers only in this squadron so if anyone doesn't like the idea, see me after the parade and I will see he gets an immediate posting to Bomber Command!"

'Neither I nor the rest of the crew liked the sound of it so we went to see him. He told us, "You are here to fly Ansons and you bloody well will. Get out!" So we got out and considered ourselves "volunteers". Fortunately, before ops started, the Air Ministry banned operational flying on Ansons so we were given Wellingtons with two .303 Brownings in the rear turret. The front turret was completely glazed over with perspex, and aerial cameras were installed.

'We spent a few nights flying the Wellingtons around the area to become fully conversant with all the landmarks. On one trip we were returning to Northolt when they had an air raid alert. All the lights, including the runway lights, were out. I suddenly spotted a runway beneath us and told Jack Haines that we were home. We came in to land and to our surprise there was a crashed plane at the beginning of the runway. We hopped over it, landed and then nearly ran out of runway. As soon as we had stopped, a Jeep roared out and we were met by some Yanks — we had landed at Hendon. We were not allowed to take off until daybreak!

'To facilitate our use as close army support, we moved to the continent as soon as a German-held airfield was captured. We transferred to Amiens and eventually moved to an airfield a few miles from Brussels. One of the airfields had a few stacks of bombs, presumably left behind by the retreating Germans. Some wise bod erected the parachute store tent near a bundle of incendiary bombs. All our 'chutes were called in for repacking and one member of the squadron went in to see if they were ready. On the way, he picked up an incendiary stick. Inside the tent he hit the centre pole with it and the marquee burned down. All the 'chutes were destroyed. We thought this would be a good opportunity for leave but unfortunately, replacements were quickly flown out.

'Our objectives were troop movements, enemy airfields and kindred targets. We carried no bombs but the bomb bays were loaded with flares to light up the scene when taking photographs. We operated singly and usually at a height of no more than 1,000 feet or so. On some days we ferried petrol from Bayeux to Amiens. We were loaded up with as many petrol cans as we could accommodate. Wellingtons could be used for practically any purpose.

'It must have been around this time that

On Christmas Eve 1944 Haines' crew flew a recce over Wegburg-Wassenberg and then went on leave. While they were away, on New Year's Day 1945, their airfield, along with many others on the continent, was attacked by the Luftwaffe in Operation 'Bodenplatte' and most of 69 Squadron's PR XIIIs were wrecked on the ground. *(RAF Museum)*

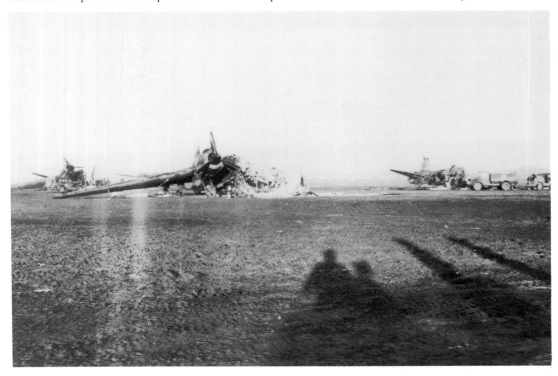

the non-flying members of the squadron were moved to another "liberated" airfield and the aircrews were left behind with some iron rations with orders to fly up in a few days' time. Meanwhile, we slept in the Wellingtons and lived as best we could.

'On 25 July 1944 we were returning towards the French coast after covering Caudebec, Pont Au Demer and La Maillery when Jerry Elston saw a Ju 88 slightly below and on a parallel course. At that time a lot of Ju 88s were being used for torpedo attacks on MTBs. Jerry gave it a burst with his tail guns. Pieces flew off it and it appeared to suffer slight fire in the engine. It pulled away, obviously damaged.

'During the op on the night of 28 July to Les Andelys, Muids, Roquette and Martet, we were doing aerial photographic reconnaissance at some bridges over the Seine to pick up troop movements. Eventually, we were caught by two searchlights, one on either side of the bank at Elbeuf. We were subjected to concentrated light flak. They had our range and I could hear flak exploding above the noise of the engines.

'Jack Haines made a quick decision as to the best way to get us out of trouble. The banks were fairly high at this point, so he put the Wellington down to skim just above the water. As we went down, so the flak merchants lowered their guns to keep on us. In their excitement they forgot to stop firing and as we skimmed over the water they were firing at each other across the river, being unable to traverse as low as we were!

'The only time that the squadron did not operate singly was on the night of 28/29 August 1944. At the request of the GOC, Canadian Army, we were to be used to drop flares all night over Caen, whilst below us were army pilots in Lysanders, directing the shelling of the city. Next day the squadron received a message of congratulations from the Canadian Army with an adjunct that "We may like a repeat performance in the near future".

'On 23 December 1944 we flew a photo-

Mk X HE508 CO-O served with 84 OTU at Desborough for almost the whole life of the unit. It arrived on 2 October 1943 (the unit formed on 1 September) and was despatched to 48 MU at Hawarden, Flintshire, on 22 June 1945 when 84 OTU disbanded. *(Michael L. Gibson)*

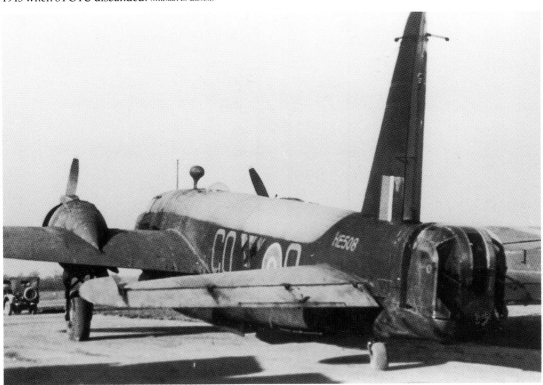

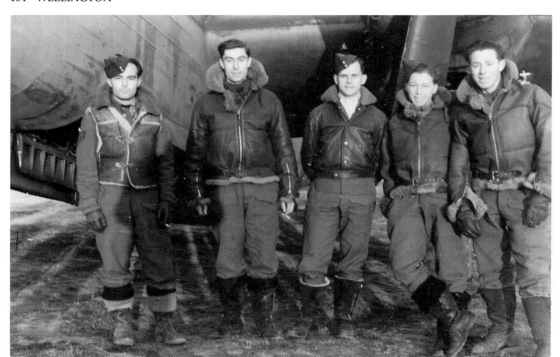

Famous Five: Left to right, Len Aynsley; Les Johnson, Air Gunner; F/O Jack Haines, Pilot; Jimmy Bourne, Navigator; Jerry Elston, Rear Gunner. Elston and Johnson shared in the Me 163 Komet 'kill' on 23 December 1944. *(Len Aynsley)*

Wellington PR XIII NC588 of 69 Squadron over Europe in July 1945. *(RAF Museum)*

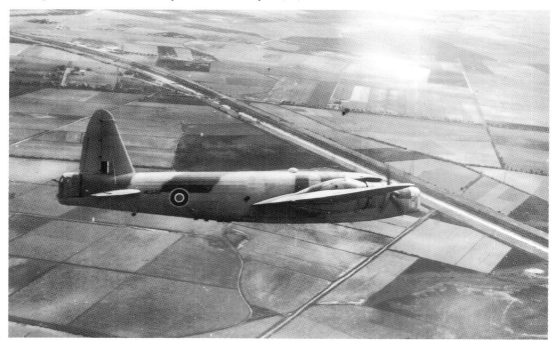

recce on Deelen. I got some fairly good photographs of German aircraft on the ground. When we got back to base we were asked to go up again virtually straight away, as another target had come up. We were the last crew back, all the others had debriefed, had a few (or many) drinks and it was thought desirable that a stone-cold sober crew should go!

'We changed to another plane which had already been tanked up and headed for Deelen (again) and Soesterberg. At Deelen, the Jerries were using rocket planes. One of them, an Me 163 Komet, attacked us. He had scarcely trained his guns on us than he was flying right past us. On his first two runs, which were made from behind, he had almost overshot us before he began firing.

'Under circumstances like these Jack Haines followed orders from Sergeant Elston, the rear gunner, who indicated which way to turn. Both Elston and Les Johnson, the other air-gunner, who had no turret to man but was used as an observer in the mid-upper astrodome, worked together. On the third

attack the Me 163 passed very close on our starboard side. Les Johnson told Gerry Elston to traverse his guns as far as possible to starboard and keep his finger on the trigger. Jerry Elston obliged. The Komet ran straight through the stream of bullets and was shot down.

'I pinpointed his crash position and I believe that the plane, or part of it at least, was found. Jack Haines was in line for the DFC for this but he made it known that it was all down to Gerry Elston, who did in fact receive the DFM. I think that this may have been the first German jet [sic] plane to be shot down by an RAF crew, but if not, it was certainly the first, if not the "only" one to be downed by a Wellington.'

It is appropriate and fitting that the foregoing account sums up the wartime career of the Wellington in Northern Europe. It says something for this remarkable aircraft that despite being designed before the war, it could still survive in combat conditions and against one of the most up-to-date fighters the Germans possessed.

Chapter 10
Desert War

A raid by two Dorniers on Norwich during the afternoon of Tuesday, 9 July 1940, was enough to alter the course of destiny for at least one nineteen-year-old boy who witnessed the horror and destruction. Wallace Gaul always intended to volunteer for the Tank Corps. The German bombing raid on his home city changed all this. Despite his reserved occupation, Gaul volunteered for RAF aircrew.

In September, while Gaul was taking the first faltering steps as an 'erk' at RAF Marham, 1,500 miles away a battle was raging in the Western Desert. When Mussolini had declared war on Britain and France on 10 June 1940, Air Marshal Sir Arthur Longmore in Cairo could call upon roughly 150 aircraft for the defence of Egypt and the Suez Canal, with about another 150 first-line aircraft scattered throughout Palestine, East Africa,

Aden and Gibraltar. However, nine of the fourteen bomber squadrons were equipped with the Blenheim I. The rest were made up of biplane fighters and bombers and seaplanes. Only a few DW I Wellingtons were in place for minesweeping duties.

Blenheims and Wellingtons, which were the only RAF aircraft with sufficient range to reinforce Egypt, had to cross the Bay of Biscay and then land at Gibraltar before making a night landing at Malta. This was clearly out of the question, so while the Wellington squadrons and OTUs kicked their heels in England, Blenheims and Hurricanes were shipped out via West Africa.

Egypt was successfully defended against the invading Italian armies and on 24 October Mussolini turned his attentions to Greece. Four days later, the War Cabinet approved a plan for Wellingtons, temporarily stationed

Wellington DWI 1 in North Africa with a forty-eight foot dural hoop energised to an auxiliary motor mounted in the fuselage to detonate magnetic mines. *(RAF Museum)*

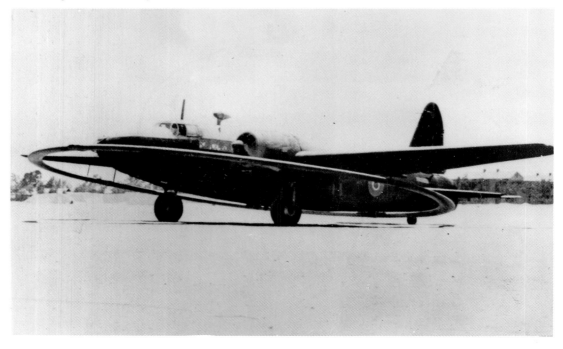

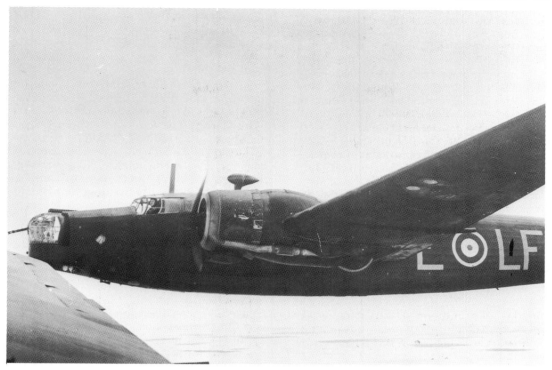

Wellington IA LF-E of 37 Squadron over Western Desert in 1940. (IWM)

on Malta *en route* for Egypt, to be used in action against Italian supply ports in southern Italy. On the night of 31 October Wellingtons bombed Naples, and for a month thereafter they were joined by others which put in raids on the Italian 'boot' prior to completing their journey to Egypt. This arrangement was disastrous for morale and at Luqa in December 1940 sixteen Wellington ICs were used to re-form No 148 Squadron, which had been absorbed by No 15 OTU in May that year.

Meanwhile, in November 1940 Nos 37 and 38 Squadrons, equipped with Wellingtons, were despatched to Egypt via Malta to help replace squadrons sent to Greece. These two squadrons helped push back the Italians in the Western Desert and were ably assisted by No 148 Squadron, which was despatched **from** Malta on occasion, to bomb targets in Tripolitania. On 7 December this squadron successfully bombed Castel Benito airfield. Achieving total surprise, the Wellingtons destroyed five hangars and many dozens of aircraft on the ground with incendiary bullets.

By 16 December the last remnants of the Italian Army had been pushed back across the Egyptian frontier. Hitler now came to the aid of his fellow dictator. Late in December, while the Wehrmacht marched into Bulgaria with intentions on Greece, Fliegerkorps X began arriving in Sicily. Their arrival was a rude shock to the British, who hit back on the nights of 12/13 and 15/16 January when Wellingtons from Malta bombed airfields on Sicily.

Fliegerkorps X could not prevent the rout of the Italian Army in Cyrenaica and early in February 1941 the last of the Italian troops surrendered. The Wellingtons had played their part with the continual bombing of the enemy but a greater test was to follow. On 12 February Rommel arrived in Cyrenaica and six days later Hitler named the General's forces the 'Afrika Korps'. Once the Germans' intentions in Greece became obvious Wellingtons of Nos 37, 38 and 70 Squadrons in the Canal Zone, and No 148 Squadron on Malta, quickly struck at the main German airfields and the port of Tripoli.

On 31 March Rommel's forces began mounting a counter-offensive and the meagre RAF forces were thrown headlong into the fight. Wellingtons of Nos 37, 38 and 70 Squadrons, 'reinforced' by No 148 Squadron, which after repeated air attacks had been forced to withdraw from Malta earlier in the month, made raids on Axis targets. By refuelling at Tobruk the Wellingtons were able to hit Tripoli in a bid to stem the flow of enemy material.

Meanwhile, replacement aircrews were heading for Egypt. On 1 October 1941 Wally Gaul, now a Sergeant rear gunner in Sergeant Jim 'Cranky' Crank-Benson's crew, left No 15 OTU at Harwell for the Middle East. Dave Clark was the Second Pilot, Jeff Jefferies the Navigator, 'Brownie' Brown the WOP-AG, and a Canadian, George Wetherhead, completed the crew as front gunner. Gaul recalls: 'The Met men predicted 10/10ths cloud over the sea. We were told, "Keep away from Brest. If you have an engine failure, make for the white beaches of Portugal. You will see them even on the darkest night." The CO added, "Take off time is 03:15. Crank-Benson will be the last of three aircraft to take off as his aircraft is faster. Good luck chaps and a safe landing."

'We taxied to the perimeter track as the first Wellington was taking off. The second followed a few minutes later. We taxied onto the runway, a final engine test, and waited for the green. Wireless transmission was out for obvious reasons. We got the green from the tower and it was "OK chaps, here we go!" Engines roared to life and we began to move, slowly at first, along the flare path. There was a hell of a swing to port, a loud thud and several gooseneck flares were blown about by our slipstream. Jim was having a hell of a job getting the kite airborne. It crossed my mind that a Wellington had recently crashed and exploded at the end of the runway but with one more "bump" we were airborne. My altimeter read 500 feet and still climbing.

'Jeff gave "Cranky" a course to set for Redruth in Cornwall. We were flying at 4,000 feet and through the break in the clouds I could see a beacon on the Cornish coast flashing the letter of the day. "Goodbye, England." I thought of those at home in Norwich tucked up in their nice warm beds, so I opened my flask of coffee and had a sip of Johnnie Walker to keep out the cold.

'When we were over the Atlantic George reported, "Flak on the port bow!" "That's Brest," said Jeff. We were flying at 9,000 feet

now and the weather was improving. At last we were above the clouds and we could see the stars. Jeff took a fix and gave Jim a new course. The sky was gradually changing colour. Dawn was near.

'We landed at Gibraltar before taking off again, for Malta, on 8 October. The Briefing Officer told us to maintain radio silence: "The Italians are red hot at three things: Singing, ice-cream and RADIO." He also told us to keep low near the heavily defended island of Pantelleria, eighty miles south of Sicily and about fifty miles north of Tunisia.

'At 08:00 hours the weather report was good. It was warm with a cool breeze blowing from the sea. We taxied out and I could see Spaniards crowding around the closed gates waving to us as we turned to the end of the strip. Jim said, "OK, everyone! Here we go." The 1,700 horsepower Merlin engines roared into life. Gathering speed, I felt the tail rise. Jim said, "Come on, old girl. Get up". The sea was getting close. At the last moment the nose lifted and we were airborne. We were climbing steadily when Jim asked me if I could see the other kite. "F for Freddie is just behind", I said, "and he's catching up." We kept the coast of Spain in sight. I had a good view of the snow-covered peaks of the Sierra Nevada mountains. As we turned away from the coast the white face of the Rock was jutting out from the blue sea.

'We set course for North Africa. Jeff said we should keep well out to sea off Bizerta because we would be fired at by Vichy French. "F for Freddie" got too close and was lucky to get away with it. George spotted Pantelleria and we descended. We were so low our props made whitecaps on the sea. It was like sitting in the back of a speedboat in my rear turret.

'We got through undetected but ran into some really bad weather. "F for Freddie" was bashing out with the Aldis lamp asking our position before we entered 10/10ths cloud and lost him. Jim tried to climb above the storm but it seemed to go to 25,000 feet. He said, "I'm going down". We descended at a fair rate and as we pulled out at 500 feet, George yelled out, "Weave, Jim. We're on top of a convoy! Jesus, that was close!" We were lucky. It was nearly always fatal to fly above our own ships as they would fire first and ask questions afterwards. Jim did a tight turn and climbed back into the clouds.

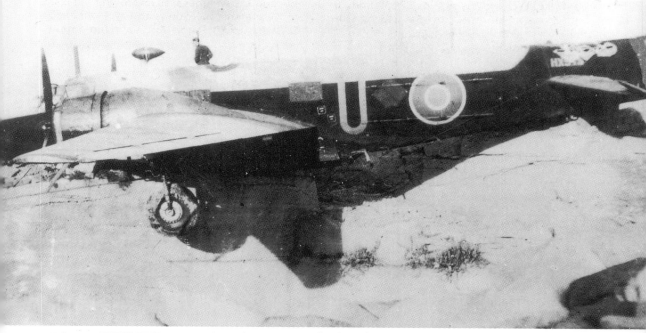

Wellington VIII HX57 U, a victim of unwelcome attention by the Luftwaffe during a bombing raid on Malta.
(RAF Museum)

'Brownie picked up Malta asking for our position. Jeff gave it to Brownie, who transmitted it. Soon Malta was in sight. As we turned on finals I had a good view of the Grand Harbour at Valletta and the cities of Singlea, Cospicua and Vittoriosa, and the airfield at Luqa. Black tarmac roads stood out in contrast to the white rock of the island. Jim made his usual good landing and we taxied to the dispersal. Eight hours had passed since we had left Gib. Even though it was late afternoon the temperature was well up into the high seventies.

'We asked if "F for Freddie" had made it. There was no sign. I thought of Mac, their rear gunner, who was rather old at 31, and of Mansell, the pilot, a dry stick; and the rest of the crew. We had trained together and had had several good "booze ups" in the "Jockey" pub near Harwell. "Well, that's how it goes," we thought.

'As we were about to board the coach a Corporal from the radio room shouted, " 'F for Freddie' has just sent out his 'indent' and is fifteen minutes from base". We prayed that he had enough fuel to get in. Then we saw the Wimpy in the distance. Mansell made an emergency landing. He only just

made it for, as they were taxying to the dispersal, both engines cut, out of fuel.'

On Friday, 10 October, Crank-Benson's crew finally set off for Egypt. Wally Gaul continues: 'Midnight came and out we went to the aircraft for final checks. The engines roared to life and we started to taxi along Saffi Strip to the peri track to wait for the green. I saw black clouds, lit up by a large flash of lightning which went right down to the sea. I had never seen anything like this before. The Met boys had said it was harmless! It was all right for them. They didn't have to fly through it!

'We taxied out to the end of the flarepath. One more check on the engines and we got the green. I felt the tail lift and after a couple of slight bumps we were airborne. Soon the flare path was out of sight and we were in the "harmless" electrical storm. Jim and Dave had a hell of a job controlling the aircraft. We were tossed about like a feather in the breeze; down 500 feet and then up 500 feet. Jim tried first to get below it and then above it but the storm reached from sea level to 25,000 feet; a height we didn't have a cat in hell's chance of reaching. The escape hatch was blown off. Most of the instruments were

U/S; it was cold and nobody spoke. The only sound was the hum of the two Merlin engines. I prayed we wouldn't lose those, like the hatch.

'After an hour we finally got into fine weather again. Jim asked for a flask of coffee up front but when I looked in the rear of the kite I saw that they had all been broken. The sun was beginning to creep over the horizon. George Weatherhead reported the coast coming up and as we turned east I had my first view of the desert. It was not as I had expected. No soft sand and swaying palm trees; just barren, rocky sand.

'Jim followed the railway line to El Daba where we were to drop a passenger. A lorry met us. "Where's this place?" we asked the driver. "Ninety miles from Alexandria and 185 miles from Cairo. Why, are you lost?" Jim took off in a cloud of dust and said he would "shoot up" the comic of a lorry driver. Jim buzzed the strip at zero height and if this didn't put the fear of Christ up him, it did me.

'Soon we were flying over the Nile Delta. Children looked up to us and waved. They were not used to Wellington bombers flying low over the Delta. I could see Cairo on the starboard side. Jim flew on to El Fayum, our final destination. The airfield was chock full with every type of aircraft imaginable awaiting transfer to squadrons. We landed, took out our gear and waited to be picked up. A breeze got up and within seconds it was blowing gale force. It was like thousands of needles cutting into the exposed parts of the body. We hurried back into the Wellington. When the sandstorm finished our gear was buried under a load of sand.'

Early in the morning of Monday, 13 October, the crew entrained for Shallufa. Wally Gaul continues: "We reported to the Middle East Pool where aircrew waited for a posting to a squadron. A lorry took us to RAF Shallufa which was HQ 205 Group. In September 1941 No 257 Wing in the Egyptian Canal Zone had been re-designated 205 Group. Nos 37 and 38 Squadrons were based here while 108 Squadron was based at El Fayid. Nos 70 and 148 Squadrons, both flying Wellingtons, were based at Kabrit.

'We spent the next few days learning about conditions in the desert at the Ground Training Unit. Flight Lieutenant Stanley, who had completed a number of ops, replaced Jim and we made a flight up to the "blue", as

the desert was known. We landed at El Daba ALG (Advanced Landing Ground) 104 and ALG 106 Fuka Satellite. The flight lasted almost five hours and we slept in the aircraft at night. On the return we landed at a couple more ALGs before returning to Shallufa. This trip was a real eye-opener for things to come and good experience for us.

'On Thursday, 23 October 1941, we were posted to 148 Squadron at Kabrit. Kabrit was a permanent station with tarmac runways, sand-coloured hangars and buildings. Wellingtons were dispersed around the 'drome. 148 was a "mobile" squadron and our living quarters were tents on the shore of the Suez Canal, near the Great Bitter Lake.

'On 25 October we flew our first operation. Dave Clark flew as Second Pilot while an experienced pilot took Jim Crank-Benson's seat. The target was Benghazi, the main port used by Jerry for supplying the Afrika Korps. We took off at 15:00 hours for a two-hour flight to one of the ALGs in the desert. We were all keyed up when, after 45 minutes' flying, one engine packed up. We had to return to base.

'Four days later Dave and Jeff were allocated to other crews. The rest of us complained to the Flight Commander, but to no avail. (This move decided the lives of four of the original crew and the death of two of them.) Pilot Officer Owen took over as First Pilot and Flying Officer Church, a Canadian, became the crew's Navigator. Crank-Benson was relegated to Second Pilot.'

On 29 October the Wellingtons attacked German shipping in Suda Bay on Crete. Gaul recalls: "We took off early in the afternoon for the one hour forty minute flight to ALG 104 to refuel, then at take-off time we set course for Crete. When we arrived over the target it was well lit up. This was the first time I had seen flak at close quarters. George said over the intercom, "Jesus Christ, look at that bloody lot!" The Skipper replied, "This is light stuff tonight. Wait 'till you see Benghazi!"

'On Thursday, 6 November, we were lazing around outside the ops room waiting for the gen when the Flight Commander yelled for a volunteer to air test "H for Harry". Mackenzie, a pilot, said he would go. They wanted one more for the rear turret. I said, "Sorry 'Mac', I haven't got my helmet". (Gaul had also left his "lucky" white and green spotted silk scarf and his mascots behind. Like almost all airmen, he was very superstitious and never ever flew without it.) One of the ground crew volunteered.

'We watched "Mac" put "H for Harry" through the test. Suddenly, he lost an engine (the Wimpy could fly on one engine safely). For some reason he turned into the "duff" engine ("Mac" was an experienced pilot who had completed a tour of ops and was waiting for the boat home to "Blighty"). He lost control and nose-dived into the edge of the Great Bitter Lake. There was just one big explosion followed by a cloud of black smoke. We all ran to the crash but we knew there was nothing we could do.

'On 12 November I flew my eighth operation, to Benghazi. Dave Clark was not "on", not having crewed up yet. Jeff was on with his new crew. This was his second. As usual we flew up to the ALG and, after we had refuelled, took off again for Benghazi. We bombed the target and were the first aircraft to land. This meant we had the pick of the "grub". The first few crews always got canned skinless sausages that were very tasty. The last to land got "bully beef".

'Soon, all the aircraft, except for one, had landed back at the ALG. We were used to this. It happened on every operation. We finished our meal and were about to turn in for the rest of the night (we slept in the kite at the ALG) when "Brownie", running towards us, said, "Jeff's crew is overdue". Sleep was impossible.

'We were told much later that the missing aircraft had been shot down over the target and several crews reported that no parachutes were seen. We were used to losing crews, all of them our mates, but when Jeff went it was different. We had lived, trained and drank together. I could see his mum and dad when the telegram arrived at his home; the same home I had stayed in for one weekend during training.'

On the night of Monday, 17 November, the Wellingtons struck at Derna. Wally Gaul's crew did not fly because their aircraft was having an engine change. On stand-down days Sergeant aircrew were assigned other duties and Gaul was put in charge of some Italian PoWs. At 16:30 hours the prisoners were transported back to their PoW camp. On the way back to Kabrit, Wally Gaul asked the driver if No 148 Squadron 'had lost any kites last night?' The driver indicated that

Mk IA T2874 W of the Wellington Flight at Luqa, Malta in 1940. On 12 January 1941, while serving with 148 Squadron, it failed to return from a raid on Catania. *(RAF Museum)*

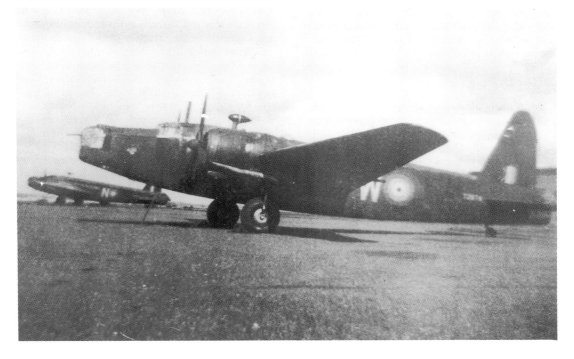

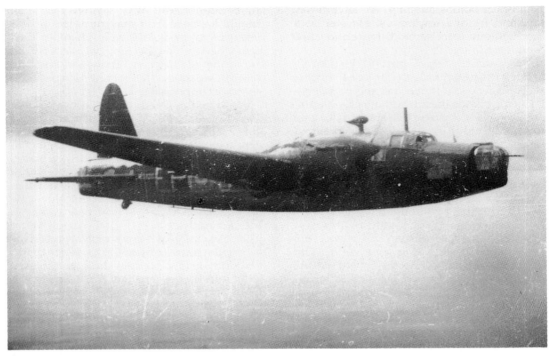

Wellington II of 104 Squadron. *(John Hosford)*

they had lost two, including one pilot who was a Flight Lieutenant with a DFC. Gaul was startled. 'We only had one pilot with the DFC and that was Dave Clark's pilot!'

'As soon as I got back I hurried over to our tent. The rest of the crew were there. As I entered, "Brownie" said, "Dave's gone. Some clot dropped a 4.5-inch flare above them as they were on a low-level bombing run. They were a sitting duck for the Jerry ack-ack. Several crews saw it happen. They had no chance of getting out or to drop their bombs. The kite exploded as it hit the deck." Jeff's bed had been taken out and all of Dave's belongings were packed on his bed. Two of the original crew had not gone. Two nights later the target was Derna; the place where Dave and his crew were shot down.

'After the briefing we took off for ALG 104; an hour's flying time from base. As usual the first thing was a meal, then time to refuel and wait for take-off. Soon we were airborne and heading for Derna where we were to bomb the airfield. When we reached the target it was fairly quiet. The ack-ack was light, so it looked like this was going to be "a piece of cake". Our skipper knew what we wanted. He said he would go in at low level and told Ron, the navigator, to drop a single stick of bombs on each run in. We made half a dozen runs over the target and when the last bomb had been released, the Skipper gave us the OK to machine-gun what was left of the airfield.

'With George in the front turret, "Brownie" on the beam guns and me in the rear turret, we let them have it. Above the noise of six Browning guns I could hear "Brownie" on the intercom shouting out, "You bastards. Take that you bastards! Go round again, Skipper; one more for Dave." As we left the target there were six very hot Browning guns! We saw two Bf 109 fighters turning to attack us. As we turned violently to port I lost sight of them. I could hear George firing from the front and then I saw tracers going away from us.

'Two nights later, on Friday, 21 November, we waited at ALG 104 for the midnight take-off time. We went over to the aircraft for a few hours' kip. All the aircraft were parked in line. Our kite was not. We were in position near the flare path as we were to be first away. I was standing in the Second Pilot's position when I noticed flak in the El Daba area. Jerry was having a "go". We could hear bombs bursting. An aircraft flew low and headed toward us. He started to machine-gun from some distance away. We were out of our kite and heading for the underground air raid shelter. George was running in front of me and, even though we were under attack, I had to smile as both his desert boots "took off". Not stopping to pick them up George dived into a slit trench with me right behind.

'Jerry had made his first run machine-gunning the aircraft that were in line, missing ours. On his next run he dropped a stick of bombs. Fires were started and the fire tender could not cope with so many kites burning. One aircraft was well alight. First the petrol tanks, then the bombs exploded, setting fire to Wimpys on the either side. Our Skipper was soon in the aircraft to taxi out of the area. Other kites were being towed to a safe distance.

'Two aircraft had been destroyed and six badly damaged. The remainder were slightly damaged but were un-flyable. One man was killed by machine-gun fire and another broke his neck when he jumped head-first into a slit trench. Several others were injured by shrapnel. Jerry had made a good job of it. November was an unlucky month for our squadron. We lost more aircraft and crews than any other month. I wondered how long my luck would last.

'On 18 December there was yet another change to the crew. Pilot Officer Owens was replaced by Flight Lieutenant (later Squadron Leader) The Honourable R.A.G. Baird. "Brownie" was replaced by Flight Sergeant "Drag" Parkin DFM. Jim was still our second pilot. George had a road accident and was not replaced on the crew. This meant we could carry an extra bomb if we did not have a front gunner.

'On 26 February the early morning sun was creeping over the horizon. As I dressed I wondered what was on today? After breakfast we reported to Ops and waited for the "gen". A voice from the Ops room said, "Ops on tonight, briefing at 12 o'clock. The target tonight is Benghazi." The "mail run" as it was called, was warming up its defences. "Navigators have a slightly different course for the run in and you may find that Jerry has brought in extra ack-ack." The Met officer added, "Right, chaps. The weather should be clear over the target . . ." (cheers and laughter from the crews — we had heard it

all before). "As I was saying, the target should be clear. You may run into 10/10ths cloud on the way." The CO added, "Well, chaps, I hope you all have a good trip. The best of luck" (cries of "we need it") "and hope to see you all safely back tomorrow."

'Briefing over, I collected two Browning .303s from the armoury and took them out to the kite where I harmonised them with the gun sight. The armourers were loading belts of ammo into the cans. Soon, everything was ready. The aircraft was towed to the end of the runway. (The Merlin was a good engine but was prone to over-heating and several crews had failed to get airborne when the engines were running before take-off.)

'The engines started and we took off without any checks. Apart from myself and the two pilots the crew were in the "rest positions" on two suspended beds (this was the norm for all take-offs and landings). The inside of the Wellington was like an oven. I was stripped down to my shorts, flying boots and helmet. I had to keep my arms well away from the metal parts of the turret, otherwise it would burn my skin.

'Just as we were climbing it started to cool off. We opened windows and hatches to let in a nice cool breeze. A few hours later we would have to dress in flying clothing as it got very cold out in the desert at night. On the way up to the ALG the pilot went aft to ride in the rear turret. It amused him to operate the controls and to test the guns. When it was my turn to fly the aircraft I told him to stop buggering about as it upset my flying! (After all, I was the Sergeant Skipper and he was only the Squadron Leader rear gunner!) All through this the Second Pilot was in his seat ready to take over in an emergency. This was unlikely as we were out of range of enemy fighters.

'After one and a half hour's flying it was back to our normal positions for the landing at the ALG. Then there was the usual mad rush to the beer tent followed by a walk to the Mess tent for a meal. Take-off time was still a few hours away so we kipped in the aircraft until we were awakened by the Skipper. "Fingers out, chaps; take-off in half an hour." We changed into our flying clothes and Mae Wests by the light from the downward ident lamp. One last drag on the cigarette, then it was all aboard for another visit to "Ben".

' "M for Mother" was the first to take off.

We were carrying extra 4.5 flares as we had to light the target for the following kites. The flight commander always got the "sticky" jobs and as we turned on to the target all hell let loose. It seemed that there were more searchlights and flak then ever. "Drag" dropped a couple of flares. (It was the Wireless Operator's job to push the flares out through the flare chute.) "Flares gone," he yelled. I watched the flares slowly drifting down, lighting up the target like day. Ships in the harbour were belting away at us. We were getting the lot and we still had to make another run to drop the bombs.

'Now the main stream was going in. Each aircraft aimed at their given target. As we turned I saw one of the kites coned in the searchlights. It looked like a silver fish as he weaved to evade the lights. All the guns below were having a go at him. Then there was one big explosion. Burning pieces of aircraft began to drift slowly earthwards. "Bloody hell!" I thought. "Yet another kite and six boys lost."

'We started the bombing run. "Steady . . . left . . . steady . . . hold it . . . steady . . . BOMBS GONE!" After a straight and level run lasting several minutes we started to weave and dive. A searchlight held us for a few seconds. I was blinded by the light. Someone shouted over the intercom, "They've got us! Get to hell out of here." The Skipper quietly and calmly said, "OK. chaps, we're going round again . . ." This time we dropped the remaining bombs and then got the hell out of it. As we left the target it was well alight. Ron said we had scored a direct hit on one of the ships on the last run in. Well, the camera would confirm it when we got back.

'After a beer and a meal I forgot about Benghazi and was soon dreaming about the boat home. 31 ops — time to come off. How much longer was my luck going to hold out? I had another go at the Flight Commander about coming off. He said, "We have a big job coming off and I know you won't want to miss it."

'On 14 April the squadron changed from Merlin-engined Wimpys to Pegasus radial-engined Wellingtons. Next day we flew an altitude test with a full bomb load to see how high the Wimpy could fly with Pegasus engines. We climbed to 15,000 feet in just over half an hour. Next day we were at it again. We reached 15,000 feet but could not

Wellington IC Z902 C of 38 Squadron in North Africa was struck off charge on 15 April 1942. *(RAF Museum)*

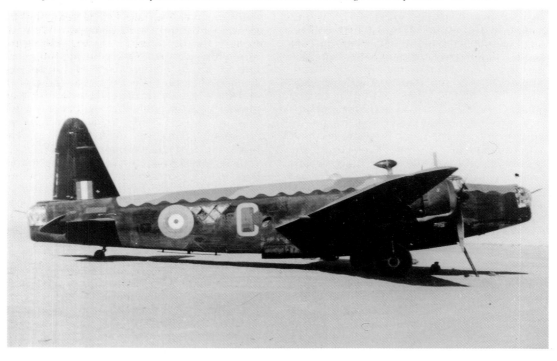

get above it. This was the highest I had flown in the desert. Our normal height was about 10,000 feet.

'Two days later we were told what the "big job" was. Air Vice Marshal Lloyd had ordered eight Wellington bombers to Malta. I was picked as the rear gunner in the Wing Commander's crew. Each aircraft would also carry a spare crew.

'On Monday, 20 April, we took off from Kabrit for ALG 106. Eight Wimpys, sixteen crews, 96 aircrew, and a few ground crews. We flew in formation as there had been an increase in enemy fighter activity in the area. A sandstorm was blowing at the ALG and made landing difficult. We stalled and hit the deck with one almighty crash. Although the aircraft was "bent up" a bit, there were no injuries. We took off again at 20:00 hours and after an uneventful flight, lasting six hours twenty minutes, we were on the circuit at Luqa. We were billeted at the Palace in Naxxar and told to stay out of sight when the raids were on.

'I woke up next morning to the sound of air raid sirens. No one bothered to get up. Then we heard the guns opening up. Although the bombs were some distance away, the palace began to shake. There were slit trenches at the rear of the building so we made a dive for them. Naxxar is on high ground so we had a good view of the bombing. The month of April 1942 will be remembered by the people of Malta. This was the month His Majesty the King awarded them the George Cross.

'On 22 April ops were on. We were taken out to the aircraft to get ready for the "big one". At last we were going to get our revenge on Jerry. Our aircraft had survived the first raid of the day. I was busy in the turret when the yellow flare went up from Luqa. Soon the sirens were wailing and I could see the first wave heading for the island. Our kite was in a sandbagged enclosure. As I wondered whether to run for the slit trench, the first bombs were falling on the airfield at Takali five miles away. Hal Far airfield was only two miles away. A lorry arrived and I was whisked away to Luqa. We made a dash to the underground shelter. The next wave was bombing the airfield at Luqa and Saffi Strip.

'On the way to the airfield another raid, on Luqa, had started. We had to scatter. Our kite was OK but the runway had to be repaired. We had lost quite a lot of kites in the bombing and the ferry crews bound for Egypt were diverted to Malta so that our squadron could take them on ops that night. (Most of the new kites were bombed the next day and the same thing would happen again.)

'A lorry took us out to our kite. A final check by the ground crew for any shrapnel damage. Everything seemed OK. The engines were started and we taxied along Saffi Strip to wait for the green. Crank-Benson, who was flying on ops for the first time as captain, made a final check on the engines. We got the green and at last we were on our way.

'Sicily is only sixty miles from Malta and the target, the airfield at Comiso, was about the same distance inland. As we crossed the coast we were greeted with heavy flak. We were flying at 8,000 feet so most of the "stuff" was bursting above us. We ran into several of these heavy ack-ack sites on the way to the target and I could see other aircraft bombing airfields.

'Searchlights probed the sky. Flares drifted down to light up the target. Light flak spiralled up and bombs exploded on the airfield. The last of the aircraft in front of us had completed their bombing. Jim elected to go in over the mountains and make a low-level run over the target. The searchlights began to fade and the flak stopped. We had the target to ourselves. Jim said, "Going in now. Here we go." Over the mountain, a steep dive and we were running up to the airfield. Then the defences came to life again. The Navigator was having a hell of a job seeing the target. Then, "Hold it steady, Jim. I can see the target now. Steady . . . bombs gone!" Ack-ack guns on the side of the mountain were having a go at us. I fired my guns in that direction but I knew it was useless. It took my mind off things down below.

'Our bombs were forty-pounders with a "mushroom" on the nose so that they scattered shrapnel across the airfield on impact. We left quite a few aircraft burning. I could still see the fires from several miles away. We ran into more flak but this was nothing compared to the target area.

'As we crossed the coast a hell of an explosion tossed the kite on its side. I told Jim there was a bloody great hole in the port side. Jim went back to take a look. He

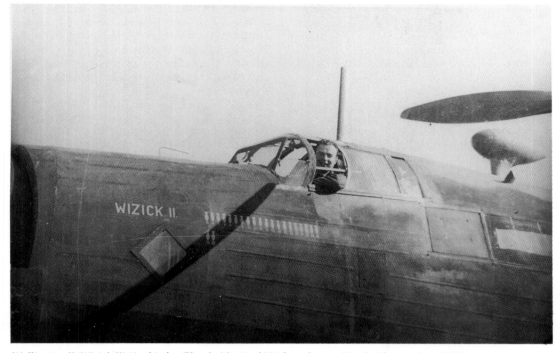

Wellington II 'Wizick II' (Arabic for 'Bloody Idiot') of 104 Squadron in North Africa early in 1942. *(John Hosford)*

exclaimed, "Jesus Bloody Christ!" Was he praying? I don't think so.

'Soon the beacon at Malta was in sight. We landed and began the long taxi to the dispersal at Saffi Strip. As usual I was the first to light up. Never had I enjoyed a fag so much before. A ground staff bod saw the damage and asked Jim, "How the hell did you get home?" "I didn't," said Jim. "The flak blew us back!" Our aircraft was U/S; two were shot down over the target; one was shot up and damaged. Total aircraft at daybreak . . . four!

'On 24 April Malta suffered a very heavy raid and our kite was hit. Two more kites were missing from the previous night's raid. The squadron was in a bad way. On 25 April we were told we were returning to Egypt. I was not sorry to hear this. I had completed 34 ops and the "old ring was beginning to twitter".

'At 17:00 hours on Sunday, 27 April, we left the Palace at Naxxar dressed in full flying kit to the cheers of the locals in the square. The *Maltese Times* gave us a big write-up about our bombing of enemy airfields in Sicily. This had raised morale no end. After briefing we had to wait for aircraft to arrive from Gibraltar.

Soon, our kite arrived. It was refuelled and the gear stowed inside. The ferry crews, who would be shipped back to Blighty by sea later, were not pleased to lose their aircraft.

'We touched down at Kabrit at 08:30 hours. As we left the aircraft we were greeted with, "Cor, you should have been here last night. We got raided by Jerry . . . one 'angar wos 'it." The Cockney driver prattled on and on. "How many kites?" we asked. "About 'arf a dozen He 111s," he said. We did not tell him that on the last raid on Malta 150 had taken part. This was the first time Kabrit had been bombed. Rommel was pushing the 8th Army back towards the Canal area, so he could bring his bombers down from the desert.'

On 6 May Wally Gaul flew his 35th op; an abortive single supply drop on Crete. Two days later he was dismayed to learn that his 36th operation was a dive-bombing raid on enemy shipping in Benghazi harbour. On an earlier raid one crew had turned off its engines as they had dived on the harbour, in an effort to fool the Italian sound locators, and had then turned them on again as they climbed dangerously away. Although they would not attempt this manoeuvre on the 8

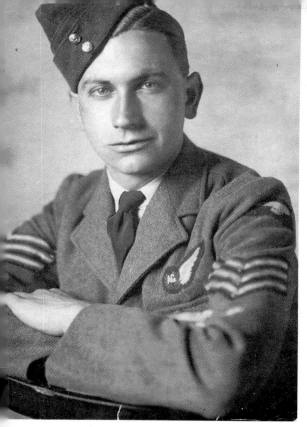

Sergeant Wally Gaul

Gaul recalls: 'We started our dive from about 8,000 feet. Wheels down, 15° of flap, engines throttled back to idling, nose down, then into a steep dive . . . bombs gone . . . pull out at 300 feet, both engines on full power. Then I opened up my two Brownings. We were the only kite over the target. At this height I stood a good chance of hitting something.

'We ran into trouble on the way back to the ALG. The Skipper asked the Navigator for our position. "No idea at the moment," he said. That's all I wanted to happen. To make matters worse one engine began to play up. The WOP/AG tried in vain to get a fix. It was daylight now and just to pile it on we ran into a ground mist. These mists occurred frequently over the desert at dawn, rising to about fifty feet. I said we could be over the salt marshes near Alexandria. I had seen these mists on several occasions. The Navigator chose to ignore me. The Skipper called me up front. The front gunner was beginning to panic. We told him to get in the rear turret. It was the safest place if we crash-landed. I saw what looked like the coast. "Over on the port, Skip," I said. We followed the coastline to El Daba and flew on to ALG 106. We had been two hours adrift in the "blue".

'I met my ex-Skipper at Kabrit and told him I would not fly with the crew again. "You won't have to," he said. "That was your last op; you're on the boat list." The next day, 11 May, was my birthday!'

May trip there was another disconcerting aspect of the operation. Wally Gaul and the skipper were at the end of their tours but the rest of the crew were on only their second trip.

Chapter 11
Mad dogs and Englishmen

While Wally Gaul departed the Middle East for a well-deserved leave before a second tour on Halifaxes, others, like Flight Lieutenant Reg Thackeray, arrived in the Canal Zone to carry on the fight against Rommel's Afrika Korps.

Thackeray, a second pilot, joined No 40 Squadron at Kabrit on Saturday, 3 October 1942, from No 2 Middle East Training School at Aqir, Palestine. The following Wednesday, 7 October, he was sitting in the right-hand seat next to Flight Lieutenant Morton, a New Zealander who was on his second tour, in Wellington IC *K* which, with seven others, made a night raid on Tobruk.

Thackeray recalls: 'It was quite a shaker after 2 METS. The bomb load consisted of four 500 lb and one 250 lb GP bombs and we had a full load of fuel (750 gallons) for the expected nine-hour trip. We got the green light from the duty pilot at 22:40 hours and thundered off the runway — a single line of "gooseneck" flares to the left. Off the end of the runway at fifty feet we flew out over the Great Bitter Lake into considerable turbulence but the wheels came up and the take-off flap was retracted as we climbed over the brightly lit German-Italian PoW camp near Fayid.

'At 4,000 feet the Captain and I changed seats and we headed due west some fifty miles south of the coastline in clear sky. There were massive cloud banks over the coast and sea and almost constant lightning. On ETA (02:45 hours) the Captain took over the controls and we turned due north — the target area was clearly denoted by the barrage of shell bursts at our height of 13,000 feet and we soon felt the "bumps" and smelt the cordite as we flew through the black puffs.

'The flashes of the guns could be seen

Wellington IL4267 of 148 Squadron during service in the Middle East (December 1940-December 1942) when no codes were used. On 29 April 1940, while serving with 15 OTU, this aircraft lost an engine in flight and crashed during a forced landing at Swindon. *(RAF Museum)*

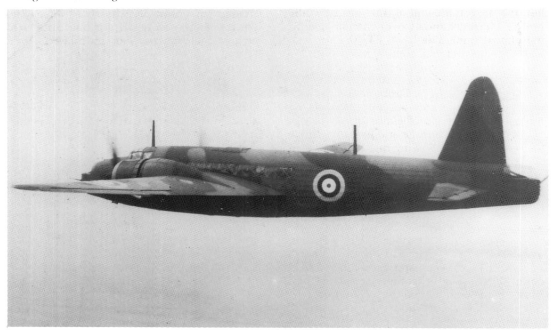

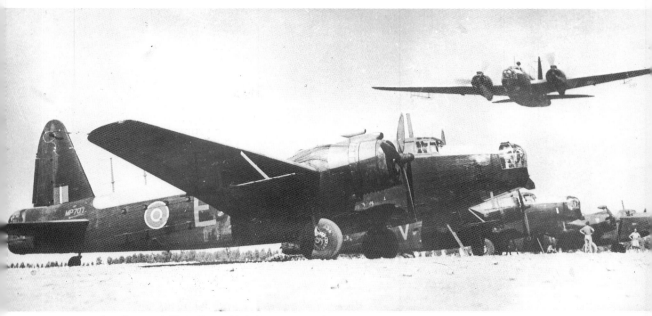

Line up of Wellington XIIIs in Egypt 1942. Nearest aircraft is MP707. *(IWM)*

through breaks in the cloud and the Captain agreed with Bill Ball, the Observer, that these should be the target. We went in straight and level at 03:15 hours but found ourselves closely engaged by predicted flak and had to lose height in evasive action. We finally dropped our bombs at 9,000 feet and left the target area at 6,000 feet at 03:55 hours. Morton handed over the controls to me almost immediately — ETA Kabrit was 07:30 hours and I was already feeling tired!

'We shared the workload. I had a "wakey-wakey" tablet and saw dawn break before we reached Cairo. The Captain made a good daylight landing and we all went off to interrogation in the Intelligence tent, followed by a breakfast of sausage and eggs. I slept all that day and the following night. One aircraft had returned early with elevator trouble and another, unable to locate the target, brought its bombs home. A Wellington which had sent an SOS failed to return. The crew walked back to our lines and rejoined the squadron early in November.

'By the end of October I had been to Tobruk four times and had been four times to attack aerodromes and the battle area in connection with Montgomery's advance from El Alamein. At this time the Wellington tour of operations was 200 hours or forty trips.

'I continued to fly as Second Pilot with a regular crew captained by Sergeant Mortimer. I did ten of my first twelve trips with him in six different aircraft. On the twelfth trip we had a full load for Tobruk of 250 lb GP bombs equipped with steel rods on the nose fuzes, about twenty inches long, designed to ensure that the bombs burst above the ground, thus causing maximum sideways blast effect. We had carried the rodded bombs on battle area trips at the time of Alamein and to attack airfields, but this was the first time to Tobruk. We were briefed to aim for the harbour buildings and dock installations, rather than shipping. The fitting of these rods necessitated the removal of the safety device from the nose fuze and no-one enjoyed carrying the bombs; a prang on take-off could be survivable if bombs were "safe" but not with rods!

'Sergeant Mortimer took off fully loaded that night as No 2 aircraft. As we climbed away we saw a flash on the airfield behind us. On our return we learned that No 3 aircraft had burst a tyre and had exploded; the pilot was on his first trip as captain. We had a very good, clear sight of Tobruk harbour and our Navigator started a big fire. This proved to be our Captain's final trip. I took over for the next one.

'Between the start of the 8th Army's advance from El Alamein and the middle of

November 40 Squadron had moved twice to see how "mobile" we could be in following the troops up the desert. In the past, the "heavies" had stayed on the Suez Canal and along the Ismailia to Cairo road, while the main battle area had shuttled back and forth along the coast between Benghazi and El Alamein. Now, 40 Squadron made a first move to ALG 222A to the west of Cairo, followed by another move to ALG 104 near El Daba via ALG 237 (otherwise known as Kilo 40 — forty kilometres north of Cairo on the main road to Alexandria).

'We all came safely together at ALG 104, close to the coast, on 12 November. The landing ground was littered with wrecked German aircraft, including many '109s. We remembered that we had put ten rodded 250 lb GP bombs and the contents of two containers of 40 lb fragmentation bombs in two sticks across the dispersal areas from 8,000 feet by the light of flares dropped for us by Fleet Air Arm Albacores, only three weeks before.

'During the following eight days we had rain showers and a sandstorm lasting 48 hours. Ops were scrubbed. On the night of 23 November I went as Skipper of my own

crew to Kastelli airfield on the western end of Crete — some 400 miles north-west across the open sea from ALG 104. We were airborne at 19:55 hours and set course on the forecast wind at a steady climb. There was 6/10ths high cloud giving a halo round the full moon. ETA was 22:20 and we crossed the coast on track at 13,000 feet. One or two heavy gun batteries were operating and we saw two or three searchlights which were ineffective.

'Circling the target area, we decided to bomb on a southerly heading across the airfield dispersals. The Navigator had an excellent sight in the moonlight and our five 250 lb bombs and two containers of 40 lb fragmentation bombs went down in one short stick. There was no flak so the bombing run until "bombs gone — jettison bars across" was straight and level. Then the nose went down, the height decreased, the speed increased and course for base was set. Our rear gunner, Sergeant Hammond, reported all bombs burst on the airfield, and we settled down with fingers crossed to cover that 400 miles of open sea again at 5,000 feet. Outside, the air temperature was just above freezing.

Sgt Cliff Mortimer's crew of 40 Squadron at ALG 104, Daba, Western Desert on 21 November 1942 with tented camp in background. Left to right, Sgt Rowley Beatson RNZAF, Front Gunner; Sgt Bert Horton RNZAF, WOP; Sgt Gordon (Reg) Thackeray, 2nd Pilot; F/Sgt Jeff Reddell RNZAF, Navigator/Bomb Aimer; Sgt Wally Hammond, Rear Gunner. *(R. G. Thackeray)*

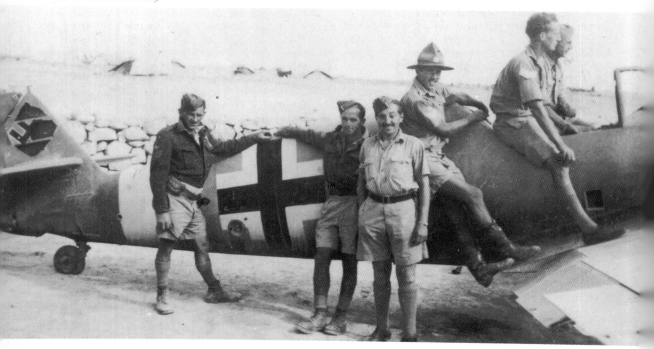

'Sergeant Stewart, my second pilot, took the controls and I went back to pump oil to the two engines — which never missed a beat! We crossed the coast at El Daba and landed at 01:15 hours. Interrogation was quickly over and we went off to an excellent breakfast of bacon and soya sausages, after we had learned that all nine squadron aircraft had attacked the target successfully and had returned safely.

'It was all good experience for our next flight three days later to Malta. Eleven aircraft were briefed for the trip and eleven reached Luqa safely. We had "L for Leather", a full crew, our kit, full tanks and an over-load tank in the bomb bay, four mechanics with their kit and tool boxes. Somebody must have checked the all-up weight, I suppose. All I know was that the run on take-off was very long and we flew west along the coast at 1,000 feet in rain. After passing Tobruk we made our final landfall at Ras el Tin and there started our run of over 500 miles to Malta. We climbed through 10/10ths cloud and came into the clear at 9,000 feet. Navigation was by D/F loop on the Malta radio beacon, supplemented by star sights using the bubble sextant and the Astrograph, a sort of overhead projector in the Navigator's compartment.

'ETA approached, we let down through the cloud and soon spotted the beacon at Luqa and the brilliant lights in the harbour at Valetta. Our approach to the runway was over the dockyards and we were glad to touch down at 07:10 hours on Thursday 26 November, just as dawn was breaking. We landed with 400 gallons of fuel left — a useful addition to the island's reserves.

'About half the squadron aircraft and crews had flown to Luqa at the beginning of November. We were shocked at the thin, haggard appearance of our friends after only three weeks on the island. Although the blocade was virtually lifted by the arrival of the "Stonehenge" convoy from Alexandria, rationing was very strict and severe.

'On Friday morning we were on the detail for a double sortie to Bizerta in Tunisia. Take-off was set for 19:30 hours. The straight line distance to the target was about 280 miles so we had a full load of 520 gallons and a bomb load of four 500 lb and eight 250 lb GP bombs, with dockside buildings the aiming point. The Met forecast was poor and the weather turned out to be very similar! The cloud base was around 1,000 feet when we went out to "L for Leather" and we were unable to start the engines owing to flat batteries on the starter trolly. It was 21:00 hours before we were airborne and we were very much the last aircraft.

'We stayed below cloud at 800 feet and skirted the well-defended island of Pantelleria, heading for the coast south of Tunis. We were climbing on track and passed over Tunis at 10,000 feet. Bizerta was under a terrific bank of cloud and the heavy flak was spasmodic and inaccurate. Searchlights were ineffective in the cloud. Just before midnight there was a break in the cloud and Jeff Reddell, our New Zealand Navigator, got a sight of the harbour. The break lasted long enough for him to bring me on to a straight and level heading at 10,000 feet and he set the "Mickey Mouse" for a single short stick.

'After "Bombs gone!" I closed the bomb doors and turned onto a reciprocal course. Almost immediately a large fire was seen and Wally Hammond, our English rear gunner, reported a large explosion. The fire remained visible for fifteen minutes as we lost height to "improve" the temperature. The oil in the constant speed units had frozen solid and it was quite some time before I was able to bring the revs under control. For long range economical cruising it was our habit to run the supercharged Pegasus XVIII engines on the highest available boost pressures but the lowest possible revolutions per minute. We were back over the Gozo radio beacon before 02:00 hours but Malta was under cloud and Luqa took some finding. By the time we had landed, it was too late to bomb up and refuel for our second sortie so we turned in for interrogation.

'Our next sorties were to Sicily — two trips on the night of 30 November/1 December to Trapani aerodrome and two trips on the night of 3/4 December to the aerodromes at Catania and Comiso. We made two more trips on the night of 6/7 December to the docks at Bizerta and La Goulette, the deep sea port of Tunis. Then we had a fruitless trip to Tunis. There was 10/10ths cloud over the target. We had flown in cloud all the way and had had a wonderful display of St Elmo's fire on the way up to 10,000 feet where we came out into a clear starlit sky. Static electricity discharged itself round the propeller tips, between the machine-guns in the turrets and on the windscreen as the

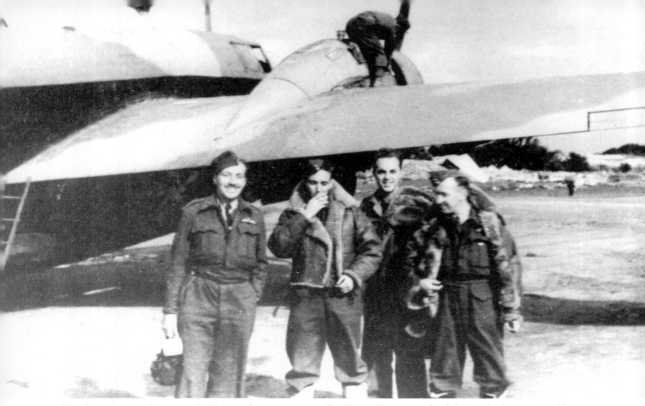

Thackeray's crew 6 January 1943, just after an air test in DV531 'V-Victor', on Saafi Strip which connected Luqa airfield with Hal Far airfield, Malta. Left to right, R. G. Thackeray, Skipper; Eric Kerbey, 2nd Pilot; Sgt Art Harvey, Front Gunner; Sgt Bert Ward, WOP. *(R. G. Thackeray)*

raindrops hit the glass! There was no sign of the target on ETA so we turned back and made a very gentle landing with our full load of bombs!

'Next morning we were told that the main port engine bearing had failed so we had to say "goodbye" to "L for Leather" which had served us so well. She had taken me to Crete, brought me to Malta and we'd been out to Sicily and Tunis on eight occasions. Our next aircraft was *DV566P*. She took us to Palermo in Sicily early on the morning of 12 December following a report of bad weather over Tunis which we had been due to visit the night before.

'We again took *P* to Tunis and La Goulette early on Sunday, 13 December. We were third off the runway at 18:20 hours and set course as usual over the tiny island of Filfla off the south-west coast of Malta. There was little cloud and we pinpointed accurately on the coast south of Cap Bon. We could see flak bursting over Tunis and a good fire at La Goulette partly obscured by light cloud.

'There was no flak over the port so we stooged around and the cloud cleared by

20:50 hours. There was a quarter moon giving good illumination of the target and we were able to go in to attack at 9,000 feet. We had four 500 lb and seven 250 lb GP bombs and decided on three sticks. Eric Laithwaite put the first stick near the electricity generating station, the second stick on the oil refinery and the third stick on two ships moored near the canal, just off the oil jetty. One ship was estimated at 8,000 tons and a fire was seen to start on this one. The fire, punctuated by explosions, was visible up to forty miles away!

'We were safely back at Luqa for interrogation at 22:55 hours. It was later confirmed that we had fired the ship and the report figured in the citation for my DFM — being a Pilot's Air Force, my Navigator has always complained that he hit the ship but I got the gong!

'We were due for a return trip to La Goulette with take-off at 00:30 hours on 14 December but we had to switch to *DV647N* as *P* had been grounded due to excessive oil consumption. All our Pegasus engines used a lot of oil — worn out by use and the sand in the atmosphere despite the Volkes air filters on the carburettor air intakes. Additional regular hours supplies had to be pumped by hand from a reserve tank carried in the fuselage. This was one of the Second Pilot's jobs and was jolly hard work at high altitude and low temperatures, which also caused high viscosity. As an example: in January 1943 *HE115N* used two gallons of oil per hour, say 145 miles! Ten gallons of oil was hand pumped — 550 strokes on a "wobble pump" — on a sortie to Tripoli.

'On take-off at 00:55 hours, the cockpit/panel lighting failed and there was a terrific juddering on the control column. It was still possible to climb very gently. There was no improvement in the situation when the undercarriage and flaps had been cleared up, so I continued, straight ahead, up to 1,000 feet and made a wide circuit and long, powered approach, leaving the flaps up until the last minute. With 3,750 lb of bombs and about the same weight of fuel I took great care to do a gentle "wheel" landing.

'Back at the dispersal it was found that the cooling gills on the starboard engine were jammed in the fully open (ground running) position and this had disturbed the airflow over the tailplane and elevator causing the "judder". I was only in the air 25 minutes! The problem was fixed quickly but the OC Night Flying cancelled our take-off since we should have returned to the island in daylight! (The *Times of Malta* reported this "Blitz on North African docks as the biggest bombing raid ever launched from Malta and the weight of bombs the heaviest ever to have been dropped in a single night by bombers operating from this island".)

'A double sortie to Tunis and La Goulette was made on the night of 15/16 December. Tunis was reached at 20:45 hours and in the moonlight we found the flak very accurate as we did our first turn. We could see many shell bursts and we smelt the cordite smoke. Eric's first stick hit warehouses and his second fell across the railway marshalling yards. We were back at Luqa by 23:00 hours and airborne again at 00:50 hours, after sandwiches. The moon had set by the time we got back to La Goulette but there was a blazing ship in the canal entrance to light the target area. The first stick fell on the harbour works and the second stick caused an explosion in the generating station. We were "home" again at 05:00 hours and found some flak damage to the starboard wing and flap.

'On Friday, 18 December, these double sorties cáme to an abrupt halt. We were briefed for Tunis and took off at 18:20 hours but as we passed between the islands of Linosa and Lampedusa, Bert Ward, our Yorkshire Wireless Operator, reported that our engine-driven generator had failed and he couldn't promise that we would have sufficient voltage in the batteries to drop the bombs if we continued to Tunis. I turned back but it was evident that the voltage would "hold" for some time and the Navigator gave me a course for Comiso in southern Sicily. We delivered our bomb load there before returning to Luqa and landing at 21:00 hours.

'Between the double sorties, the aircraft were marshalled in a line alongside the runway for refuelling and bombing up, whilst all the crews took a breather and had a snack. Because of our generator failure in *HX382M*, we had switched our kit, bombsight etc, to *DV512J* and were preparing for take-off at 23:30 hours. At 23:00 the sirens sounded and shortly afterwards a concentrated dive bomber attack was made on Luqa. The squadron lost seven aircraft destroyed and three damaged. After this, every aircraft was put away in protected dispersals along the Saafi Strip which ran across the island to Hal Far, the fighter aerodrome. The Second Pilot performed this arduous taxying chore after the trip, whilst the Captain, Navigator, Wireless Operator and gunners proceeded to the Intelligence Section for interrogation.

'There were no casualties to air or ground crew during the raid. Most of us literally went to ground in slit trenches and shelters on the airfield. We were all very scared to be so directly on the receiving end and very lucky to survive.

'On 21 December five aircraft were available to operate against Tunis, and ten aircraft took off for Tunis (or Sousse as the alternative) at 18:10 hours on 25 December. The weather forecast was dreadful — heavy cloud up to 12,000 feet. We had "N for Nuts" *HE115* and didn't see anything on ETA at Sousse or Tunis so we brought our bombs back, as did most others. We felt relieved that we had not had to bomb on Christmas Day. (One crew ditched but were picked up by Malta ASR at dawn.) We had a tasty meal in the Officers'

Mess on Luqa main camp before turning in at 00:30 hours on Boxing Day.

'Attacks on Sousse, Sfax, Comiso, Palermo and Tripoli followed during January 1943 and became almost routine. Some were more difficult than others. One night our bombs fell out, due to an electrical fault, when the bomb doors opened and undershot the target (Sfax harbour) and fell in the town. Another night we lost an engine over Tripoli but managed to limp back to Malta (200 miles) losing oil from the "good" engine. Then, on 22 January, we flew back to Egypt for leave and did not return to Malta.

'On 7 February I was told to muster my crew, organise transport to Fayid and find an aeroplane and fly it to ALG 1 where we should find 40 Squadron and other squadrons of 205 Group. I was given Wellington *BB478*, straight out of a major inspection and with no identification letter. She later became C and we took her to Trapani and Palermo later that month.

'ALG 1 was at Magrun, thirty nautical miles south of Benghazi. It accommodated parts of 37, 40, 104 and 108 Squadrons in a large tented camp, with 70 Squadron away to one side. Within a couple of days 40 and 70 were on their own, the other squadrons having moved up to a complex of airfields at Gardabia, near Misurata, some 100 nautical miles east of Tripoli, which had just been occupied by the Eighth Army. ALG 1 became waterlogged and after the sand had settled 40 Squadron joined them at Gardabia.

'The first few days at Gardabia were spent air-testing aircraft, swinging compasses and making other general preparations for the resumption of operations. The Wellington squadrons in Algeria were using the Hercules-engined Mks III and X, whilst 37, 70 and 108 were re-equipped with these versions. All their Mk ICs (with the Pegasus XVIII) went to 40 Squadron. 104 Squadron had always used the Mk II with Merlins and, to ease the maintenance problems, had always operated from the same airfield as 462 Squadron, RAAF, which flew some elderly Halifax Mk Is. Thus, we had plenty of aeroplanes and I was fortunate to be given the new Mk IC I had brought from Fayid.

'On 20 February she took us to Sicily. We were briefed to attack port installations at Palermo and had a load of six 500 lb "rodded" bombs. This trip turned out to be one of our more interesting ones. Visibility

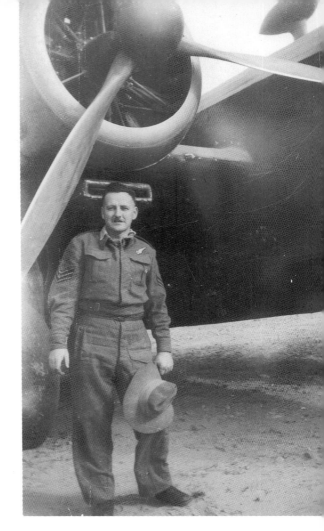

Sgt Observer R. 'Bob' J. Williams, RAAF, of 40 Squadron at Gardabia East (Misurata) in February 1943. *(R. C. Thackeray)*

on take-off was poor and we did not see the flashing beacon at Homs to get a good pinpoint on the coast. Soon afterwards, we found ourselves sandwiched between two layers of cloud, so our Australian Navigator could not calculate the course by reading the drift from flame floats dropped into the sea, nor could he use his bubble-sextant to get position lines from the stars. On top of this, we had a generator failure, so I ordered the radios and lighting to be used for essentials only.

'We pressed on across Sicily, seeing nothing, until we should have been over Palermo. Still nothing. So we turned south and within minutes we were engaged by a heavy flak battery. Coming down to 9,000

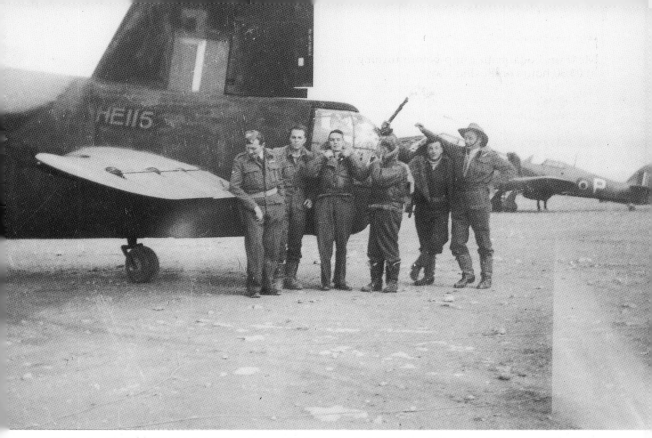

Wellington IC HE115 'N-Nuts' of 40 Squadron which forced landed at El Adem (Tobruk) on 23 January 1943 with a stopped port engine, during a flight to Egypt after a three-month stint on Malta. On landing, the port fuel tanks, pipe lines, filters and carburetter had to be cleared of forty gallons of water which had got into the tanks on Malta! Left to right, Flt Sgt R. G. Thackeray, Sgt Art Harvey RCAF, Sgt Eric Kerbey; Sgt Bert Ward, Sgt Taffy Ball and Sgt Bob Williams RAAF. *(R. G. Thackeray)*

feet we found a break in the cloud and recognised Trapani harbour below us — our first pinpoint for four and a half hours and some sixty nautical miles from our primary target! We had a clear sight of the docks, so our bomb load was put down in one stick. We were well in range of the light flak by now and evasive action took us down to 6,000 feet before we were clear of the defended area. I saw an indicated airspeed of 280 mph at one time and we were not a little shaken up by the time we were back on the straight and level.

'Our Navigator now had a good and accurate pinpoint and was able to estimate a new value for wind speed and direction and, re-starting his air plot, he got us back to the North African coast (east of Tripoli, via Malta) very accurately. The whole trip had taken us eight hours and we learned when we went to interrogation that all aircraft had been recalled about the time that we were at

Trapani becuse of weather conditions — our radio was dead by that time. Several of 37 Squadron's aircraft landed in Malta and two aircraft crashed on landing. Quite a night, one way and another!

'Two nights later we were again briefed for Palermo and had a completely successful trip, bombing the oil tanks from 12,000 feet by the light of a nearly full moon. Other crews were less lucky though, and no fewer than thirteen aircraft diverted to Malta with flak damage. Warrant Officer Massey's crew from 40 Squadron was lost.

'Two nights later C was ditched by Flying Officer Smith on his way back to base from an attack on Gabes. The port engine failed while the aircraft was over the sea east of the isle of Djerba and the captain made a successful landing in the area. All the crew took to the 'j'-type dinghy; land was reached in four days and they all got back to base with the help of friendly Arabs.

'When my name appeared on the detail on 25 February for my 40th trip, I was down to fly "D-Dog" (*HF904*). The target was to be Gabes West Landing Ground, in an effort to reduce Luftwaffe support for the Afrika Korps, dug in on the Mareth Line. Four aircraft were due to take off but only three made it: D, X and B; Q was unserviceable. Our load was 4,500 lb, the maximum, made up of eighteen 250 lb GP bombs with nose rods. I had signed Form 700 for a fuel load of 320 gallons — heavy load/short distance to the target — but the gauges showed 520 gallons. Assuming this to be because of sticking floats in the tanks the position was accepted and we started to run down the runway just after midnight.

'It was not long before the first and second pilots knew that D was overloaded but since the desert runway was, more or less, unlimited in length, and obstacles of any height were virtually non-existent, I just got the tail well up and watched the airspeed build up to 95 mph, hoping the tyres would stand the load. Eventually, she "bounced" into the air and stayed there, so it was "up undercart" and climb straight ahead. About four miles south of the airfield we had reached 150 feet and a slow turn brought us back over base to set course at 400 feet. Not a very good start, but we were up to 5,000 feet in 75 minutes and at 11,000 feet on ETA target. The landing ground was not visible through the haze so we pinpointed the town on the coast and did a timed run. We knew we had found the target when we were engaged by heavy flak — the first run was not straight and level and the second was made at 9,000 feet. Sergeant Williams, our Australian Observer, had a good sight of the airfield and the eighteen bombs went down in one long stick.

'Further heavy and accurate flak caused us to abandon "straight and level" for the camera and photoflash and we were all glad to be clear of the target area and on course for base at 7,000 feet. Oil was visible behind the starboard engine nacelle, so we realised the flak had been really close. A direct course back to base was plotted and since this took us close to Tripoli, which was crammed with Eighth Army Staff and supplies, we put the IFF set on to "distress" and hoped the engine would keep running. I thought we could always divert ourselves to Tripoli airport if a real emergency developed. It did not, but we were diverted by radio to Gardabia Main and found that we were being treated as "hostile" since our IFF was not functioning. As a result of this we had caused an air raid alarm in Tripoli. We had been in the air over six hours on our assumed fuel load, so we were officially "overdue" as well as "hostile". However, since we got back safely no action was taken in respect of the overloading.

'This proved to be my last operational trip. I was declared "tour expired", took leave of my crew and a few days later flew back to Cairo. My forty operations had totalled 206 hours of night flying. Six weeks later I was back in the UK, later converting to Hercules-engined Mks III and X. These marks were just arriving at Gardabia when I left and 40 Squadron was given all the Mk ICs whilst the other squadrons got the Hercules, so 40 Squadron was the last to operate the IC.'

Chapter 12
African adventure

On 8 November 1942 the Allies landed American and British troops ashore on the coast of French Morocco and all objectives were quickly taken. Once Air Marshal Sir W. Welsh, KCB, had established a permanent headquarters for Eastern Air Command at Maison Carrée, outside Algiers, he realised that night bombers should be despatched from England without further delay.

On 26 November, just as the bombing of Germany was gaining momentum, an urgent request was received from North Africa for two squadrons of Wellington night bombers to be urgently sent to Algeria. As a result, both Nos 142 and 150 Squadrons were ordered, at short notice, to each prepare thirteen crews and a ground echelon, 100 strong, for shipment to North Africa. The understanding was that they would be on detachment for only three months.

Some thirteen specially 'tropicalised' Wellingtons arrived at No 142 Squadron's base at Waltham, near Grimsby. Similiarly, another thirteen 'tropicalised' Wellingtons arrived at No 150 Squadron's base at Kirmington in Lincolnshire. On 9 December 1942, Nos 142 and 150 Squadrons, ill-equipped and with no provision for replenishment, flew to Portreath, their advance base, leaving those who were left behind to merge with the home echelon of No 142 Squadron to form No 166 Squadron.

At Portreath, bad weather delayed the Wellingtons' departure. They finally left England on 19 December. All the crews were experienced; some were on their second tour. The universal thought was that operations in Africa would be 'a piece of cake' compared to flying night bombing raids over the Ruhr.

Blida airfield. Wellingtons, Blenheims and Bostons can be seen at various dispersal sites in the vicinity of the control tower. *(Rupert Cooling)*

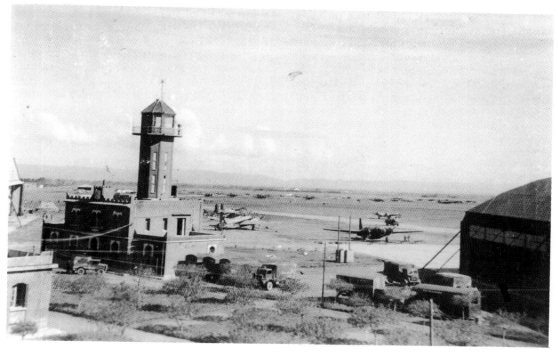

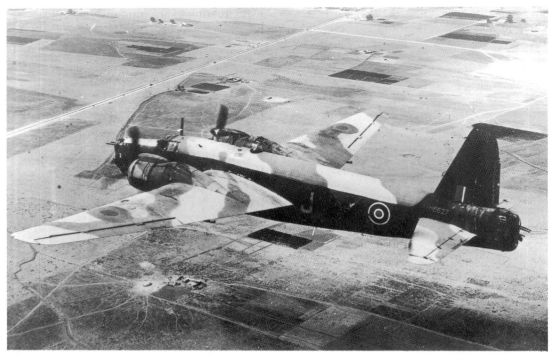

Wellington X HE627 J in flight over North Africa in 1943. *(RAF Museum)*

The Wellingtons refuelled at Gibraltar before carrying on to Blida, 35 miles south-west of Algiers. (Blida is located under a fir and evergreen covered range of the Atlas Mountains which rise to a height of 6,000 feet.) The airfield had been built during French colonial days and boasted several large hangars, barrack buildings and work-shops, which had once accommodated up to 8,000 British and Americans. Although it had a fairly well drained terrain the airstrip was very muddy and two of the Wellingtons crashed on landing.

Two squadrons of Wellingtons would only make a small impact on the land battle but any bombers were welcome at this time. The Wellingtons carried out a diversity of missions, ranging from the flying of supply drops to beleaguered French troops, anti-submarine patrols, leaflet raids and fighter and searchlight co-operation duties.

The Tunisian campaign was a severe test for Allied forces. It would drag on from January until May 1943, largely due to the very effective generalship of Field Marshal Rommel and his highly trained Afrika Korps. Another factor in the campaign was the weather. Heavy rain prevented the first

operation being flown until the night of 28/29 December when eight Wellington IIIs were despatched to bomb Bizerta docks.

Flight Lieutenant Ronnie Brooks, DFC, had a hang-up with his 4,000 lb 'cookie' over the target while flying at 11,000 feet. Arthur Johnson, the bomb aimer/front gunner, recalls: 'I had just got the target beautifully into my bomb sight when I found the release gear had packed up. I tried three times to get the bomb away but it wouldn't drop. When I went to the bomb bay I found the couplings underneath the bomb had iced up.'

Johnson and the Navigator, Flight Sergeant Jim Oldham, tried to unscrew the couplings but the ice was too thick. Oldham then got an axe and made a hole in the bottom of the fuselage big enough for him to put his head and shoulders through. With Johnson holding his legs, Oldham then hung through the fuselage and chipped away at the ice until he tired. Johnson then took his place. Flight Sergeant Chuck Delaney, the Canadian rear gunner, also had a try.

The Wellington cruised around the target for about twenty minutes while the three men hacked at the ice. Fairly heavy flak was coming up all the time the airmen were chipping at the ice. Once the bomb was free of ice Johnson went back to his bomb sight and, at the right moment, shouted to the other two airmen to let the bomb go. Delaney and Oldham gave a lusty push with their feet and the 4,000-pounder hurtled down onto Bizerta, exploding near a barracks.

During January bad weather continued to dog operations but 231 sorties were flown. Bizerta came in for heavy punishment, being bombed on no less than 22 occasions that month. The Wellingtons often used the concrete runway at Maison Blanche as an advanced base and landing ground when their airstrip at Blida was put out of commission by the weather.

On 1 January 1943 Wellingtons of No 142 Squadron, each carrying a 4,000 lb 'cookie', mounted an operation on the docks and oil storage tanks at Bizerta. At briefing, crews were informed that the port, which was the main supply facility for the Afrika Korps, was heavily defended. The Met report was as follows: 'Light NE wind. 10/10ths cloud throughout, cloud base 2,500 feet — variable height. Icing index high in cloud.'

Norman Child recalls the operation: 'We took off at 02:29 hours, set course for the Maison Blanche beacon and then time ran to the turning point thirty miles off the coast. We turned on course for Bizerta and checked our position with back bearing. We climbed to 6,000 feet for minimum "cookie" height and flying in cloud. Radio navigational aids were very poor so we relied on dead reckoning.

'Through a small break in the cloud the rear gunner reported surf below and we were crossing the coast and drifting inland. The winds had obviously strengthened from the north and we were close to Philippeville. There was much turbulence. The Atlas Mountain range was only twenty miles inland. We changed course to port and climbed rapidly to try and break cloud for a star shot. We climbed to 13,000 feet and still we were in cloud. The aircraft was beginning to ice up rapidly. The position was serious. We could not climb above cloud and the weight of the ice was too much. The airspeed fell off.

'The target was only twenty miles to starboard. We decided to make a shallow descent to the target area. Searchlights ahead were shining through the cloud. The aircraft

was vibrating badly and the flying speed was just above stalling. We selected a dropping position in the centre of the searchlight ring and released the "cookie". With a lightened load the aircraft was climbed another 1,000 feet and we broke cloud at 14,000 feet. The ice crystalized and broke up, great chunks being flung off the props. We got a good astro fix and set course for base, maintaining our height.

'We homed onto Maison Blanche beacon and descended rapidly through the cloud, icing up again. The cloud base descended to 1,500 feet and the warmer air broke up the ice. With a sigh of relief we crossed the coast and flew up the valley on the Blida beacon. We had been airborne for six hours 15 minutes.'

On the night of 14 January the weather was instrumental in the loss of two Wellingtons. Twelve aircraft were detailed to attack Bizerta and the Met report indicated (wrongly as it turned out) that conditions would be perfect. At the target conditions were indeed ideal and three blockbuster bombs burst successfully in the dock area. However, half way back to Blida the formation ran into a violent thunderstorm with 10/10ths cloud at all heights.

Returning aircraft were forced to circle Blida and Maison Blanche hoping for a break in the clouds to enable them to land. Six eventually managed to put down at Maison Blanche and four more touched down at Blida. Flight Lieutenant Vincent, DFC, was forced to beach his Wellington near Djidjelli and he and his crew, including Squadron Leader Carmichael of Coastal Command, managed to clamber to safety. The seas were running so high that the Wellington broke up within minutes before any items of equipment could be saved.

Wing Commander J. D. Kirwan, DFC, CO of No 150 Squadron, carrying Flight Lieutenant Summers, the Int/Ops Officer, to report on the flak at Bizerta, arrived over Blida only to find the cloud base down to the deck. To avoid hitting the mountains, the pilot turned out to sea again. For upwards of an hour he skimmed along the line of breakers. Once, he caught a fleeting glimpse of Maison Blanche, only to lose it when over the aerodrome. After eight hours in the air the petrol gave out and at 01:00 hours the crew baled out over the Atlas Mountains. All of the crew landed with leg injuries and slight

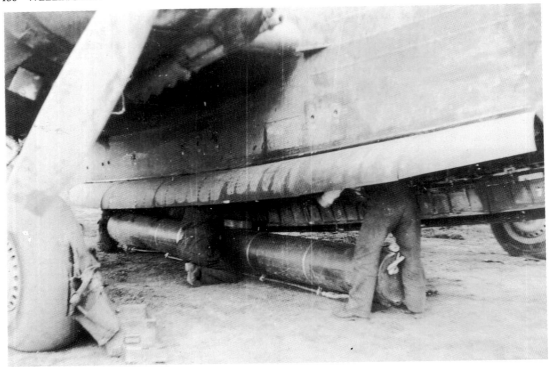

Overload tanks being fitted to a Wellington of 142 Squadron at Blida for a raid on Trapani. *(Rupert Cooling)*

concussion but relatively unhurt in wild mountainous country.

Four nights later, on 18 January, Squadron Leader J. F. H. Booth and crew were among those detailed to attack the docks at Bizerta. Dropping two sticks of bombs, they circled offshore to observe the effect of the main attack. Then, in bright moonlight, and with no cloud cover, they were attacked very determinedly by a Ju 88 night fighter. On the first attack the starboard engine was set on fire making the Wellington easy prey for the Ju 88 crew, anxious to finish off their quarry. The night fighter made three further attacks, knocking out the hydraulic system, rear turret, air speed indicator and flaps, and setting a portable oxygen tank on fire.

After delivering a fourth attack the fighter formated several hundred yards to starboard. An attack was then made from the front turret of the Wellington, which resulted in the fighter breaking off the engagement. When the fighter had broken off the engagement Squadron Leader Booth ordered the crew to come forward to prepare to bale out.

LAC J. Skingsley, acting as Flight Engineer, with great gallantry and complete disregard for his personal safety, ignored his parachute pack and attacked the blazing oxygen bottle. Being unable to put the fire out, Skingsley picked up the blazing bottle in his bare hands, carried it to the escape hatch and threw it out. He then proceeded to assist in lightening the machine by jettisoning all the equipment that was not screwed down. Squadron Leader Booth managed to bring the Wellington home for a crash landing and he was later awarded the DFC. By his actions, Skingsley undoubtedly saved the aircraft and lives of the crew. He was awarded the DFM.

The night of 21/22 January proved quite eventful too. Three distinct operations were undertaken. Bizerta Sidi Ahmed aerodrome was attacked by five Wellingtons of No 142 Squadron and they registered two hits on the hangars and three on the runway. Meanwhile, five Wellingtons of No 150 Squadron attacked a torpedo bomber base at Elmas aerodrome in Sardinia. The Wellingtons were obviously not expected because the airfield lights and those at three satellites nearby were blazing brightly. Flight Lieutenant Donald Dunn could not believe his luck and he and his four crews put the airfield out of action for 48 hours.

The following day the Wellingtons were called upon to assist the Eighth Army's advance into Tunisia with a bombing raid on enemy aircraft at Medenine, 500 miles distant. Later reconnaissance photos revealed that a number of aircraft had been destroyed on the desert air strip.

On the night of 31 January the Wellingtons attacked Sicily for the first time. Trapani, on the western end of the island, a port much used by the Axis to tranship war material to Rommel's forces in Tunisia, had been reconnoitered and found with a considerable amount of shipping along the quays and four skulking destroyers in the harbour. The night proved exceptionally dark and made bombing results difficult. However, three large fires were started and photos later revealed that the docks and adjoining warehouses had been well hit.

February opened with a second raid on Cagliari Elmas aerodrome. The weather, which had been bad, now deteriorated considerably. In spite of every effort, including daily briefings and bombing up, operations were possible on only eleven nights during the month. Bizerta was attacked on seven occasions. These constant raids on the Tunisian port helped stem the flow of supplies getting through to the Afrika Korps.

On 22 February the Wellingtons suffered their first casualties. Sergeant A. M. Jensen (No 142 Squadron) and crew failed to return from a raid on Bizerta. Three nights later, in bad weather, No 150 Squadron lost Pilot Officer J. G. Swain, DFC, and crew while returning from another operation to Bizerta. The aircraft flew into the cloud-covered mountainside about ten miles east of Blida aerodrome.

In the middle of February Wing Commander J. D. Kirwan, CO of No 150 Squadron, returned to England suffering from the effects of an injury sustained while baling out of his aircraft on the night of 15 January. He was succeeded by Wing Commander. A. A. Malan, who had previously commanded a Blenheim V squadron in North Africa. Other changes, at top level, were also made. With the continued advance of the Eighth Army, a change in command and disposition of Allied Air Forces in North Africa was made. Mediterranean Air Command under Air Chief Marshal Tedder came into being and,

under him, General Spaatz took command of the North-West African Air Force, comprising all the Allied air units from Tunisia to Morocco. On 19 February the Wellington squadrons came into the North-West African Strategic Air Force (NASAF) under the command of Major-General James H. Doolittle, USAAF, famous for his air racing days before the war and his leadership on the B-25 Mitchell raid on Tokyo from the deck of the carrier *Hornet* in 1942.

Doolittle wasted no time getting to know the units in his new command. On 22 February he flew down to Blida and went with Flying Officer Roberts to see for himself the bombing of Bizerta docks by night. The General was able to witness a well executed attack, with the majority of bombs going down in the space of two minutes. The goods station was hit and oil tanks were left burning. The fire could be seen for up to fifty miles away.

On the night of 12 March Prince Bernhard of the Netherlands and other high ranking officers attended the briefing for a raid on marshalling yards at Tunis. On 24 March Air Marshal Tedder visited Blida and addressed the crews. Morale began to soar with the arrival of badly needed replacement crews. However, during the first three months of the campaign no Wellington spares were received at Blida. Maintenance was kept up by robbing unserviceable and crashed aircraft and an average serviceability of 85 per cent was maintained.

With the Eighth Army now in Tunisia, the Wellingtons were detailed to give direct assistance to the advancing troops. In spite of the bad weather (rain fell almost incessantly during February and March) attacks were made on enemy landing grounds, hidden away in olive groves. Despite the weather the Wellingtons managed to fly 115 sorties in March, ending with a trip on the 'mail run' to Bizerta and back.

On 17 April twenty Wellingtons were detailed to attack Tunis docks and marshalling yards. During the raid a burst of flak under Sergeant Chandler's aircraft pierced the petrol tank. With difficulty, Chandler succeeded in reaching the neighbourhood of Algiers Bay, where both engines cut. With the intercom failing the aircraft had to be ditched without warning to the crew. They were thrown in all directions.

With the aircraft rapidly filling with water,

Chandler scrambled through his escape hatch. The bomb aimer was thrown over the main-spar and went out through the astrodome. The rear gunner, standing near the flare chute at the moment of impact, was knocked down and picked himself up to find water up to his shoulders: he went through the astrodome closely followed by the Navigator, who had no recollection of what happened. The W/Op hit the door of the cabin and was shot out in front of the aircraft.

They all then helped each other into the dinghy, where they lay completely exhausted. For 36 hours they drifted, always within sight of land. A C-47 and five vessels, which all came close, failed to have their attention attracted by the firing of Very cartridges. Eventually, they were picked up by the Polish destroyer *Blyskowila*, returning to Gibraltar after a few days for repairs. Flown back from Gibraltar, after a few days spent in recuperation, the crew were soon back on operations.

On 19 April Group Captain 'Speedy' Powell, DSO, OBE, of *Target for Tonight* fame, arrived from England to co-ordinate Nos 142 and 150 Squadrons' efforts and to form them into a Wing. Area bombing was to be replaced by precision bombing and a move nearer the front lines was imminent. The squadrons moved to Fontaine Claude, fifteen miles from Batna, to take up station as part of No 330 Wing.

On 6 May twenty Wellingtons were detailed to take off from Fontaine Claude for a raid on Trapani. However, malfunctions and the inability of some crews to find their aircraft in the dark, meant that ony thirteen actually managed to take off. It was hardly an auspicious debut. Worse was to follow. En route thick cloud and violent thunderstorms forced the remaining aircraft to abort. Ten Wellingtons landed back at Fontaine Claude, one put down at Biskra, 'the Garden of Allah', and another landed near Guelma. Sergeant H. Venning, DFM, in the remaining aircraft, ran out of petrol and crash-landed on a desolate stretch of the coast. None of the crew suffered any lasting injuries from their adventure.

Tunis fell on 7 May and the Axis Powers were finally cleared from Africa on the 13th. With no targets in the desert left to bomb, the Wellington crews turned their attentions to Sicilian and Sardinian ports. In the course of a single week Palermo was attacked twice

Wimpy under wraps for protection from the desert sandstorms in Tunisia, 1943. *(Harold Hamnett)*

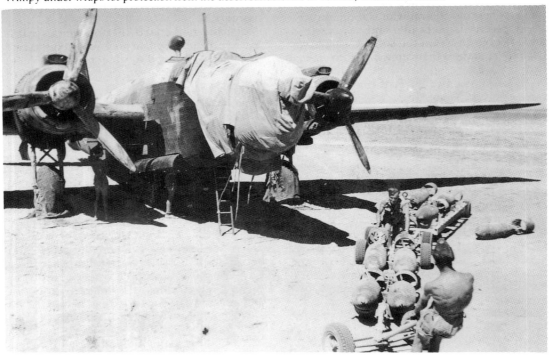

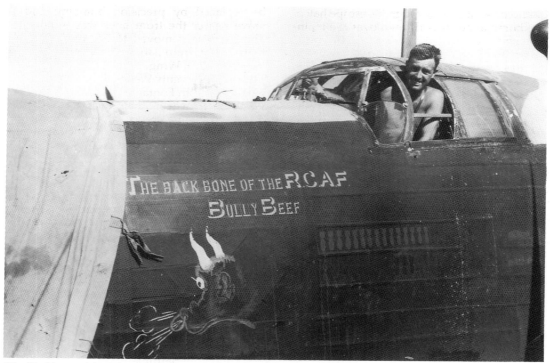

The 'Backbone of the RCAF: Bully Beef' of 424 'Tiger' Squadron at Kairouan-Zina in July 1943. *(Harold Hamnett)*

and Naples, Alghero, Cagliari, Marsala and Trapani were each visited once. On the first raid on Palermo the railway station and the docks received direct hits and several fires were left burning. On the second visit it was the power station that came in for particular attention.

On 16 May crews made the long-awaited visit to Rome. However, the Wellingtons dropped nothing more sinister on the eternal city than a million leaflets, while the heavy stuff was used on the Lido di Roma seaplane base at the mouth of the Tiber, eighteen miles away. Leaflets, or 'Nickels' had proved relatively successful in the desert. On one occasion, 7,000 Italians, each bearing a 'laissez-passer', had given themselves up in one day.

On the night of 17/18 May 1943 Major-General James H. Doolittle flew with No 142 Squadron to see for himself the results of a raid on Alghero in Sardinia. In the middle of May, Wing Commander Bamford handed over command of No 142 Squadron to Wing Commander A. R. Gibbes, DFC, RAAF. On 25/26 May, the Wellingtons moved to the holy city of Kairouan. Shortly after their arrival, the Luftwaffe dropped three bombs, all of which missed the airfield by a wide margin.

The fortified island of Pantelleria (which lies approximately half way between the east coast of Tunisia and the south-west of Sicily) attracted the attention of the planners in May 1943. Both islands were proving a stumbling block to the invasion of Sicily from North Africa. Pantelleria was teeming with 11,000 Italians who had sufficient food and water to withstand a long siege. Underground hangars had been constructed on the airfield and a small harbour was suitable for fast motor torpedo boats.

A variety of aircraft bombed Pantelleria around the clock. On the night of 23 May it was the turn of No 142 Squadron. Rupert 'Tiny' Cooling, who had been posted to No 142 from No 9 Squardon in March 1943 and was now pilot of "Y-Yorker", recalls: 'It was a two and a half hour round trip; the first wave took off at sunset, the second somewhat before midnight, while the last was timed to cross the Tunisian coast, homeward bound, at first light. It was an easy target to find; one would scarcely overlook an island of some sixty square miles however dark the night, particularly with a peak topping 2,000 feet in the centre.

'The Italians helped too. Approaching, one was aware of a darker mass against the reflective blackness of the sea. Then a searchlight or two would spring up and grope uncertainly in the darkness. A thin hosepipe of light flak, pink, apple-green and white, might rise like a charmed snake, then vanish. The harbour was easily identified. The coast was distinctive and a course over the headland towards the peak ensured passing over the port, the town, and the airfield. A right turn through ninety degrees put the aircraft

Ground crew pose for the camera in front of 'Al's Sugarbox' of 142 Squadron which proudly sports fourteen operations symbols on its nose. Left to right Electrician, Dave (who hopped a ride on 10 June 1943 with Rupert Cooling) and Smudge. *(Rupert Cooling)*

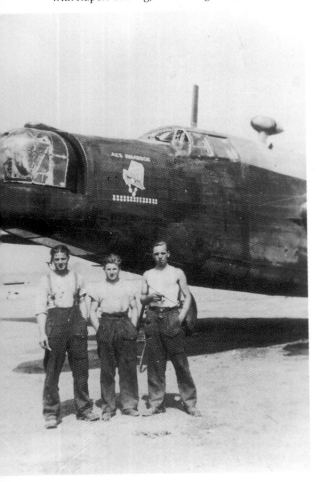

on course for base. There might be a few thumps of heavy flak, a scatter of brief embers flowering against the sable coverlet of darkness; but in general, the crews were all happy. If only the Italians would hold out long enough, they might get their tour of forty ops completed in record time. Compared with Palermo, Messina, Catania, Naples, it was a doddle; in the vernacular, "a piece of piss".

'The scale of operations was gradually stepped up until the aircraft were doing three sorties nightly; the crews two on one night and one the next. From 29 May to 11 June 1943 Pantelleria was visited every night by the Wellingtons, 225 sorties being flown in twelve nights. As a fitting climax NASAF staged 1,000 day sorties, to which No 330 Wing added 45 at night, some of the 21 serviceable aircraft making two and even three flights.

'At briefing, on Thursday, 10 June, we were on the mid detail. No 330 Wing were putting in forty sorties; the other Wellingtons of No 205 Group were aiming for fifty. Something like 160 tonnes of bombs were to fall on Pantelleria that night. "The culminating point of an interesting experiment," as Group Captain Powell put it. There might even be signals from the ground to indicate surrender. The Navigator asked, in mock seriousness, if we should land to take formal possession!

'Just after midnight, "Y-Yorker", refuelled, with another 6,000 lb of bombs winched into her belly, was ready. We climbed aboard. Dave (a ground crewman who was being smuggled aboard to experience for himself a raid over Axis territory) stood beside me as I started up the two Hercules engines and then ran them up. There was not a tremor on the tachometers as we tested each magneto in turn. Revs and boost were spot on. Chiefy Sword disappeared towards the adjacent dispersal: Dave dived down the back. The ladder came up; the door thudded shut. Smudge heaved away the chocks and "Y-Yorker" rumbled towards the flare path.

'A green light winks in the darkness; we line up with the flares on our left, stretching away into a wall of darkness. Fifteen degrees of flap, cowling gills closed, brakes held on. Advance the throttle levers and the Hercules bellow with restrained power. The Wellington trembles, eager to be airborne. Brakes off, control column pushed towards the instru-

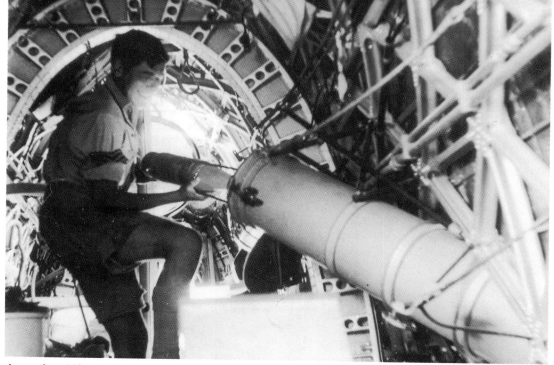

It was the wireless operator's task to throw out flame floats, flares and photo flashes. Here, Sgt Harold Bean demonstrates how it should be done. *Rupert Cooling)*

ment panel and ''Y-Yorker'' surges forward, lifting her tail into the plume of dust behind us. The flares accelerate to pass beyond the wing tip, there is a brief bump; the wheels touch once again; the last flare speeds by as the altimeter slowly starts to unwind. Bill, standing beside me, snaps down the detente and lifts the stubby undercarriage lever. Green lights on the instrument panel go out and are replaced by red as the wheels fold back into the engine nacelles. We are on our way.

'It was almost an hour later that Bill went down into the nose to set up the bombing panel. Dave stood beside me, peering into the darkness. In the distance, a photo flash exploded, throwing the rugged outline of the island into sudden silhouette. If this was to be an experience, we might as well show Dave something of the country. I turned slightly to starboard to pass south of the island for a run up the east coast before swinging left over the target. As we crossed the coast, there appeared on our port side what looked at first like a flare but which grew suddenly larger, then larger still, emitting coloured stars as it fell slowly towards the surface of the sea. Suddenly, it was recognisable. The golden filigree of a Wellington's

geodetic wings and fuselage, gyrating like a sycamore seed, slid slowly towards extinction in the water beneath. This was definitely not part of the programme.

'Somewhat shocked, we turned to line up on the harbour. Bill's voice came up over the intercom, ''Bomb doors open. Left. Left. Steady. Right. Bombs gone!'' There was a sharp jolt as ''Y-Yorker'' shed her load. ''Photo flash away'', Beanie (Sergeant Harold Bean, the Wireless Operator) called out over the intercom as he launched the flash through the flare chute. We held steady, awaiting the bright burst of light which would give us our picture. Then it was hell-bent for home. The compass needle had barely settled between the grid wires when the voice of the rear gunner sounded in our earphones. ''There's another kite going down in flames behind us.''

'Dave slipped out, as planned, after we landed and taxied to dispersal. Shag Sword had his doubts as to where he had been, but said nothing. Squadron Leader Roy Chappel (Intelligence Officer, No 104 Squadron, one of our sister units) wrote in his book, *Wellington Wings*, of the night of 10 June: ''Several of our crews reported encounters with single-engined fighters, probably Fw 190s, over the

Pantelleria area. Single-engined fighters are unusual at night. Two of our aircraft are missing: 'X-X-Ray' . . . and 'W-William' (Sergeant Eason and crew) who were on their last operation before completing their tour. What cruel luck!"

'Three of "X-X-Ray's" crew landed safely by parachute on Pantelleria: the other seven were lost. Had "Y-Yorker" not been carrying Dave on his sightseeing mission; had we not decided to make a circuit of Pantelleria and come in from a novel direction, then "Y-Yorker" herself might well have been the fighter's second success, lurking in the deceitful cover of darkness on a too well established approach path where hazard had been so lightly dismissed.'

Pantelleria surrendered to the British 1st Infantry Division on 11 June. Another fortified island, that of Lampedusa, capitulated unconditionally after one raid by the Wellingtons! The way was now clear, once the last of the landing craft had arrived, for Operation Husky, the Allied invasion of Sicily, to begin.

Meanwhile, No 330 Wing had been reinforced by four squadrons of Wellingtons from the Middle East, and the arrival at Kairouan/Zina in Tunisia of Nos 420 'Snowy Owl', 428 'Tiger', and 425 'Alouette' Squadrons of the RCAF, from England. Fred Wingham, pilot of Wellington 'V-Victor' (later re-christened 'V-Virgin'), No 420 Squadron, recalls: 'On 26 June we flew our first raid. We took off and headed for Kelibia Point, on the eastern tip of Tunisia, and crossed the Sicilian Channel for Sciacca, on the west coast of Sicily. It was not a very good trip, as seven of our 500-pounders failed to release. We made several runs over the target but despite all our efforts we could not get rid of them. Nevertheless, we did manage to land safely at base. Beacons always helped guide us home but at 2,000 feet on a warm night one could literally smell Kairouan!

'Three nights later, on 29 June, we carried a mixed load to Messina; they all went in one stick on the docks and quayside. All our raids now seemed to be tactical. We bombed docks and airfields and railways. On one

Fred Wingham and the 'gang' all smiles in front of 'V-Virgin', their tour completed. Left to right (back row), P/O J. H. Cressman RCAF, Navigator; Sgt Eddie Hanratty RCAF, Bomb Aimer; Flt Sgt Fred Wingham, Pilot; Sgt J. Owen, WOP; ground crew technician, RCAF. *(Fred Wingham)*

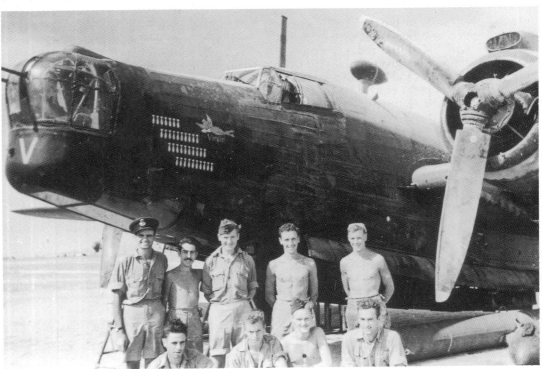

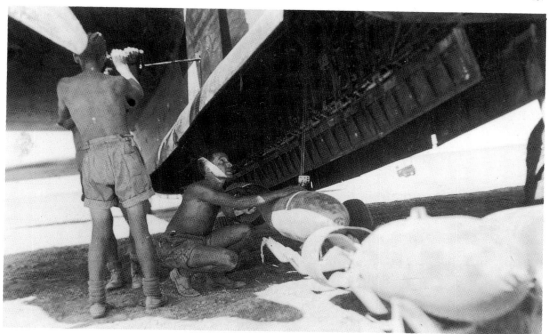

Hot work as armourers hoist 250 lb bombs into the bomb bay of a 424 Squadron Wellington X in Tunisia, 1943.
(Harold Hamnett)

occasion we bombed a village to fill the streets with rubble to delay the German transport.

'The climax came on the night of 9 July. We were given another Wellington which was fitted with Mandrel radar jamming equipment. I was also given an additional gunner because we would be on a long stint. We were sent to a point between Malta and Sicily. It was daylight in the early hours of 10 July when we got there. We set up and flew to and fro, using Mandrel to jam enemy radar. At this point the invasion of Sicily started. Other Wimpys were on other beats and we covered the whole south coast of Sicily.

'As darkness fell I could see Malta lit up like day with the action of the ships moving out. In the dim light of the night sky we could see the gliders being towed away to the dropping points and we saw some coming back. We were airborne for eight hours and ten minutes; rather a long stint.'

Wingham's original Wellington was returned to him and further operations were flown in it, to Corsica, Sardinia and Italy. 'V-Virgin' caused many a raised eyebrow as Fred Wingham recalls: 'The squadron padre was a jolly soul and one day he looked at the beautiful, voluptuous female painted on the side and declared, "She's far too broad in the hips for a virgin!" '

In September all three Canadian squadrons moved to Hani East ALG for further operations before flying home to the UK at the end of October. In December they all converted to the Halifax. The establishment of airfields in Italy that same month enabled the remaining Wellington squadrons of No 205 Group — Nos 37, 40, 70, 104, 142 and 150 — to move to airfields in the Cerignola area of southern Italy. The night bomber force had assumed quite formidable proportions and the tide in the Mediterranean Theatre was now turning in the Allies' favour.

Chapter 13
Mediterranean missions

Crews were pleased to exchange the dust and heat of the North African desert for what they thought would be better conditions in the lush green vine groves of southern Italy. This did not prove to be the case. Camp comforts were more or less non-existent and weather conditions were often poor. Over northern Italy they could be fatal, as Roy Gristwood, a navigator of No 142 Squadron, which shared Cerignola III with the 15th Air Force, recalls: 'On 24 November, during an attack on a ball-bearing factory in Turin, we were preparing to descend through "cloud" when "Mac" McNab, the gunner, shouted a warning to our Australian pilot, Flying Officer Lyn Clarke, that the "cloud" was the snow-capped Alps! The Group sustained heavy losses with many aircraft running into the Ligurian Alps south east of the target area.'

During the Anzio landings in February 1944, No 205 Group harrassed enemy troop movements behind the German lines, sometimes twice nightly. Roy Gristwood recalls: 'On the nights of 15 and 16 February we attacked troops and motor transport seen on the move in the area. Bombing was made visually from 4,000 feet. The operations were short — only just over three hours at the most — and no opposition was ever met, although some crews reported seeing fighters. They were probably other Wimpys stooging around.

'On 24 February we attacked the Steyr-Daimler-Puch aircraft factory at Steyr, Austria. We were unable to make a landfall on the north Adriatic coast because of cloud. Crews were further frustrated because a lake, which was an inland turning point, was frozen and snow-covered which made it

Flash photo of Fiume torpedo factory taken from 7,300 feet on the night of 21/22 January 1944 from F/O Clarke's Wellington of 142 Squadron. *(Roy Gristwood)*

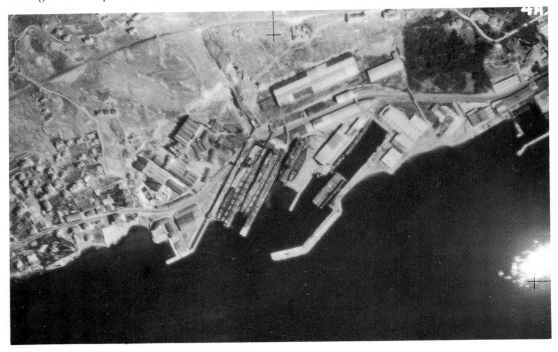

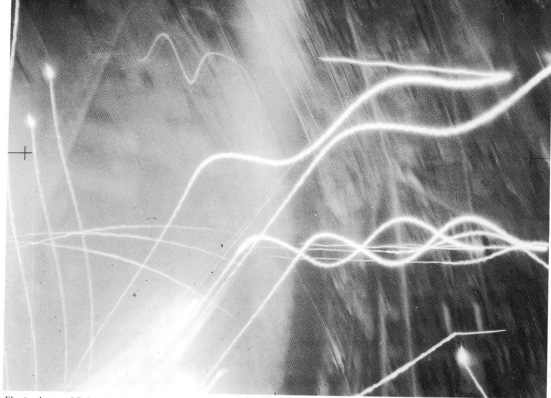

Flash photo of flak taken from 11,500 feet over Budapest on the night of 3/4 March 1944 from F/O Clarke's Wellington of 142 Squadron. *(Roy Gristwood)*

indistinguishable from land! The winds in the Alps are totally different from the Adriatic, so as far as we were concerned we could not positively identify the target. We saw some bombing fifty miles west, so we "joined in". Intelligence subsequently identified this as a minor railway town many miles west of Steyr.

'Some crews assumed that they were bombing Steyr, so they set off on homeward courses from their false position. Sergeant Armstrong's crew mistook the coast of north-west Italy for the coast of north Yugoslavia. When fuel ran low they baled out over Corsica. Believing this to be northern Italy, they hid in the hills for several days until they were winkled out by the Free French. Some aircraft even landed in Sardinia. Many aircraft were lost.'

On the night of 15 March Gristwood flew the 27th operation of his tour when No 142 Squadron visited the marshalling yards at Sofia. It was the first of three he made to the Bulgarian capital. 'On the first trip we carried 54 flares to illuminate drops for bombing aircraft. We had to stooge around the target

providing illumination by periodic flare drops and this meant a longer flight time than normal bombing drops.

'Sofia was still lit up as we arrived over the city but they soon went out. They were replaced by about fifteen searchlights with light and heavy flak moving into action. Conditions over the target were perfect, but on our return the cloud base was down to 400 feet at Cerignola.

'After we landed and had been debriefed, we were breakfasting in the tent lines, about 1½ miles from the actual airfield, when we heard an aircraft very low overhead and coming in to land. A Wellington from a neighbouring squadron flew in out of the low cloud (now lower than ever) and landed *between* the lines of tents. The crew climbed out with their hands up — believing they had landed on an island off Yugoslavia! It was another example of how the dangers were not always flak or the Luftwaffe but the weather and lack of effective navigational aids.

'On the next night it was Sofia again with the situation reversed. We carried nine SBCs (small bomb containers) totalling 800 four-pound incendiaries. This time there was 10/10ths cloud over the city but we had been told that "authority from the highest source" had been given to bomb through cloud if necessary. Apparently Churchill had not forgotten the Bulgars for some misdemeanours during the First World War!

'A week later, on 24 March, we went to Sofia again with another cargo of 54 flares. Sofia was again under 10/10ths cloud so we could not identify the marshalling yards. The flak was the heaviest to date. They were learning.'

On 29 March Flight Sergeant Walker's crew arrived at Foggia to join No 150 Squadron. Les Hallam, the air bomber, recalls: 'We were told that *MF238* would be the aircraft we would be using on operations, but this did not turn out to be the case. Our Wimpy went into a pool for replacements required by the squadrons. Amendola airfield was used by American B-17s, flying daytime missions and by 150 and 142 Squadrons; both of whom were equipped with the Wellington X. From

our tented camp site we had about a half-hour ride on the transport trucks to the airfield. Officers were quartered in a farm-house and other farm buildings.

'Our Skipper did two trips with other crews before we did our first op as a crew on 15 April to marshalling yards at Turnu Severin. Even at this stage of the war things were a bit "Fred Carno" with regards to direction of attack. A lot of aircraft were victims of collisions over the target rather than to enemy action. We were not at a very great height for our first op and the place was a blazing inferno when we bombed. We could feel the heat from the fires as we went over the target.'

By April 1944 the powerful Mediterranean Allied Strategic Air Force was playing a vital role in the conduct of the war. While the vast aerial fleets of 15th Air Force bombers and fighters pounded targets by day, the RAF Wellingtons and Liberators struck under the cover of darkness, stoking up the night fires. On the night of 3 April Roy Gristwood had flown the 32nd operation of his tour with

Clarke's crew in April 1944, Italy: Left to right, Ron Groves, WOP; 'Red' Fisher, Bomb Aimer; Roy Gristwood, Navigator; Lyn Clarke, Pilot; John McHale, Gunner. *(Roy Gristwood)*

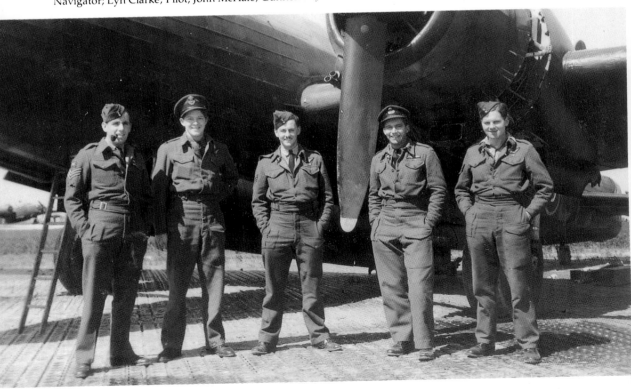

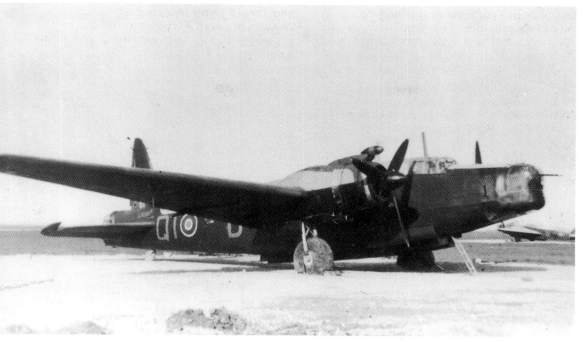

Wellington X LN387 of 142 Squadron pictured at Cerignola III, Italy, in April 1944. *(Roy Gristwood)*

a visit to the Manfred Weiss factory at Budapest. Once again his Wellington was used for target illumination and the long trip to Hungary meant a reduced load of 36 flares to accommodate an overload fuel tank in the bomb bay. Gristwood recalls: 'This was the first night raid on Budapest and followed a daylight raid by the USAAF. We were the leading crew of illuminators and *LN503* was the first aircraft over the city. We and other flare carriers lit it up for the bombers leaving fires raging below. There was flak and plenty of searchlights.

' "Red" Fisher, our New Zealander bomb aimer, fell sick and we flew with "odd" bomb aimers for a few sorties. When "Red" came out of sick bay he flew some extra sorties with different crews to "catch up" with us. He wanted to finish his tour at the same time as us, naturally. On a further attack on Budapest — one we did not go on — he flew and did not return. We assumed he was lost over the target but his crew may not have been very experienced and it could easily have been a navigational error (all our sorties were flown without any radar aids). We were probably the last of the dead reckoning dinosaurs in the European Theatre. Gee was installed at Foggia during March-

April 1944 but only the replacement aircraft and crews coming out from the UK were equipped and trained to use it.'

Clarke's crew completed the 36th operation of their tour on the night of 3 May with a trip to the marshalling yards at Bucharest. Gristwood recalls: 'It was an easy one! There was only light flak over the target but we got holed over Nis in Yugoslavia on the way home. Nothing vital was hit — an engine out would have been serious with the mountains still to be crossed but we got back safely. Thirty-six trips and only hit once within hours of finishing — a lucky tour for us all, except "Red".'

On 6 May it was No 150 Squadron's, and Flight Sergeant Walker's, turn to bomb Bucharest. Les Hallam recalls: 'This was one of our great moments. On our way back, the wireless operator spotted an enemy fighter, coming in to attack from the rear. The rear gunner let him have it and down the fighter went in flames. Its destruction was later confirmed. This was the first such success recorded for 150 Squadron. Flight Sergeant Walker got the DFC and the rear gunner was awarded the DFM.

'On 27 May we attacked the Germans in retreat at the Viterbo road junction in northern

Italy. Being only a short trip, only three to four aircraft took part at a time, but there were three or four take-off times through the night so, as far as the Germans were concerned, it amounted to an all-night attack.

'On 1 July we laid mines in the River Danube near Belgrade. This was a very scary experience. At 200 feet the river banks rose above us on either side and one slip by the Skipper and we would have been goners. On the second mining operation, on 30 July, there was action from the guns from one side of the Danube. As I was down in the bomb hatch in the nose of the Wellington there were red tracer bullets flashing past. We got away safely, but some aircraft from 250 Group were lost on this trip.'

On 2 July, No 150 Squadron moved to Regina airfield near Foggia. Les Hallam recalls: 'The runway was a mud track through the field and the control tower was a wooden building on stilts. By this time some Halifaxes had joined us as Target Indicators. They dropped the red or green flares onto the target and if we dropped our load on these, then as far as the squadron was concerned, the raid was a success. On 21 July we raided the oil refinery at Pardubice. It was a success as far as we were concerned, but all we had done was to more or less wipe out the population. The American B-17s had to destroy the oil refinery by daylight bombing.'

One of the new arrivals in Italy in the summer of 1944 was Jack Weekley, a Navigator, who had completed an OTU tour on Wellingtons at Quastima, Palestine, before being posted to No 150 Squadron at Regina. Weekley flew his first operation on 16 July when the squadron raided the Smederevo oil refinery in Yugoslavia. Each Wellington carried nine 500 lb bombs and the main aiming points were the boiler house and cracking plant. Three days later the squadron bombed another oil refinery, this time at Fiume in northern Italy. Both targets put up an intense barrage of light and heavy flak respectively.

On 24 July Weekley's Wellington made a solo six-hour leaflet, or 'Nickel', raid on Piacenza near Milan. Weekley recalls: 'The idea was to drop the leaflets about seven miles away and allow the prevailing wind to scatter them over Milan. The bomb bays and the interior of the aircraft were stuffed with leaflets. Some were printed in German, and others in Italian. One of the stories was about D-Day and the invasion.

'On target, we opened the bomb doors and let half of the leaflets go. Then we circled round, throwing leaflets out of the astrodome, while one crew member pushed leaflets out of the flare chute. It was estimated that we carried about half a million leaflets and so we circled for some time but saw no fighters or guns.'

The diversity of operations continued. On 26 July three aircraft of No 150 Squadron, each with nine containers in their bomb bays, made a supply dropping trip, code-named 'Lambley', to partisans in northern Italy. The crews dropped on a light which replied to their downward coded signal. Jack Weekley saw a flare from an enemy aircraft nearby but the Wellington crews encountered no opposition.

On 3 August the Wellingtons of No 150 Squadron turned their attention to a target in southern France — the marshalling yards at Porte les Valances. It was a long flight — some eight hours — and a bomb load of only six 500 lb and two 250 lb bombs could be carried. The remaining bays were taken up with an overload petrol tank because of the length of the trip.

Four days later, on 7 August, the squadron loaded up each of its available Wellingtons with eighteen 250 lb bombs for a five and a half hour round trip to the Szombatheley fighter aerodrome in Hungary. Jack Weekley explains: 'The object of the raid was to neutralise the 'drome to help a daylight raid next day by the American 15th Air Force. Some of our bombs were set for instantaneous detonation; others carried a six to 24 hours' delay. This was a typical mixed load for aerodromes.

'It was a bright moonlit night and a squadron of night fighters seemed to be airborne, waiting for us. We were one of the first to bomb. As we came out of the target another Wellington was only a few yards on our starboard side. Suddenly, it burst into flames and fell in three pieces. In the flames of the burning aircraft we saw a Ju 88 break away underneath us, so close we could see the aircraft markings. As we flew on we saw a number of aircraft going down.'

On the night of 13 August Wellingtons of No 205 Group bombed Genoa. The following night No 150 Squadron returned to France loaded with six 500 lb and two 250 lb bombs in their bomb-bays and fitted with overload petrol tanks for the seven-hour round trip. Other aircraft carried incendiaries. Their target was the port installations at Marseilles. Jack Weekley recalls: 'En route to France we flew over a large convoy. This was the invasion of southern France. As we neared the target we could see the fires of Toulon, bombed in the afternoon by the 15th Air Force. We were met with heavy and light flak.'

On 17 August the Wellingtons bombed the submarine pens and harbour installations at Marseilles, as the American 7th Army were to make their landing in southern France the next day. On 18 August the Wellingtons raided an aerodrome at Vanence/La Tresoreria. Most aircraft bombed individually with the aid of ground markers. Unfortunately, the markers were dropped in the wrong place and most bombs fell miles from the target. It was scant reward for a long, eight and half hour trip, requiring two overload petrol tanks in each Wellington.

Les Hallam flew the 38th and final sortie of his tour on 20 August 1944 when No 205 Group raided the Hermann Göring AFV

works at St Valentin in Austria. Their route took them on a track between Linz and Steyr, a heavily defended zone. The crews were met by a barrage of searchlights and intense flak.

On 22 August, Wellingtons of No 150 Squadron attacked the Miskolk marshalling yards in Hungary to hinder German supplies reaching the Russian front. Two nights later the marshalling yards at Bologna in northern Italy were bombed. Jack Weekley recalls: 'There was a change of time on target following the briefing but for some reason we were not told and so we were flying in the Po Valley in the target area for about half an hour all on our own. When the markers did go down we bombed successfully.'

On the night of 25 August it was Italy again as the Wellingtons struck at marshalling yards, this time at Ravenna. 'It was another disaster for us,' reflected Jack Weekley. 'There was an electrical fault on the aircraft. As soon as the pilot operated the bomb door switch, which was also the master switch, the whole bomb load of nine 500 pounders fell. As the bomb doors had not had sufficient

Wellington 'W' 'Madame X' of 'B' Flight, 150 Squadron, on 20 August 1944 just prior to the crew's final op of their first tour, to the AFV Works at St Valentin, France. Left to right, Ives (R-AG); F/O Hindle, Navigator; P/O Walker, RNZAF, Skipper; F/Sgt Les Hallam, Air Bomber; Sgt Henderson, WOP. *(Les Hallam)*

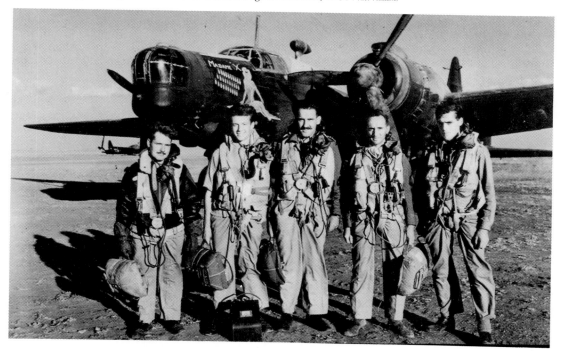

time to open fully, the bombs smashed through them. For a moment we thought we had been hit. The bombs fell well short of the target and we had a draughty journey home.'

On the night of 27 August the Wellingtons went in search of troop concentrations in the Pesaro area of northern Italy, each armed with a mixed load of 500-pounders and 250-pounders. The large bomb load meant that each Wellington had to carry a reduced fuel load so flight planning for the three hour forty minute round trip was critical. Wellingtons of No 205 Group crossed the target area three to four at a time to prolong the raid. Next day, light bombers pounded the area and that night, the Wellingtons returned to carry out the same procedure as the night before. This time the bombing took place only about half a mile in front of the Allied lines where the Polish Army was about to advance. In all, this night and day bombing was kept up continuously for 72 hours.

The Wellingtons resumed raids on marshalling yards at Ferrara and Bologna in northern Italy. The Hungarian and Rumanian railway system was especially important to the Germans and came under constant Allied aerial bombardment, while the Russians effectively deprived the Germans of the use of the Lwow-Cernauti railway. The only alternative route linking Germany with the grainlands of Hungary and the oilfields of Rumania was the River Danube, capable of carrying 10,000 tons of war material daily. By mid-March 1944 the Danube was carrying more than double the amount carried by rail. Even a temporary halt would seriously hamper the German war effort and in April 1944 No 205 Group began 'Gardening' operations, 'sowing' the waterways with mines.

At first the 'Gardening' sorties were only flown when there was a full moon as the aircraft had to fly no higher than 200 feet and even heights of forty and fifty feet were reported. On the night of 8 April nineteen Wellingtons of No 178 Squadron and three Liberators dropped forty mines near Belgrade. Over the next nine days 137 more mines

Despite hopes to the contrary, weather conditions in Italy were very often wet and landing strips were sometimes turned into swamps. Living accommodation was often rudimentary and improvised, as this photograph of spartan living conditions at Foggia shows. *(Anderson)*

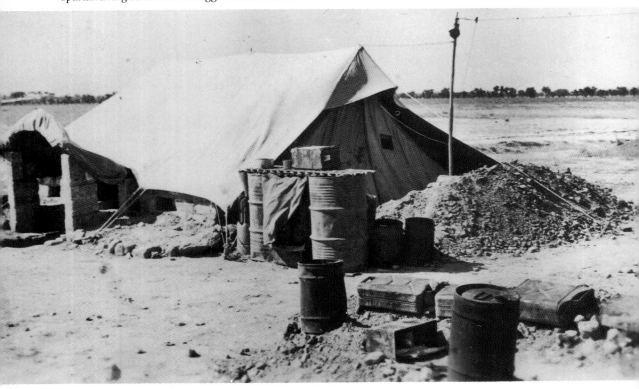

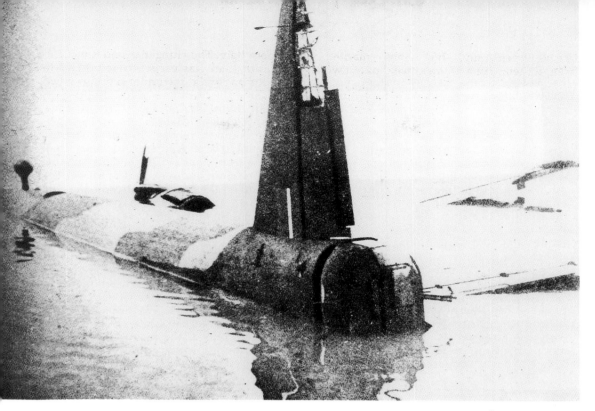

Watery grave for LN858 which was shot down during a raid on Budapest and crashed on Lake Balàton, (or the 'Plattensee', as the Germans called it) the largest lake on continental Europe. *(George Puuka via Hans-Heiri Stapfer)*

were dropped, and in May the total number dropped had risen to over 500. The effect on the supply route was catastrophic. Several ships were sunk and blocked parts of the waterway. By May coal traffic had virtually ceased. Canals and ports were choked with barges.

No 'Gardening' sorties were flown during June, but on the night of 1 July 53 Wellingtons and sixteen Liberators dropped 192 mines in the biggest operation of the mining campaign. The following night another sixty mines were dropped. By August 1944 the volume of matériel transported along the Danube had been reduced by seventy per cent. 'Gardening' sorties continued throughout September and October. Jack Weekley's mining operation took place on the night of 6 September and involved a round trip of five hours forty minutes. 'We mined the Danube about thirty miles south of Budapest. About four aircraft would be detailed to do the mining operation. There would be a raid on at the same time and the mining aircraft would fly some of the way in the main stream and then break away.

'Mining operations could only take place on about three nights a month when the moon was full because it was a low level night attack. The aircraft carried two 1,000 lb Mark V parachute mines. These had to be dropped at a height of about 180 feet, or less. As it was moonlight and the height was so low the aircraft were targets for every ground weapon imaginable. The area chosen was a long narrow island in the middle of the Danube, which divided the river into two narrow channels. The aircraft concerned were briefed to mine a particular channel. As mining was done regularly, the enemy knew more or less when the operation would take place. Generally crews only did one such trip — one they did not look forward to.'

On the night of 4 October, eighteen Wellingtons and four Liberators flew the final mining operation and dropped 58 mines in to the Danube in Hungary, west of Budapest, north of Gyor and east of Esztergom. In six months of operations, 1,382 mines were laid by Wellingtons and Liberators of No 205 Group in eighteen attacks.

In mid-September 1944 heavy rainfall stopped operations as the earth and grass strips soon became heavily waterlogged. When conditions improved, on 26 September, the target selected was the Borovnica railway viaduct in northern Yugoslavia, which the enemy were using for troop and supply trains to Greece. Jack Weekley recalls: 'We bombed with eighteen 250 pounders. There was some heavy flak but a 4,000 lb "cookie" bomb was seen to hit the centre span of the viaduct.

'At this time 150 Squadron was broken up. The air and ground crews were posted to Nos 40 and 104 Squadrons, the other Wellington squadrons at Foggia Main. Two other squadrons, 37 and 70, were based at Tortorella. So, 150 Squadron "came home on paper" and was re-formed at Hemswell on Lancasters. My crew was posted to No 104 Squadron at Foggia in October.'

Also in October 1944, Sergeant 'Tubby' Gaunt's crew were posted from No 77 OTU Palestine to No 37 Squadron at Foggia. Their first four operations were almost uneventful. Each time, they were scheduled to drop supplies to Tito's partisans in Yugoslavia. Normally, the canisters were dropped in daylight from 3-4,000 feet without parachutes. Sergeant Maurice 'Scats' Sandell, the air bomber, recalls: 'It was a strange experience to be shot at horizontally by small arms fire from sides of valleys. One time we had a freeze-up and we couldn't release the containers in the bomb bay. Eventually, the mechs had to chop them out with axes. "Tubby" didn't like going round a target again.

'On another occasion, we dropped supplies to Italian partisans at Pecorra in northern Italy. It was like a Hollywood movie. They lit fires for us to go in. We had been briefed to avoid Udine where German jet aircraft were based. Another place to avoid was Pola (now Pula) on the Istrian coast of Yugoslavia which was one of the main sites for anti-aircraft batteries. It was a funny sort of war. We supplied pockets of partisans on one side

The mass of pipes, geodetics and the narrow walkway leading past the Elsan toilet to the tail are clearly shown in this interior view of the Wellington. *(Rupert Cooling)*

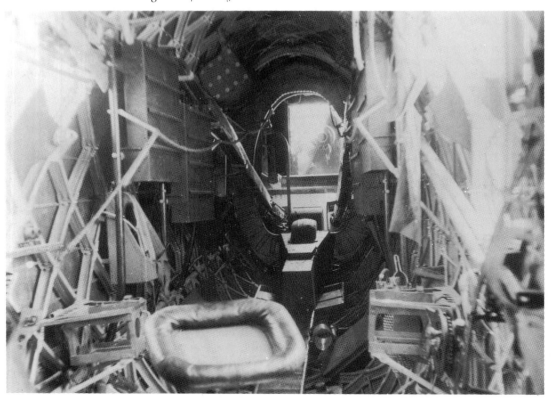

of a mountain range and bombed the enemy on the other.'

During November 1944 operations were predominantly aimed at dropping bombs on targets in Yugoslavia, involving a dozen Wellingtons at a time. On 23 November No 37 Squadron attacked German troop concentrations at Uzice, each Wellington carrying six 500 lb bombs and a dozen 250 pounders. Gaunt's Wellington received five flak holes but returned safely to Foggia.

The Wellingtons did not carry a front gunner. This task was carried out when needed by the air bomber, as Maurice Sandell recalls: 'I would sit or stand beside "Tubby" most of the time and only went into the front if asked. Flying in the front turret was so remote it was like flying with no wings. The front turret was so small I had to be helped out. Flying in the tail turret was much better.

'The bomb aimer's job in a Wimpy was the best job in the Air Force. On return trips I occasionally used to fly the aircraft. Then "Geordie" Hazleden, our "rough tough" tail gunner, who would tear down German night fighters with his bare hands if all else failed, would have a spell. I also helped out with map reading. One day "Jock" Scanlon got lost. According to his reckoning, a crossroads would soon show up and give us an opportunity to get a "fix". It came and we flew over it. The Germans peppered us with 88 mm shells. "Jock" got his "fix" all right!

'My main task, of course, was bomb aiming. Although the bomb sight at OTU was an early type with manual drift wires, in the squadron we used an electric bomb sight. I fed the wind speed, height and various information into it from data provided at briefing and by "Mac" McMememy, our Wireless Operator, and "Jock" Scanlon, the Navigator. This would alter the angle on the glass plate with an illuminated cross for bombing. I would then select the sticks of bombs to be dropped using my bomb selector box, or "Mickey Mouse" as it was called. Normally, there were four or five bombs in a stick. The 500 pounders would be dropped first and then the 250 pounders.'

On 4 December 1944, Gaunt's crew flew the last of ten operations with No 37 Squadron. The squadron then re-equipped with Liberators, or 'Spam Cans', as the RAF called them, and Gaunt's crew was among those transferred to No 70 Squadron, where they continued to operate the Wellington. On 19 December they flew the first operation with their new squadron, to Matesevo-Konilas in Yugoslavia. Two days later they took off at 13:35 hours for a three-hour round trip to bomb a bridge at Mojkovac in Croatia. 'Scats' Sandell admitted to a 'hairy' feeling on take-off for they were carrying a 4,000 lb 'cookie'. Sandell felt they were not flying a Wellington but rather a 'cookie with wings'. The object of the operation was to prevent German troops reaching the partisans' area.

Unfortunately, both Gaunt's Wellington, and a second which also carried a 'cookie', missed the bridge. However, Gaunt's crew were relieved to see the massive bomb go. As Maurice Sandell pointed out: 'At least when a "cookie" was gone, it was gone; there was no question of it hanging up.'

The war did not stop for Christmas. On Christmas Day 1944 Tubby Gaunt's crew flew a daylight supply dropping operation, code-named 'Crnomelj', to the partisans in Yugoslavia. 'Scats' Sandell recalls: 'We strung along in a bomber stream in broad daylight just as if it was in the middle of the night. Good job there was no opposition. Supply dropping by daylight was a colourful sight. Supplies of guns, medicines, ammunition, clothes etc, were dropped using a different coloured parachute. This enabled the partisans, who could be seen quite clearly on the outskirts of the drop site, to grab some of each kind of supply and get away as quickly as possible.

'The next night we made another supply drop, code-named "Cazma" in Yugoslavia. This time we flew with the Flight Commander as pilot.'

On Boxing Day night, No 70 Squadron was despatched to Casarsa in northern Italy was to bomb a railway bridge. Pathfinders went in first and lit up the bridge with target indicators. When the Wellingtons arrived over the target, in moonlight, they could see quite clearly red flares at one end of the bridge and green flares at the other. Each aircraft carried a mixed bomb load of nine 500 pounders and four 250 pounders which were to be dropped in 'Blitz time' along the length of the bridge.

Each Wellington flew singly over the target in trail and released its bombs but without success. 'At least,' thought Maurice Sandell, 'we will not run into each other this way.' As each stick of bombs dropped a photo flash, timed to go off when the bombs exploded, lit

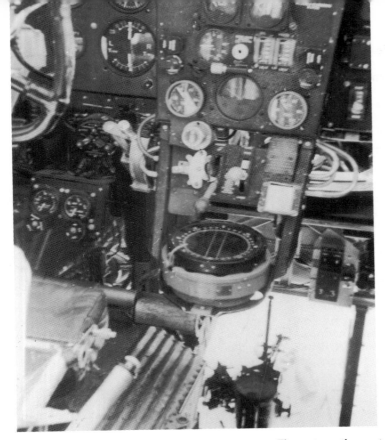

Pilot's position above the bomb aimer's compartment. The seat was the most comfortable that most pilots ever encountered, mainly because it had adjustable armrests and soft pads to give support under the knees.
(Rupert Cooling)

up the area like day while a camera, activated when the bomb release was pressed, snapped the scene below. The photo flash brought back bad memories for Maurice Sandell. Wellington fabric and fire were partners in death and at OTU more crews had been lost from accidents with photo flashes than anything else.

On 8 January 1945 'Tubby' Gaunt's crew awoke in their primitive tents pitched among the wine groves and set off for the Mess hut for breakfast. At briefing, the Wellington crews learned that the day's operation would be a supply drop to partisans in the Ljubljana region in Yugoslavia. Although this did not present the same dangers as a trip to Ploesti or some other oil target, there were other dangers, mostly from the elements. The briefing officer warned that bad weather could be expected over Yugoslavia. The ceiling would be about 16,000 feet and the safety height over the mountains only 10,000 feet.

No 70 Squadron's crews began taking off around 11:25 hours. 'Tubby' Gaunt's crew pressed on across the Adriatic, which was covered in thick cloud. 'Scats' Sandell recalls: 'We went into storm clouds and got tossed around like a "pea in a drum". The instruments went haywire. At one time our Wellington stood on her tail, then went nose down. Everything hit the ceiling. Mud, which was always trudged into the aircraft, splattered everywhere. We were icing up. It got so bad that the flapping motion of the wings stopped with the weight of ice. There was a "twang" as bits of ice spun off the prop blades and hit the fuselage.

'We never found the target and our supplies had to be brought back. Eventually, we broke cloud. Through the small clear gap on the windscreen "Tubby" and I could see the "white horses" of the wave tops on the sea. "Tubby" exclaimed, "We've made it, 'Scats'!" However, it was not the sea. The "whitecaps" were in fact snow drifts of fir trees clinging to the sides of mountains. We were still over Yugoslavia!

'We took up our crash positions. "Tubby" flew right up a valley, losing height rapidly. Suddenly, we hit. A tree took the starboard wingtip off and we went through a line of hedgerows. "Tubby" had made a lovely crash landing and this was the only time I had seen a Wimpy crash not end in flames. This is probably because our Wellington had broken her belly and snow had poured in until it was knee deep. I was sitting on a little flap seat next to "Tubby" who was strapped in. I blacked out. When I came to, I could see "Tubby's" forehead denting the windscreen. I could hear the "drip, drip" of petrol spilling onto the snow. I opened the escape hatch and said, "After you, Tubby!"

' "Geordie" had his legs jammed under the servo-feed in his rear turret. We got him out and jumped into the waist high snow. For the first time we noticed armed men and women dressed in green uniforms with little red stars on their forage caps. Luckily, we had landed among partisans. Immediately, some women came over and began collecting the dripping petrol in tins. They wanted to go inside the aircraft but we told them it was too dangerous. The partisans wanted the machine-guns and they were stripped from the turrets. The supply canisters probably contained explosives but they took them anyway. They took everything they could get their hands on.

'A Yugoslavian, who had worked as a lumberjack in Canada, told us that this side of the valley was controlled by the partisans. The other side was controlled by Chetniks!

'The partisans set us on our way. We passed through various groups and British missions. Eventually, on 7 February, we reached the British military mission at Zara (now Zada) on the coast and were put aboard HMS *Columbo*, a depot ship, for the night. Next day, we sailed for the Allied repatriation centre at Bari aboard HMS *Wilton*. As No 70 Squadron members, our war was over. We were repatriated home from Naples by ship.'

In January 1945 No 70 Squadron, at Tortorella, had begun re-equipping with Liberator VIs, as had No 104 Squadron at Foggia Main. On 21 February No 205 Group flew the last of its operations using Wellingtons. Pola naval base was selected as the target, as Jack Weekley recalls: 'We attacked in daylight. As usual, we flew night bomber stream tactics with no effort to formate. There was fighter escort in the target area, which was heavily defended. We were about the second or third aircraft to go in. The Wellington in front of us was hit and went down.

'Behind us a Liberator was hit. It went down on fire and broke up. We saw three parachutes go down right to the target area. One of our bombs hit the ammunition dump and in seconds there was a huge pall of smoke up to hundreds of feet (later the film in our camera proved it was ours). We were so fascinated that we went round again for another look. It was stupid in view of the opposition and more so when we got back and the CO told us we had finished our tour.'

While Jack Weekley was going home, others, like Les Hallam, returned to Italy and No 150 Squadron in March 1945, for a second tour on the ever faithful Wellington X. 'I have often wondered whether 205 Group helped us beat the Germans or did a better job of putting the Iron Curtain countries in worse trouble by helping the Russian advance and their eventual take-over of those countries. Perhaps ops were easier, compared with the home-based "big boys", but the air and ground crews had to endure much more primitive living conditions and lower food standards.'

Chapter 14
Maritime operations

Apart from service with Coastal Command, Wellingtons also served in the maritime role throughout the Mediterranean, Middle East and Far East Theatres. It will be remembered that No 458 Squadron, RAAF, left England at the end of January 1942 to take up a torpedo-bomber role in the Middle East. Wing Commander Mulholland led three Wellington ICs, which had been fitted with 'tropicalised' Bristol Pegasus engines, off from Stanton Harcourt. The flight to Malta via Le Havre, a distance of some 1,460 miles, was made without mishap until the formation reached Malta. Mulholland overshot the island and he and his crew perished when they were brought down by enemy night fighters. The other three Wellingtons touched down at Luqa safely.

On 27 February 1942 the second formation of Wellingtons left England for the Middle East, flying the first stage of their journey from Portreath to Gibraltar before continuing to Malta. The first No 458 Squadron Wellington to land in Egypt touched down at Kilo 26, a landing ground halfway between Cairo and Alexandria, on 1 March. the rest of the squadron flew in over the next few weeks and ground personnel arrived from their previous base at Holme-on-Spalding Moor, mostly by sea.

Training in the new role of a torpedo-bomber unit followed, but it was a 'conventional' load of 250 pounders and armour-piercing bombs that were dropped when the first operation was flown, on the night of July 25/26. A single Wellington, piloted by Sergeant Ian Cameron, took off from Abu Sueir and dropped its bombs on enemy positions in the Qutefryca area.

By September 1942 the full complement of No 458 Squadron had arrived in the Canal Zone and the unit was now based at Shallufa, flying torpedo bombing operations. The squadron, together with two other Wellington squadrons, Nos 38 and 221, formed No 248 Wing of No 201 Group. No 221 Squadron had arrived in Egypt in January 1942 with a brief to use their ASV sets to locate enemy convoys for torpedo-armed 'Fishingtons' of Nos 38 and 458 Squadrons to carry out the actual attacks.

No 38 Squadron had served in the Middle East since November 1940. At Shallufa during the latter part of 1941, the squadron had added minelaying sorties to its list of activities. In December 1941, a pressing need for torpedo-carrying aircraft with sufficient range and the ability to carry more than one weapon at a time, led to trials being conducted using modified Wellingtons as torpedo-bombers. The nose turret was removed to improve pilots' vision forward, the bomb bay was modified to hold two torpedoes and, later, long-range fuel tanks were fitted.

On 20 December 1941 Wing Commander John Chaplin, the CO, made the first practice drop of two torpedoes and his success was followed by a series of dummy torpedo drops by Chaplin's crews. In February 1942 the whole squadron ceased to become a purely bomber unit and the 'Fishingtons' were transferred to No 247 Wing, No 201 Naval Co-operation Group. There began a period of operations exclusively against Axis shipping.

Chaplin found that the best method of attack was to approach the target at eighty feet and drop their two tin fish from 1,000 yards distance. Mostly, attacks were carried out at dusk or by moonlight to minimise the threat of flak and detection by enemy fighters. In March, with the installation of long-range fuel tanks, attacks were made on shipping as far afield as Patras (Patrai) in Greece. In May, the first successful torpedo attacks were made on an enemy convoy, resulting in two hits and one ship beached. The squadron now had detachments based in Malta, Palestine and along the Western Desert.

On the eve of the Battle of El Alamein on the night of 1 November 1942, the 'Fishingtons' of Nos 38 and 458 Squadrons were used against enemy shipping north-west of Tobruk. The next day a German destroyer was bombed by two of No 458 Squadron's Wellingtons.

Anti-submarine patrols and minelaying operations in the Gulf of Sirte were carried out during the remainder of the month.

Some of the squadron's Wellingtons were sent on detachment to outlying bases in the desert and even further afield. On 17 January Wing Commander Johnson, the CO, and twelve Wellingtons flew to Malta and landed at Luqa to begin torpedo strikes on Axis shipping. The 'Fishingtons' flew in all kinds of weather, including severe electrical storms, which caused losses of men and machines. During two months, February and March 1943, the squadron flew over 1,250 operational hours.

May 1943 saw the start of several moves for Wellington torpedo-bomber units. No 458 Squadron moved to LG91, Amiriya, with further moves to Benghazi, Misurata and Tripolitania. Meanwhile, at the eastern end of the Mediterranean, No 36 Squadron, equipped with Wellington VIIIs, flew into Blida from India, where it had been engaged in maritime duties, to begin anti-submarine duties in the Mediterranean.

During June 1943 No 458 Squadron was largely based at Protville, near Tunis, and, together with No 38 Squadron, joined in the offensive aganst enemy shipping in the Mediterranean. During the summer of 1943 Wellington Mk VIIIs with ASV radar entered service with No 38 Squadron. The 'Goofingtons', as they were known, proved very effective hunter/killer aircraft; the squadron's first success in this role occurring on 26 August when an enemy tanker was torpedoed and sunk.

By September Wellingtons of No 458 Squadron were attacking targets in Corsica and Italy. Maritime reconnaissance operations were exceptionally long and tiring, involving searches throughout the vastness of the Mediterranean. On 13 September a No 458 Squadron Wellington, with a single eighteen-inch torpedo aboard, logged a total of ten hours twenty minutes' night flying time on instruments during a search in the area Sardinia-Genoa-La Spezia-La Rocca. On 26 September, one of its crew discovered and depth-charged a U-boat, forcing it to surface

Wellington XII of 221 Squadron with ASV radar, Malta, January 1944. *(Grp Capt M. J. A. Shaw)*

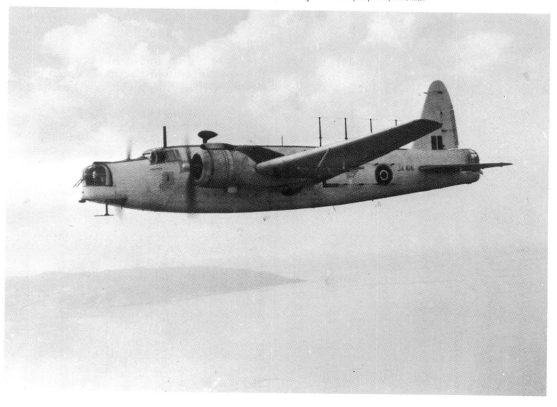

and leaving it in a damaged condition. Two days earlier No 294 Squadron had been formed at Berka equipped with a mixture of Wellington ICs and XIs and a few Walrus II amphibians for ASR duties.

Despite successes, losses were high and in the UK volunteers were called upon to train in the dangerous art of torpedo bombing. In July 1943 Ernie Payne was posted to No 7 OTU at Limavady. 'I joined Flying Officer "Mac" McGaw's crew flying in Wellington Is and IIs. McGaw volunteered us for torpedo work and in September 1943 we were posted to 1 TTU at Turnbury for a seven-week intensive course. We started with low flying over the

Sergeant Pilot (later Major) Steve Oliphant.
(Steven Oliphant)

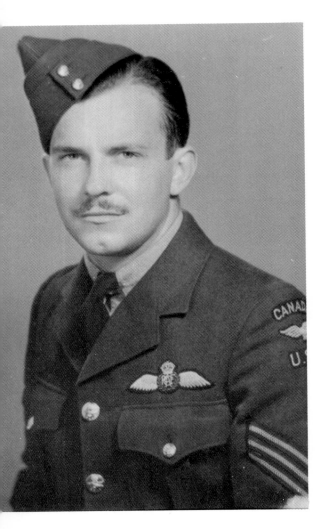

sea by day and night (with the assistance of flares). The object was to keep the plane at fifty feet above the water. We then did simulated attacks on designated ships, using first a camera that operated when the bomb doors opened, and later, a torpedo with a dummy warhead.

'At night the method was to first find the ship using ASV then, if it was a moonlit night, the skipper would lose height and make his attack, using the moon to silhouette the target. If there was no moon, two sticks of 4,100 candlepower flares were dropped at right angles to each other so that whichever way the ship turned it would still be silhouetted.

'There were many incidents; the fifty feet above the sea at night being one of the main problems. Too high, the torpedo bounced (as one of the ships found out), too low usually resulted in prop damage, or, as happened on more than one occasion, the Wellington hit the sea. When we were lumbering down the short runway at Turnbury in a Wellington I with a 2,000 lb torpedo on board we wondered more than once if we were going to make it.'

Stephen A. Oliphant, an American pilot serving in the RCAF, did his torpedo training on the Wellington at Abbotsinch. 'How the hell we were supposed to know what fifty feet was at night is beyond comprehension. We lost one crew with the exception of the tail gunner when a pilot misjudged the prescribed fifty feet and dug in. Also, when a torpedo is incorrectly dropped it can come up out of the water looking for the joker that dropped it. Guess that could be called a self-inflicted wound. Twice, I saw a captain of a destroyer wait until he saw our dummy torpedo drop and then haul his ship over so hard that our torpedo missed by a country mile.' Fortunately, neither man ever saw action on torpedo-dropping Wellingtons. Ernie Payne was posted to a Warwick unit and Stephen Oliphant joined the USAAF shortly after completing training.

Meanwhile, Wellingtons were carrying out maritime operations in the Gulf of Oman and Indian Ocean. On 12 September 1943 No 621 Squadron had formed at Port Reitz, Kenya, and personnel were sent out from England. One of them was Sergeant Pilot Henry Fawcett. A constable in the Sheffield City Police Force when war broke out, Fawcett had wanted to join the RAF since his first flight in an Avro Avian from York racecourse at the age of thirteen. In 1941 the Home Office decreed that any police officer who wanted to become a pilot or navigator could join the RAF. Fawcett enrolled and subsequently passed out as a pilot.

After training in the UK and Rhodesia, Fawcett was posted to No 3 OTU at Cranwell as a Sergeant Pilot. At this time Ju 88 night fighters were shooting down Wellingtons in the area. After one week Henry Fawcett was sent to No 78 OTU at Haverfordwest. Squadron Leader West, a regular since 1937, who had completed two operational tours and a third tour as an instructor, became the pilot. The new crew completed Ferry Training at Talbenny and in August 1943 made operational sweeps out over the Bay of Biscay in brand new Wellington XIIIs.

West's crew received their overseas posting to No 621 Squadron on 6 September 1943. They left Hurn and flew their Wellington XIII, grossly overloaded with fuel and spares, to Cairo via Fez and Castle Benito. Then they flew west, to Khartoum, Djouba, Nairobi and on to their final destination at Mombassa; a total flight time of some 35 hours fifteen minutes. At Mombasa, West's crew flew anti-submarine patrols over the Indian Ocean. On one ten-hour search they looked for an aircraft which had gone down in the sea. They also dropped supplies to survivors from a shipwreck who had managed to swim ashore on the African coast. They were picked up the next day by another aircraft.

The September anti-submarine patrols and convoy escort duties gave way to reconnaissance of a different kind on 21 November. Inland of Mogadishu, Somalia, the Wellington crews carried out a 'Tribal Recce'. Fawcett recalls: 'A group of marauding tribesmen had been pillaging and raping and we were sent out to find them. It was fantastically hot and bumpy. We found the tribe and dropped signals to the Army. Next day an Aussie crew went out in their Wellington and against orders, strafed them from their gun turrets.'

In December 1943 No 621 Squadron moved to Khormaksar, Aden. West's crew were one of several sent on detachment to Bendiskassim, south of Aden, where the Wellingtons continued flying anti-submarine patrols over the Indian Ocean for some months. By February 1944 its sister unit at Khormaksar, No 8 Squadron, and No 244

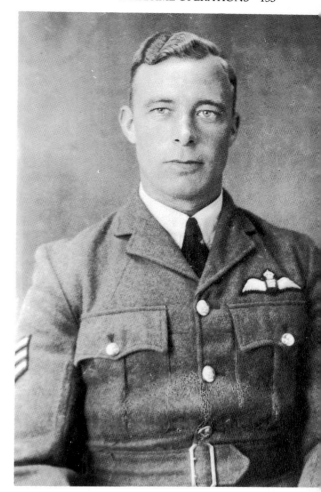

Sergeant Pilot Henry Fawcett. *(Henry Fawcett)*

Squadron at Sharjah, had begun conversion to the Wellington XIII. Both squadrons were engaged in anti-shipping and maritime reconnaissance over the Indian Ocean and the Gulf of Oman respectively. No 8 Squadron had been in Aden since May 1942 and No 244 Squadron had been at Sharjah since 1943, with a detachment at Masira.

Not all operations were anti-shipping, as Alan Smith, a WOP-AG of No 8 Squadron, recalls. 'On one occasion we transported the Sultan of Muscat, with his bodyguards, from Ras al Hadd to Salala on our way back to Aden. The Sultan sat at the Nav table and I looked after the two near-naked bodyguards aft of the bomb bay. After we had been flying for an hour my Canadian skipper, "Red" St Henri, shouted "What the hell is going on

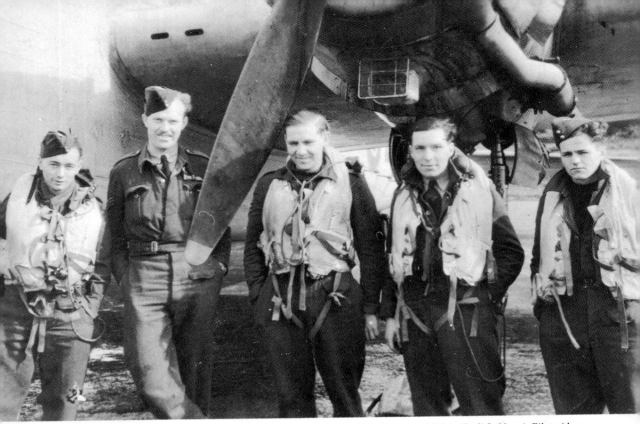

'Red' St Henri's original crew in 8 Squadron. Left to right, F/Sgt Mathews, 2nd Pilot; 'Red' St Henri, Pilot; Alan Smith, WOP-AG; Bob Beetenson, WOP-AG; Tom Richardson, WOP-AG. *(Alan Smith)*

back there?'' The aircraft was starting to weave about. I found the problem. One of the bodyguards was winding his toes around the wires leading back to the twin tabs. I gently persuaded him to untangle himself!

'Accidents were not uncommon at Aden. One night Flight Sergeant Mac McGiveney was landing at Khormaksar and taxied over a "goose neck" flare. He set the tyre alight and in a few minutes all that was left was a Wimpy skeleton — the quickest crew evacuation on record.'

Meanwhile, on 4 October 1943, in the Mediterranean Theatre with the Allied campaign in Corsica reaching a successful conclusion, the Wellingtons of Nos 38, 221 and 458 Squadrons bombed the last remaining evacuation port at Bastia. Two days later the Australians were posted to Bone to begin anti-submarine operations. Although orders stated that their torpedo gear must go with them to Algeria, the squadron would in future be armed only with depth charges.

A number of anti-submarine and air-sea rescue operations were carried out during November-December. In November 1943 No 203 Squadron in North Africa exchanged its Martin Baltimores for Wellington Mk IIIs and moved to Santa Cruz for maritime operations over the Indian Ocean.

On the night of 11/12 December Wellingtons of Nos 36 and 458 Squadrons, each armed with eight depth charges, together with Venturas of No 500 Squadron, flew cover for an Allied convoy of 53 ships. A U-boat was attacked and kept submerged north of Cape Bugaruni until early afternoon on the 13th when it was the recipient of more depth charges, this time from a destroyer of the Royal Navy. With batteries running low and foul air making breathing difficult, the German Commander was forced to scuttle his craft.

During December 1943 new Mark XIV Wellingtons, fitted with Leigh Lights, began equipping the maritime squadrons in North Africa. Training was badly hampered by torrential rainstorms which turned airfields into muddy swamps. By now detachments had been sent further afield. A No 458 Squadron detachment was based at Grottaglie,

Italy, while detachments from Nos 14, 500 and 458 Squadrons were stationed at Ghisonaccia on the eastern side of Corsica.

Anti-U-boat operations were carried out from the island until mid-April 1944, several aircraft having been lost through ditchings. Other detachments were sent to Malta. The U-boat had now become the main threat to Allied forces in the expanse of the Mediterranean. Accordingly, No 38 Squadron had dropped its torpedo role and had reverted to a normal maritime reconnaissance unit, although on occasion, its crews still carried torpedoes.

On the night of 2 February 1944 the 4,300-ton MV *Leopardi*, with four destroyers in escort, was located by six Wellingtons. The Wellingtons attacked, amid intense anti-aircraft fire, with bombs from 5,000 feet and torpedoes from fifty feet. The *Leopardi* exploded and sunk, but two aircraft, including the one which launched the final torpedo, were shot down. Seven days later, a Ju 52

was shot down from the rear turret of a Wellington engaged on offensive operations in the Aegean, and, during April, two Ju 52s were shot down during a return flight from minelaying operations in the harbour at Rhodes.

The difficulties the enemy faced in supplying its forces in the Aegean were reaching impossible proportions and the maritime Wellingtons added to them by moving ever closer. On 23 May 1944 No 458 Squadron moved from its North African base at Bone and took up residence at Alghero on Sardinia. The first operation was carried out on the night of 13/14 June when ten Wellingtons were sent on a search west of the island for U-boats, but without success. By now the Leigh Light Wellingtons not only provided illumination for the Beaufighters of No 272 Squadron, RAF, but were fitted with Mk IX bomb-sights for bombing strikes on targets in northern Italy.

Although shipping targets were getting

An Arab boy and his donkey get in the picture with Wellington XIII HZ879 'Johnny 2' at Relizane, Algeria, in November 1943. This aircraft was flown to Kilo 40, Cairo, where it was turned over to Middle East Command and the crew were assigned another Mk XIII and ordered to report to 8 Squadron at Aden. *(Alan Smith)*

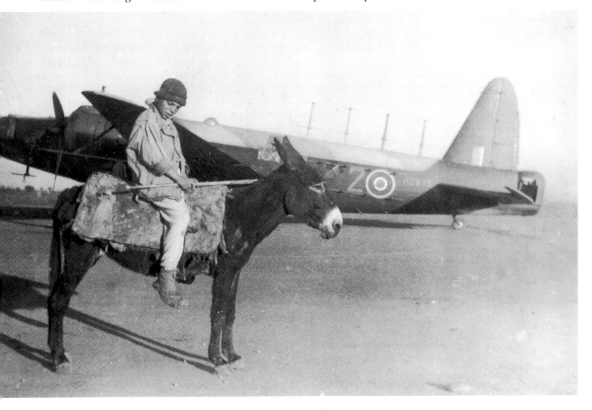

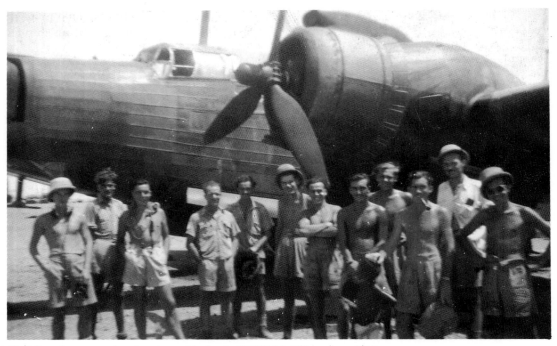

No 8 Squadron crews in relaxed mood in front of JA201-M at Riyan, June 1944. *(Alan Smith)*

rarer, on occasions the enemy appeared in relatively large numbers. On an earlier raid, on 1 June, Wellingtons of No 38 Squadron spotted a convoy of three merchantmen escorted by three destroyers and four corvettes. They shadowed the force until, low on fuel, they were forced to return to base after dropping their bombs in vain. The next day a strike force sank two of the merchantmen, one destroyer and two corvettes. Five enemy aircraft were also shot down during the action. That night the squadron was out in force, bombing and torpedoeing in Candia harbour where the remnants of the convoy had sought refuge. One Wellington was shot down.

The failure of this convoy to reach its destination with the bulk of its supplies marked the beginning of the end for the Germans in the Aegean. On the night of 29/30 July Flight Lieutenant Rubidge, a South African pilot in No 458 Squadron, searched in vain for shipping targets near La Spezia and Nice, so he turned his attentions to the shipyards and factories at Pietra. No hits were made and the Wellington crew had to ward off light flak and attacks by two night fighters. They landed safely back at Alghero after some five hours forty minutes in the air.

In August 1944 Henry Fawcett, late of No 621 Squadron, was posted to No 38 Squadron at Benghazi as a Wellington Skipper. His Second Pilot was 'Alex' Alexander while the Navigator was a Scot, Sergeant 'Jock' Nimmo. His WOP-AG was Ernie Brown, an ex-professional footballer with Newcastle United, while Jack Dougary, his brilliant nineteen-year-old radar operator, had been a cub reporter in Fife. The final member of the crew was Bill McLeod, the rear gunner.

Fawcett's crew operated from a forward base at En Shemir where they flew anti-submarine patrols and convoy escorts by day and night. In addition, the maritime Wellingtons flew minelaying and leaflet dropping operations and even dropped spikes onto airfields in Crete to hamper Ju 52 operations.

On the night of 12 September the Wellingtons of No 38 Squadron struck at Maleme airfield on Crete. The German defences assisted the RAF crews by inadvertently turning on the lights, mistaking the Wellingtons for Junkers Ju 52s. Each Wimpy dropped twelve 200 lb bombs straight across the runway from 8,000 feet. The bombs were fitted with timed delay fuzes which caused the bombs to explode at half-hour intervals to deny the Germans the use of the airfield for 24 hours.

The Wellingtons came under heavy fire as Henry Fawcett recalls: 'One piece of flak as big as a turnip went through one side of the front turret and out the other. Another piece went through the fuselage making a pencil hole through the "king post" on the empennage. Fortunately, it did not drop off. The air stream peeled off about thirty feet of fabric. Dougary, who was a bit of a comic, took the hot-air tube and stuck it down the front of his flying suit. He still complained of cold in the 140-knot wind.

Seven nights later, on 19 September, No 38 Squadron mounted a maximum effort against the SS *Corona*, which lay at anchor in Porto Lagos in the Aegean. Each Wellington carried eleven 200 lb bombs but the raid was not entirely successful. Henry Fawcett recalls: 'My bombs missed by half a mile but they set a naval barracks on fire.'

In September 1944 No 458 Squadron had also moved to Italy. They alighted at Foggia, with the main elements moving north to Falconara where they shared the airfield with No 454 Squadron, RAAF, with No 450 Squadron, RAAF, based nearby. On 14/15 September No 458 Squadron flew its first operation from Falconara when Warrant Officer Priest sank a 2,000-ton ship. On 15 September No 36 Squadron flew its last maritime operation. Three days later the squadron completed the first leg of the journey to the UK to join Coastal Command, finally arriving at Chivenor on 26 September.

On 4 October No 38 Squadron dropped leaflets on Crete and Rhodes. Henry Fawcett recalls: 'The whole fuselage was filled with leaflets. We circled right around Crete pushing out these bundles. It was on flights like this that we used to get torchlight signals from freedom fighters in the hills. Even if we could read morse they were in a foreign language.'

On raids like this opposition from Ju 52s could be expected. Normally, this three-engined transport provided little danger but they were capable of firing a very heavy gun from a side door. Fawcett recalls: 'On one occasion three Ju 52s formated on our tail. McCleod spotted them. He shouted, "The aircraft with three engines!" Then he opened up and away they went.'

The Aegean conflict drew gradually to a close and at the end of September an advance party from No 38 Squadron had left Berka III for the Delta, where they boarded a ship for Piraeus. The party was ultimately based at Hassani airfield near Athens which had recently been vacated by the Luftwaffe. By 14 November the whole of No 38 Squadron had installed their Wellingtons on the airfield. Greece proved a welcome change of climate after 23 months in the desert, but on 28 November part of the squadron was posted to Grottalgie, near Taranto, and the Italian Theatre of Operations, while the remainder of the squadron found itself confined to base as civil war broke out in the recently liberated country.

By December 1944 No 38 Squadron was stationed at Kalamaki. The Greek Civil War was beginning to get into full swing, so on 6 December the remaining Wellingtons, packed with tents and supplies, took off and made the three-hour flight to Grottalgie amid small arms fire and artillery. The squadron spent Christmas 1944 in tents and billets situated on muddy fields. In addition to bombing operations, its tasks, as part of the Balkan Air Force, included dropping supplies in Greece and Yugoslavia.

On January 1945 the Wellingtons made the thirty-minute flight to Bari where they loaded up with supplies to drop to the partisans in Yugoslavia. At Bari, Henry Fawcett broke the tail wheel. 'Taxying in what I thought was deep rutted mud turned out to be baked hard. An oleo went through the turret. The throttle on the replacement Wellington had become disconnected and the pilot who brought her in did a very worthy single-engined landing.'

In the New Year the snows receded and operations began again with renewed vigour. On the night of 3/4 January four of No 458 Squadron's Wellingtons and six Beaufighters of No 272 Squadron mounted an armed reconnaissance off Pola. One of the Wellington pilots spotted a 2,000-ton oil tanker and, dropping a mercury flare, called in the 'Rockbeaus' to attack. The fighters badly damaged the ship and stopped it in her tracks.

On 25 January 1945 No 458 Squadron flew to Gibraltar to resume anti-U-boat operations in the Mediterranean. A period of Leigh Light training followed and then on 13 and 14 February anti-submarine patrols were mounted between Cape St Vincent and Lisbon. With the sea almost entirely devoid

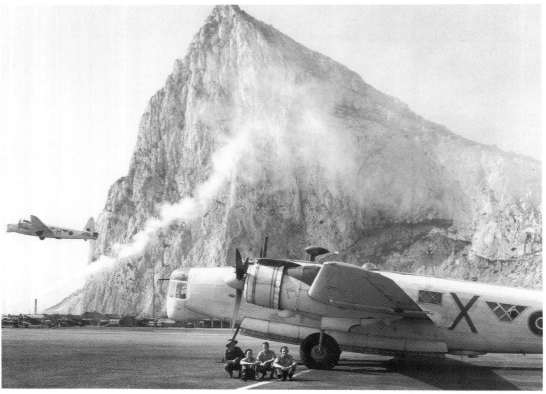

Wellington XIV 'H-Harry' of 458 Squadron (RAAF) takes off from Gibraltar with 'X-X-Ray' in the foreground, in February 1945 on an anti-submarine patrol. *(Australian War Memorial)*

of enemy shipping the Wellington crews were now virtually on a training status, although convoy patrols of seven hours' duration were still the order of the day as the war drew to a close.

At this time it was decided that a detachment of seven Wellingtons would be maintained at Rosignano, near Leghorn, for anti-shipping strikes in co-operation with Naval coastal forces in the Gulf of Genoa. Part of No 38 Squadron was despatched to Rosignano while the rest of the squadron was to operate from Foggia on similar operations along the coasts of Venice and Trieste in the northern Adriatic.

On 6 February No 38 Squadron flew its Wellington XIIIs to Blida, near Algiers, where it swapped them for the Mk XIV. This version was equipped with the very latest radar and radar altimeters, accurate to one foot, which registered the height of the waves. For operations low over the sea this meant that the pilot could set fifty feet and keep in the 'traffic lights' (amber). If the

needle went into the red, the Wellington was too low. Green meant they were too high.

On 21 February the squadron flew an armed reconnaissance over the Genoa-La Spezia area off the west coast of Italy. Their quarry was German shipping. Most of the enemy's larger vessels were either disabled or sunk so the squadron's targets were by now primarily barges, small coasters and E- and F- boats, although on the western side of the Gulf of Genoa, where there was much greater freedom of action so far as shore installations were concerned, the occasional KT ship was also found.

At this stage of the war the Germans were forced to move their supplies in barges along the west coast of Italy by night because by day their road convoys were mercilessly attacked and strafed by Beaufighters. The barges were often escorted by E-boats which developed a technique of firing vertically when Wellingtons were overhead.

The Wellington crews also employed a technique, whereby one aircraft flew a course

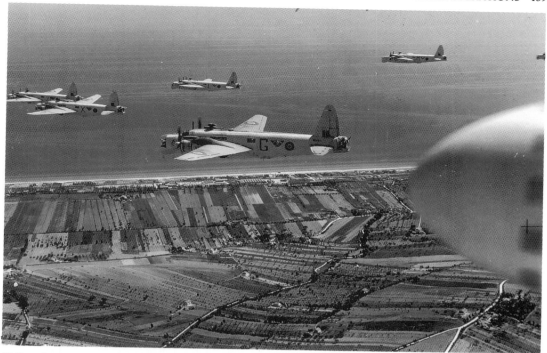

38 Squadron Wellington XIVs over Ancona in 1945. *(Henry Fawcett)*

8,000 feet in a straight line while another flew a head-on course in the opposite direction at 5,000 feet. Henry Fawcett recalls: 'I remember one Wellington that swished past over the top of me at fifty feet!' The Wellington crews worked in close co-operation with the Royal Navy MTBs in the night attacks on barges. To Henry Fawcett the MTBs, with their three Merlin engines, were 'magnificent little beasts'.

Success depended on the close co-operation of the Wellington and MTB crews. One night Fawcett's crew were to be accompanied by a Chief Petty Officer from the Royal Navy. 'Before the Petty Officer ventured on an actual operation he wished to fly a practice flight first. We took him up on an air test. This usually involved a flight up the coast, a few turns around the leaning tower of Pisa, return and then a beat-up of the beach where the lads were. I quite forgot about the Chief Petty Officer. Quite green, he went off at lunch time and I never saw him again.

'On the night of 27 February we hit one of these "glorified" barges. Hits didn't do much damage so we aimed for bomb pressure damage. Usually, we dropped sticks of 250 lb bombs to go off at thirty feet above sea level.

On this occasion, two hit. I went into a steep turn and all I saw was a tiny bit of burning debris. The barge was gone in seconds.

'On 21 March Jack Dougary, the radar operator, found a convoy of five ships. We went safely out to sea and came in at 1,000 feet. We homed in on the ships, which were sailing along like a ghostly convoy, climbed to 8,000 feet and dropped through the thick cloud. I had no idea where our bombs went. We came in and found the convoy again. Flying level, we flew alongside and my gunners strafed the ships. There was no response at all. The first sighting report had been sent off and a second Wellington was coming in. I climbed very fast into the cloud, just as our starboard engine stopped near La Spezia. We had to fly for an hour on one engine back to Rosignano. Next day we discovered that the engine had partially seized climbing to 8,000 feet so rapidly.

'On 2 April at Falconara near Ancona, we hit miniature U-boats, crewed by six-man sabotage teams. One was surfaced and abandoned. We went back to refuel and and re-arm, returned, and got another contact. It was the six survivors. We flew around while a Walrus picked them up. Next day

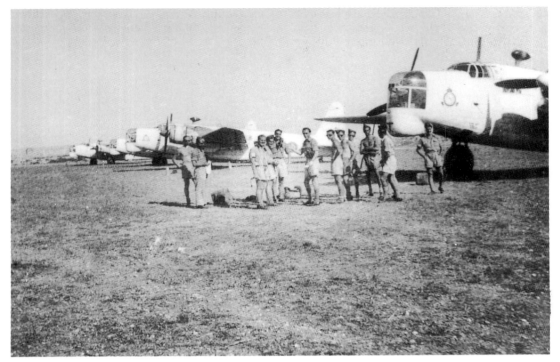

Wellington XIVs of 38 Squadron on Malta, 17 July 1945. *(Henry Fawcett)*

Beginning of a new era; Vickers Warwicks of 38 Squadron, which began equipping with the type in Malta in 1945. *(Henry Fawcett)*

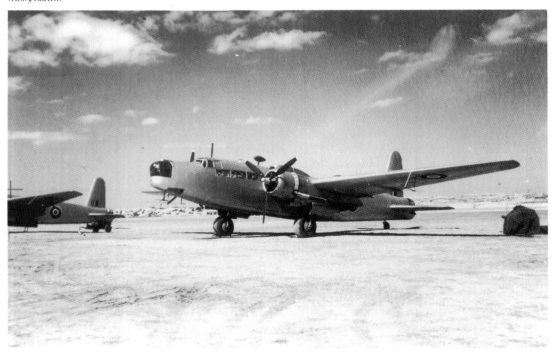

we dropped nine 250 lb depth charges on another. We saw plenty of planks, oil and dead fish but we received no credit for sinking the boat this time. We made no mistake on 10 April when we sank a 1,000-ton barge.

'On 23 April we attacked a small convoy with eleven 250 lb bombs but missed hitting any ships. Then it was leave to Sorrento for two weeks. We returned to the squadron to begin mine spotting. Off Yugoslavia we flew at fifty feet for four hours fifty minutes. In that time the Navigator plotted fifty mines.'

The detached flight of No 38 Squadron was transferred to Falconara and the entire squadron was able to celebrate VE-Day together. On VE-Day, No 458 Squadron flew the last official anti-U-boat operation, altlhough a number of ASR missions were flown throughout the rest of the month. After all the excitement, in June, No 458 Squadron was disbanded. In July 1945 No 38 Squadron transferred to Malta and exchanged its Wellingtons for Warwicks for ASR duties. On 25 August 1945 No 221 Squadron was disbanded in North Africa.

Once again, the Wellington had proved its worth in a diversity of roles from minelaying and supply dropping, to bombing operations, torpedo-bombing and anti-submarine work. These relatively unknown maritime operations carried out by the Wellington squadrons undoubtedly contributed to the downfall of the German naval and air forces in the Mediterranean Theatre of war. The same could also be said of their involvement in all other theatres of the war.

Truly, the Wimpy was a geodetic giant.

* * *

Post-war service

With the end of hostilities Wellingtons soon all but completely disappeared from the RAF inventory, as L. W. Collett, an RAF regular since 1938, recalls: 'At the end of the war hundreds and hundreds of Wellingtons were flown to Little Rissington (not far from Cirencester) for disposal. They were better than the ones we had at Wellesbourne and we used to go and rob bits and pieces off them to maintain our serviceability.'

Several Wellington Xs were revamped by Boulton Paul for extended service as crew trainers with Flying Training Command.

Wellington T10 MF628 is now on permanent display at the RAF Museum, Hendon. *(RAF Museum)*

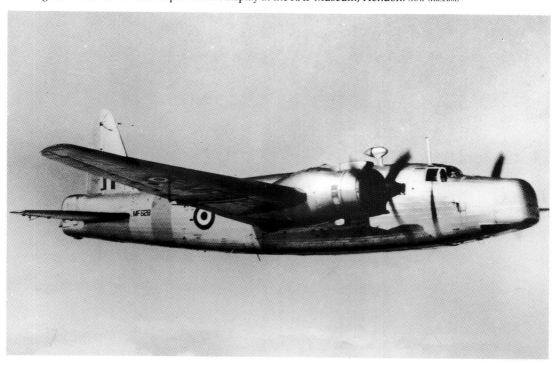

This version was known as the T 10 (one of which is on permanent display at the RAF Museum, Hendon) and earned the distinction of being the last Wellington in RAF service. The last Wellington T 10 was finally struck off charge in 1953. Both the T 10 and the T 19 were superseded in the Air Navigation Schools and at 201 Advanced Flying School at Swinderby by the Vickers Valetta T 3 and the Vickers Varsity respectively.

It was the end of an era. For seventeen years the Wimpy had earned the undying affection of its air and ground crews. During the Second World War no other British bomber was built in greater numbers, and the 11,461st and final Wellington, a T 10 built at Squires Gate, Blackpool, was delivered on 13 October 1945. No other RAF bomber saw greater and more widespread service. The Wellington's place in aviation history is thus assured.

Further reading

419 (Canadian) Squadron Unit History Blida's Bombers, Squadron Leader Eric M. Summers, MM, 1943

Bomber Command War Diaries, Martin Middlebrook

Bomber Squadrons of the RAF, Phillip Moyes, Macdonald 1964

British Bomber Since 1941, The, Peter Lewis, Putnam 1967

East Anglian Crash Logs, R.J. Collis, unpublished

Famous Bomber Aircraft, Martin W. Bowman, Patrick Stephens 1989

History of RAF Mildenhall, A, Dr Colin Dring, Mildenhall Museum Publications 1980

Royal Air Force 1939-45, Denis Richards and Hilary St G. Saunders, HMSO 1974

Story of another Loch Ness Monster, The, Robin Holmes, The Loch Ness Wellington Association Ltd

Index

Aachen 51
Alconbury 74
Aldergrove 36
Angell, Sqdn Ldr E. E. M. 40, 44
Antwerp 70
Aqir, Palestine 118
Aynsley, Len 101-5

Baird, Sqdn Ldr, The Rt. Hon. R. A. G. 113
Balch, LAC 17, 26-29
Baldwin, Air Vice-Marshal Jackie 23
Ball, Bill 119
Bamford, Wing Cmdr 133
Barton Bendish airfield 13, 20
Bassingbourn, RAF 35
Benbecula 41
Benghazi 111-114, 151
Bennett, Wing Cmdr 65
Berlin 53, 56, 63, 66, 71
Berners Heath 17
Bernet, W/O, DFM 92
Bernhard, Prince 131
Berry, Eric 63-65
Biddle, Gord, RCAF 41-43
Billancourt 73
Binbrook 69, 73, 76
Bircham Newton 40
Bizerta 121, 129-131
Black, Sqdn Ldr 58-59
Blida airfield 127-128, 131, 158
Booth, Sqdn Ldr J. F. H. 130
Borley, Flt Sgt 18
Boscombe Down 16-17
Bottomley, Air Commodore Norman 23
Bowhill, Air Chief Marshal Sir F. 35, 37
Breighton 70
Bremen 46, 61, 65, 77, 79, 84, 95
Bremerhaven 91
Brest 66, 70
Briden, F/O 29
Brooklands 27
Brooks, Flt Lt Ron, DFC 94, 128
Brough, Flt Lt J. F. 22
Brown, Stuart 98
Bruce, Sgt Don 80-90
Brünsbuttel 14-15, 17
Buckley, Wing Cmdr 52
Buckley, F/O 16
Budapest 139, 145
Burn airfield 99
Burnell, F/O 48
Burtt-Smith, Sgt Jim 91-93
Bury St Edmunds 23

Cameron, Sgt Ian 150
Carmichael, Sqdn Ldr 129

Carton-De-Wirate, Lt General 9
Cartwright, Sgt James 74-75
Catt, Sqdn Ldr R. G. E. 22
Cerignola III 138-139
Chamberlain, Neville 13
Chambers, F/O 44
Chambers, Flt Lt 41
Chandler, F/O John 19
Chandler, Sgt R. F. 65-67
Chandler, Sgt 131-132
Chaplin, Wing Cmdr John 150
Chester, Vickers factory 3
Child, Norman 93-94, 96-97, 129
Chivenor 37, 39, 42
Churchill, Winston 21
Clark, Sqdn Ldr Anthony W. J. 61-62
Clark, Dave 108, 110-112
Clarke, F/O Lyn 138-141
Cobb, John 61
Collett, L. W. 161-162
Cologne 58-60, 66, 68, 76-77
Coltishall, RAF 29
Cook, F/O B. G. 67
Cook, Sgt E. R. 61
Cookson, Sqdn Ldr Sawry 60
Cooling, Rupert 'Tiny' 49-51, 133-136
Cooper, F/O 22
Coote, P/O 58
Cousens, Sqdn Ldr 84
Crank-Benson, Sgt Jim 108, 113
Croft RAF airfield 97-99
Croppi, Noel 95-96, 101

D'Ath-Weston, P/O E. H. 91-93
Dalton, RAF 97-99
Davidstowe Moor 40
Day, Eric 3-5
Debach 66-67
Deeth, George 42-43
Delaney, Flt Sgt Chuck 128-129
Dick, LAC G. 48
Dishforth, RAF 79, 97, 99
Dixon-Wright, Wing Cmdr 85
Doolittle, Maj-Gen James H. 131, 133
Dorken, Fred 40
Dougary, Jack 159
Douglas, Sgt 49-51
Downey, Flt Sgt 23
Driffield, RAF 66, 75
Duguid, Flt Lt A. G. 21, 24
Duisburg 84-86, 90
Dunn, Flt Lt Donald 130-131
Düsseldorf 95, 98

East Moor, RAF 99
East Wretham, RAF 74

Edwards, Air Vice Marshal, RCAF   75
El Alamein   119, 150
El Fayid   110
Elliott, Don   69
Elliott, Flt Lt R. P.   65
Elston, Gerry   104-5
Emden   63, 70, 75, 80-81
Esbjerg   16
Esling, Sgt Ron   84-90
Essen   74, 77
Everatt, Sgt G. H.   76

Farnborough, RAE   3
Fawcett, Sgt Henry   152-153, 156-157, 159-161
Feltwell, RAF   13, 24, 29, 52, 56
Field, Grp Capt R. M.   51
Fifteenth Air Force   138
Finlayson, P/O W. J.   56
Firestone, Harvey   41-43
Fisher, Red   141
Fiume   138
Fletcher, Sgt   57
Fox, Charles   9-10
Fox, Douglas   71
Frankfurt-on-Main   94
Franks, P/O   63
French, Sgt Jack   91-92
Frizzell, Sgt W.   91-93
Fulton, Wing Cmdr John, DSO, DFC, AFC
  75-76, 79, 93

Gardabia   124-126
Gardening sorties   144-145
Gaul, Wally   106, 108-117
Gaunt, Sgt 'Tubby'   146-149
Gee, Sgt Tony   69
Gelsenkirchen   58
Genoa   70
Gibbes, Wing Cmdr A. R., DFC, RAAF   133
Gill, P/O Alan   93-94, 97
Gilmour, Sgt Jock   50
Goad, Jack   82
Goodwin, F/O   63-65
Graham, Ken   42-43
Grandy, George   42-43
Grant, Flt Lt Peter   15, 23, 29
Gray, Sgt George   59
Griffiths, Wing Cmdr J. F.   22
Gristwood, Roy   138-141
Guthrie, Sqdn Ldr   20, 29

Haddock, Gordon   44
Haines, P/O Jack   101-2
Hallam, Les   140-143, 149
Hamburg   46-47, 56, 66, 75, 79, 91, 93
Hamm   67
Hammond, Wally   121
Hampton, F/O Trevor A. 'Happy'   59-62
Hancock, P/O Bill   84
Hankins, P/O Hank   53
Hannover   18, 65, 101
Harcus, Sgt Len   91-93

Harris, Air Marshal Sir Arthur   36, 73-77
Harris, Sqdn Ldr Paul   15, 21-23, 29
Harwell, RAF   13, 108
Heathcote, P/O G. C.   17, 26, 28-29
Heligoland   21
Helmore, Grp Capt   37
Hemswell, RAF   4, 146
Hendon, RAF   162
Hetherington, Flt Lt E. J.   22-23
Hirszbandt, Flt Lt   77
Hitchmough, Bill   56
Holme-on-Spalding Moor   70, 72
Honington, RAF   13, 19, 29, 34-35, 49, 70, 74-75
Husky, Operation   136

Jarman, Sqdn Ldr L. E.   29
Jenner, Sgt Alfred   57-58, 63-65
Jensen, Sgt A. M.   131
Johnson, Wing Cmdr   151
Johnson, Arthur   94, 128-129
Joubert, Air Marshal Sir Philip   35, 37

Kabrit   110-111, 115-118
Kairouan/Zina   133, 136
Kalsruhe   52
Kassel   93-94
Kay, Sqdn Ldr Cyrus   52
Kellett, Wing Cmdr Richard   21, 23, 25, 29
Kemp, LAC   17, 28-29
Khormaksar, Aden   153-154
Killelea, Sgt Eddie   80, 82
Kirmington airfield   127
Kirwan, Wing Cmdr J. D., DFC   129, 131
Kitely, Sgt   58
Kitson, Sgt   17

Lamb, Sqdn Ldr Lennox   17-20
Lampedusa   136
Larney, Sgt Joe   52-53, 56
Leconfield, RAF   99
Leeming, RAF   93, 97
Leigh, Sqn Ldr H. de B.   37
Leipzig   22
Lemon, F/O   26, 29
Lewis, P/O   23
Lilley, LAC   29
Limavady   44
Linton-on-Ouse airfield   99
Little Rissington   161
Lloyd, Air Marshal Hugh Pugh   16, 115
Longmore, Air Marshal Sir Arthur   106
Lossiemouth   31
Lübeck   75
Luqa   115

MacDiarmid, F/O I. R., DFC   62
MacFarlane, Geoffrey   6-8
Macrae, F/O   27
Magdeburg   56
Maison Blanche   128-129
Malan, Wing Cmdr A. A.   131
Maleme airfield   156-157

Malta   115-116, 121-122, 151, 155
Mannheim   57, 66, 100
Mansfield, The Rt. Hon. Terence   69-71, 76-77, 79
Manston   96
Margerison, Sgt Bill   80-90
Marham, RAF   13, 16, 20-21, 49, 67, 70, 80-90, 93, 96
Martlesham Heath, A&AEE   2
Massey, W/O   125
Masters, Sgt Eric   58, 65-66, 68-69
Mathews, Sgt O. A.   68
Maydown, RNAS   44
McFarlane, P/O 'Spanky'   56
McGiveney, Flt Sgt   154
McGraw, F/O   152
McKee, Sqdn Ldr Andrew   22, 29, 49
Messina   136-137
Methwold, RAF   13
Middleton, St George, RAF   97
Milan   52, 96, 142
Mildenhall, RAF   13, 18, 69-71, 73, 76, 79, 93
Mitchell, Sgt Alex, RCAF   98
Modin, Grp Capt   52
Molesworth   70, 75
Mooney, Flt Sgt Del   80, 82-90
Mortimer, Sgt   119
Morton, Flt Lt, RNZAF   118-119
Mount Farm airfield   17
Mulholland, Wing Cmdr N. G., DFC   70, 150
Mönchen Gladbach   70
Münster   69, 93

Netheravon, RAF   16
Newmarket airfield   13, 23, 57-58
Nicholas, Sgt David   74
Norrington, Sgt W. C.   80-82
North Coates, RAF   27
Northolt   101
Norwich   106
Nürnberg   22, 71

O'Callaghan, Flt Lt Robert   75
Oakington   65
Oboe blind bombing device   7
Ogilvie, P/O G. S.   63
Ogilvie, Sqdn Ldr   65
Oldham, Flt Sgt Jim   94, 128-129
Oliphant, Stephen A.   152
Owens, P/O   113

Palmer, P/O   63-65
Pandeveswar   9-10
Pantelleria   108, 133-136
Parkin, Flt Sgt, DFM   113
Pattison, Flt Lt   76
Payne, Ernie   152
Pierse, Air Marshal Sir Richard   73
Pelmore, P/O Milton   67
Pendleton, Sgt   74
Petts, Sgt Frank   14, 16-20, 23-25
Pfeiffer, Leutnant Rolf   61
Pickard, Grp Capt Percy, DSO, DFC   52

Pierson, R. K.   1
Powell, Grp Capt, DSO, OBE   132, 134
Predannack   40-41
Priest, W/O   157
Purdy, Sgt   17

RAF Units:
   No 1417 Flight   37
   No 1 Group   70
   No 2 Group   12, 14, 93
   No 3 Group   12, 14, 16, 23, 34, 46, 52-53, 71, 76, 93
   No 4 Group   12, 98
   No 6 Group (RCAF)   97-98, 100
   No 18 Group   31
   No 201 Group   150
   No 205 Group   110, 134, 137-138, 142-145, 149
   No 3 OTU   153
   No 6 OTU   8
   No 7 OTU   152
   No 11 OTU   35
   No 15 OTU   13, 17, 57, 107-8, 118
   No 16 OTU   95
   No 18 OTU   8
   No 20 OTU   13
   No 22 OTU   95
   No 77 OTU   146
   No 84 OTU   103
   No 3 PRU   65
   No 44 Squadron   71
   No 66 Squadron   19
   No 1 TTU Turnbury   152
   No 247 Wing   150
   No 248 Wing   150
   No 257 Wing   110
   No 330 Wing   132, 134, 136
Ramshawe, Sgt   17, 29
Rawlings, F/O Arthur   40-41, 45
Richardson, Sgt Joe   80-81
Roberts, F/O   131
Robertson, Sgt   17, 27-29, 33-34
Roosevelt, President Franklin D.   14
Rostock   75
Rotterdam   70
Rowley Mile, Newmarket   13, 18, 57
Rubidge, Flt Lt   156

St Henri, 'Red', RCAF   153-154
St Pierre, Sqdn Ldr Joe   79
Saich, Sgt J. C.   70
Saint Nazaire   82
Sandell, Sgt Maurice   146-149
Sapiston   19
Savard, Flt Lt Logan   79
Saxelby, P/O   56
Second Tactical Air Force   10, 101
Scanlon, Jock   147
Shallufa   110, 150
Sharjah   153
Sharpe, P/O Douglas   66-67
Shepherd, Sgt Robert   52-54, 56
Singerton, Albert   75

Singerton, Reg 74-75
Skingsley, LAC J. 130
Skipton-on-Swale, RAF 97, 99
Skitten 38
Smith, Alan 153-154
Smith, Arthur 63-65
Sofia 139
South Cerney, RAF 16
Spaatz, General Carl 131
Spiers, F/O J. H. C. 29
Squires Gate 3, 9, 162
Stanley, Flt Lt 110
Stavanger 47
Stewart, Flt Lt J. B. 21
Stewart, Sgt 121
Steyr, Austria 138-139
Stradishall, RAF 16, 52
Stuttgart 99
Suda Bay 110
Summers, Capt J. 'Mutt' 1
Summers, Sgt E. T. 'Slim' 20-21
Swain, P/O J. G. 131
Swinderby, RAF 162
Sywell, RAF 8

Tedder, Air Chief Marshal Sir Arthur 131
Telling, Sgt 70
Tempsford, RAF 6
Thackeray, Flt Lt Reg 118-126
Tingley, Fred 67
Tobruk 118
Topcliffe, RAF 99
Torkington-Leech, F/O 20
Torrens, Sqdn Ldr David 63
Tortorella 149
Tunis 121-123, 131-132, 151
Turner, Flt Sgt 18

Upper Heyford 95

Venning, Sgt H., DFM 132
Vincent, Flt Lt, DFC 129

Waalhaven 49-50
Waddington, RAF 71
Walker, P/O, DFM 140-141, 143
Waltham, RAF 93-94, 127
Ward, Sgt James, VC 69
Warren, Sgt R. 61
Waterbeach, RAF 63, 65, 72, 94
Weekley, Jack 142-147, 149
Wellington Squadrons:
  No 8 153
  No 9 13, 15-16, 18, 23, 27, 30-31, 34, 35, 47, 49,
    63, 70, 74, 100, 133
  No 10 (RAAF) 37
  No 12 69, 100
  No 14 42, 45, 155
  No 15 55
  No 36 42, 44-45, 151, 154, 157
  No 37 13, 23-24, 26, 29, 107, 110, 124, 137,
    146-147

No 38 13-14, 16, 19-21, 34, 47-49, 55, 107, 110,
  114, 150-151, 154, 156-158, 161
No 38 (Special Duties) 100
No 40 118, 120, 124-125, 137, 146
No 57 55-56, 100
No 69 10, 101-4
No 70 107, 110, 124, 137, 146-7
No 75 (New Zealand) 13, 32, 46-47, 54, 67, 69,
  93, 100
No 99 2, 9, 12, 13-14, 18, 22, 46, 51-52, 57-58,
  62, 65, 68, 72-73
No 101 100
No 103 100
No 104 71, 101, 112, 124, 137, 146, 149
No 108 110, 124
No 109 6-7
No 115 5, 13, 20, 21, 47, 66-67, 70, 80-90, 93
No 142 93-94, 96-97, 101, 127, 129-131, 133,
  137-140
No 148 17, 107, 110-111, 118
No 149 13, 15-18, 21, 23-24, 29-30, 46-48, 50-52,
  54-55, 59, 63, 69, 71, 77-78
No 150 100, 127, 129, 131, 137, 140-142, 146
No 156 74, 100
No 158 100
No 166 100, 127
No 172 37-40, 44-45
No 178 144
No 179 38, 40, 42
No 196 100
No 199 100
No 203 154
No 214 13, 48, 52, 75
No 215 9-10, 13, 32-33
No 218 55, 73
No 221 36, 150-51, 154, 161
No 244 153
No 272 155, 157
No 300 (Masovian) 55, 100-101
No 301 (Pomeranian) 55, 100
No 304 (Silesian) 36-37, 40, 45, 55, 78, 100
No 305 (Ziemia Wielkopolska) 5, 55, 77,
  100-101
No 311 (Czech) 36, 39, 55, 75
No 405 (Vancouver) 66, 75
No 407 (Demon) 39, 40, 41, 45
No 408 97
No 415 (Swordfish) 39-40, 42
No 419 (Moose) 68, 73, 75-76, 79, 93, 97, 99-100
No 420 (Snowy Owl) 97, 136
No 424 (Tiger) 97, 99-100, 133, 137
No 425 (Aloutte) 77, 97, 99-100, 136
No 426 (Thunderbird) 97, 99-100
No 427 (Lion) 97-98, 99-100
No 428 (Ghost) 97, 99-100, 136
No 429 (Bison) 99-100
No 431 (Iroquois) 99-100
No 432 (Leaside) 99-100
No 450 (RAAF) 157
No 454 (RAAF) 157
No 458 (RAAF) 70, 72, 150-151, 154-158, 161
No 460 (RAAF) 70, 75, 100

No 462 (RAAF)   124
No 466 (RAAF)   99-100
No 524   40, 42, 45
No 544   38
No 547   38-40
No 612 (RAFA)   39, 40, 45
No 621   152-156
Welsh, Air Marshal Sir W., KCB   127
Weybridge   4
Wick   41
Widdowson, Sqdn Ldr R. P.   69
Wilhelmshaven   13, 23, 25, 29, 58, 91
Williams, Bill   48, 54
Williams, Sgt R. J., RAAF   124, 126
Wingham, Flt Sgt Fred   136-137
Wyton, RAF   15